U0295745

阅读上海医院建筑
著者：乔争月
摄影：乔争月　张雪飞

鸣谢：

郑时龄　唐玉恩　李乐曾　常　青
高　晞　陆　明　杨　震　卢永毅
钱宗灏　华霞虹　张晓春　殷　浩
黄钰婷　刘文韬　陈　贤　陈乔丹
Peter Raven

机构：
上海市档案馆
上海市政府新闻办公室
上海图书馆
上海市文化和旅游局
上海市医学会
中国医药工业研究总院
上海市徐家汇藏书楼
上海市建筑学会
同济大学校史馆
上海申康医院发展中心
上海市静安区文化和旅游局

Shanghai Hospital Architecture
Author: Michelle Qiao
Photographer: Michelle Qiao, Zhang Xuefei

Acknowledgements:

Zheng Shiling, Tang Yuen, Li Lezeng,
Chang Qing, Gao Xi, Lu Ming, Yang Zhen
Lu Yongyi, Qian Zonghao, Hua Xiahong,
Yin Hao, Zhang Xiaochun, Huang Yuting,
Liu Wentao, Chen Xian, Chen Qiaodan,
Peter Raven

Shanghai Municipal Archives Bureau
Information Office of Shanghai Municipality
Shanghai Library
Shanghai Culture and Tourism Bureau
Shanghai Medical Association
China National Pharmaceutical Industry
　　Research Institute
The Xujiahui Library
The Architectural Society of Shanghai,
　　China
History Museum of Tongji University
Shanghai Hospital Development Center
The Culture and Tourism Bureau of Shang-
　　hai Jing'an District

阅读上海医院建筑

乔争月 著
Michelle Qiao

上海三联书店

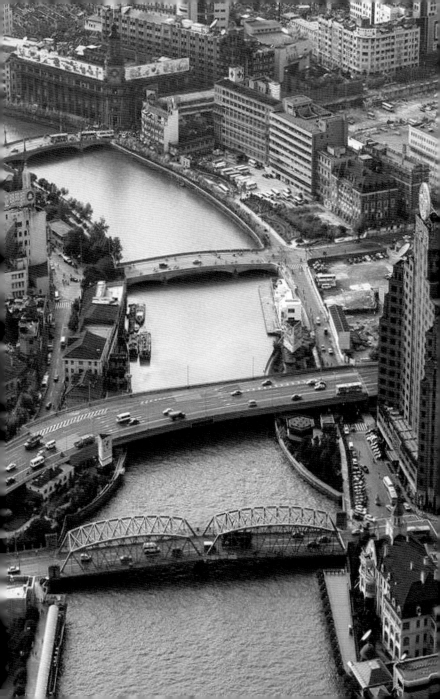

目录

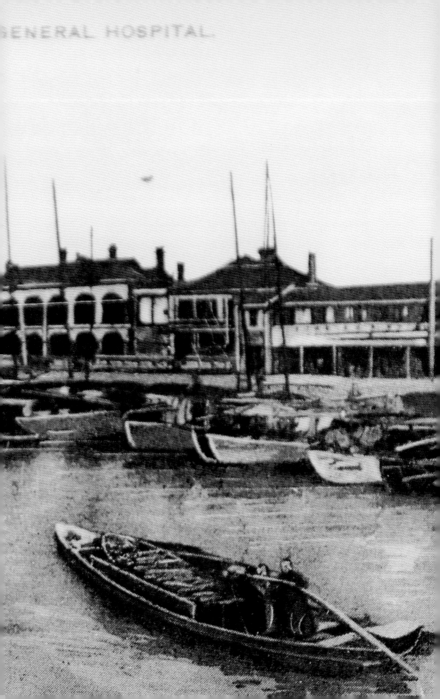

Contents

读《阅读上海医院建筑》

我国古代就有"医院"一词，其实质是一种政府机构，例如历朝宫廷的太医院，真正执行医疗功能的场所如"疾馆""病坊""安济坊""养病院""药局"等。公共卫生与医疗机构的出现意味着城市公共服务体系的进步，随着中世纪城市的建设，欧洲出现了医院建筑，自公元6世纪至今，医院建筑已经有将近1500年的历史。医院建筑的发展是近代上海社会现代化进程的一个重要标志，象征着上海社会的现代转型。据《上海卫生志》记载，1910年时，上海仅有19所医院，到1936年增至108所。自1844年在民宅开设第一所近代意义上的医院——华人医院（仁济医院的前身），直至1949年，上海曾有过近300家西医院，考虑到城市的人口规模和空间范围，

这是一个惊人的数字。许多医院建筑仍深藏掩映于医院的庭院深处，保留至今，并延续着昔日的医疗功能。

《阅读上海医院建筑》的作者乔争月是关于上海的历史和历史建筑的专栏作家，发表了诸多文章和专著，对介绍、认知和研究上海的历史建筑做出了卓越的贡献，在中国文化和建筑遗产的各种活动中都是显赫的演讲嘉宾。《阅读上海医院建筑》是她的又一部新著，深入研究特殊的建筑类型，以建筑来认识医院，作者感叹这是调研难度最大，也是收获最大、感受最深的专题。建筑类型的研究是建筑历史的重要领域，涉及建筑的功能、技术和风格的演化，尤其是目前关于近代建筑的研究多集中在博物馆建筑、交通建筑、办公楼、商业

建筑、教堂、学校、工业建筑、住宅等建筑类型方面。她对医院建筑的专题研究有着重要的意义，也为上海的历史建筑保护提供了重要的参照。

医院建筑研究是一项综合性的跨学科和门类的课题，《中国建筑》杂志曾经在1934年4月刊登文章论述医院建筑设计，阐述了文化的发展必然会引发医院建筑的建设，说明医院建筑已经为近代城市社会所关切。文章细数医院建筑设计的复杂性，医院建筑设计涉及现代科学技术的应用，医疗观念的进步，以及必须具备现代设备的知识。近年来已经有许多学者从医疗社会史、医疗卫生制度、现代医疗空间和医学教育等领域进行研究，

乔争月从中外文报刊、档案和文献中寻找史料，进行现场勘察和考证，收集到许多珍贵的史料和图片，挖掘出不少极富价值的档案资料，有许多图片还是第一次得到披露。《阅读上海医院建筑》顺着时间的脉络，讲述了30所延续至今的医院和医院建筑，包括教会、公立和私立的

医院、专科和专属医院、疗养院等，实际上这30家医院又引申出许多相关的其他建筑、景观、人物和故事，展示更广阔的画面。作者告诉我们那些鼎鼎大名的医院的辉煌历史，也叙述了霖生医院那种不再是医院的医院建筑，公惠医院那种昔日的住宅，以后成为医院建筑的建筑，书中也介绍了颜福庆医生的旧居，以及一些昔日的住宅今天成为医院的故事，揭示它们跌宕起伏的前世今生。这些医院可能是我们日常接触频繁的场所，但平素却熟视无睹，我们的精力往往集中在医院看病的各种程序中，几乎很少有人去探寻医院中的那些历史建筑，了解医院的历史，追溯无数杰出的医院捐助人、创办人、医生和建筑师。

上海的近代医院建筑也是近代建筑的缩影，完整地展现了近代上海医院建筑的风貌，形成规模可观、空间多样、设备先进、服务各类患者和疾病的多元样貌，成为现代城市的公共建筑类型。书中记载了许多我们熟悉或鲜为人知的医院，叙述了那些医

学界和建筑界先驱们的奉献，告诉我们一个个感人的故事。尤为重要的是医院建筑倡导的现代主义建筑，堪称现代建筑的典范。书中记载了英国建筑师事务所马海洋行、匈牙利建筑师邬达克、俄国建筑师李维、英国建筑师事务所德和洋行、德国建筑师汉堡嘉、法国建筑师赉安等的作品，以及中国近代著名建筑师庄俊、董大酉、奚福泉、基泰工程司等的医院建筑作品，还有更多作品的建筑师还有待考证。

书中介绍庄俊设计的孙克基产妇医院是医生与建筑师密切合作的范例，功能完备，建筑造型完全摒弃装饰，表现出简洁实用的"国际式"风格，表明了庄俊的功能主义主张："务以求切实用为要着。"董大酉设计的市立医院及卫生试验所融合医疗、研究和教学三大功能，作为上海的医学中心，是华界第一所公立医院。医院的原设计由九个部分组成，建筑造型为简洁的现代风格，医院最终建成的建筑实际上只是规划方案中的一幢主楼。奚福泉的虹桥结核病疗养院受德国1926年建造的魏特林根疗养院的启示，将空间作为特定疗法中"医疗设备"的一部分参与到治疗中，使得空间不再仅仅承担隔离的功能，这座建筑被誉为上海最具代表性的一座现代主义建筑。中山医院大楼由基泰工程司设计，是兼具教育功能的教学医院。整体造型以五层高的巨大体量的西式现代建筑作为病房楼主体，顶部架设官式歇山屋顶。

虽然本书介绍的医院只能说是近代医院建筑中的冰山一角，更多的医院建筑还有待深入的调查和考证，由于历史的演变，这幅上海近代医院建筑的拼图还有大量的空白，还有许多建筑正在进入人们的视线。医院建筑的研究是一项跨学科和学术门类的综合研究，随着时间的推移和医院历史研究的深入，近代医院建筑的全貌也必然会越来越清晰。

关注医院建筑也是关注城市的社会发展、公共服务和医疗卫生事业，关注现代城市生活和现代科学技术，关注城市的价值取向，关注历史建筑的保护。这本书让我们拓宽视界，其中的每一所医院，每一座建筑，每一个人都是一部历史，历史成为过去的集体记忆注入建筑之中。历史守护着社会的心灵，关注历史意味着文化的自省意识，关注历史实际上是回望过去，观望当下，展望未来。

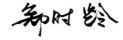

2023 年 6 月 17 日

Reading *Shanghai Hospital Architecture*

The term "hospital" existed in ancient times in China, which was actually a kind of government institution, such as the Imperial Hospital in the court of successive dynasties and the places that really performed medical functions, such as "Jiguan" (Sick House), "Bingfang" (Sick Place), "Anjifang" (Safe and Relief Place), "Yangbingyuan" (Health Hospital) and "Yaoju" (Pharmacy Bureau) etc. The emergence of public health and medical institutions meant the progress of urban public service system. With the construction of medieval cities, hospital architecture emerged in Europe, which has a history of nearly 1500 years since the 6th century AD. The development of hospital architecture is an important symbol of the modernization of Shanghai society and signifies its modern transformation. According to the Annals of Shanghai Health, there were only 19 hospitals in the city in 1910, but the number increased to 108 by 1936. From 1844, when the first modern hospital, the Chinese Hospital (the predecessor of Renji Hospital) was opened in a private house, until 1949, there were nearly 300 Western hospitals in Shanghai, a staggering number considering the size of the city's population and spatial scope. Many of these old medical buildings are still hidden deep in the courtyards of local hospitals, preserved to this day, and continue to serve their former functions.

The author of *Shanghai Hospital Architecture*, Qiao Zhengyue (Michelle Qiao), is a columnist on Shanghai's history and historic buildings. She has published numerous articles and monographs, made remarkable contributions to the introduction, knowledge and study of Shanghai's historic buildings and has been a prominent speaker at various events on China's cultural and architectural heritage. *Shanghai Hospital Architecture*, another of her new books, delves into special building types and uses architecture to understand hospitals, a topic that the author exclaims is the most difficult to research, but also the most rewarding and deeply felt. The study of architectural types is an important field of architectural history, involving the evolution of the function, technology and style of buildings, especially the current research on modern architecture is mostly focused on buildings that serve as museums, transportation, offices, shops, churches, schools, industries, residences and other architectural types. Her thematic study of hospital architecture is of great significance and provides an important reference for the conservation of historical buildings in Shanghai.

The study of hospital architecture is a comprehensive and interdisciplinary and cross-genre subject. *The China Architecture* journal once published an article on hospital architectural design in April 1934, explaining that the development of culture would inevitably trigger the construction of hospital architecture, indicating that hospital architecture had already been a concern for modern urban society. The article detailed the complexity of hospital architecture design, which involved the application of modern science and technology, the advancement of medical concepts, and the necessity of having knowledge of modern equipment. Many scholars have been studied in recent years in the fields of medical social history, health care systems, modern medical spaces, and medical education.

Qiao Zhengyue has searched for historical materials from Chinese and foreign newspapers, archives and documents, conducted site surveys and examinations, collected many precious historical materials and pictures, and unearthed many extremely valuable archival materials, with many pictures being disclosed for the first time. *Shanghai Hospital Architecture* follows the chronology of 30 hospitals and hospital buildings that continue to this day, including mission hospitals, public and private hospitals, specialized and exclusive hospitals and sanatoriums etc. In fact, these 30 hospitals lead to many other related buildings, landscapes, people and stories, showing a broader picture. The author not only tells us about the glorious history of those famous hospitals, but also former hospital buildings that are no longer hospitals such as the Lin Sheng Hospital, the former residence that became a hospital such as the Large

Building in Hsiai Lane and the former residence of Dr. Yan Fuqing, as well as the stories of some residences that became hospitals today, revealing their ups and downs. These hospitals may be places that we come into frequent contact with on a daily basis but are plainly familiar with. Our attentions are often focused on the various procedures of hospital visits, and few of us explore those historical buildings in hospitals to learn about their history and trace the countless distinguished hospital donors, founders, doctors and architects.

Shanghai's modern hospital buildings is also a microcosm of modern architecture, which showcases a complete scene of modern Shanghai hospital architecture. They form a diverse pattern of sizable scale, diverse spaces, advanced equipment, and services for all types of patients and diseases, becoming a public building type in the modern city. The book chronicles many familiar or little-known hospitals, recounts the dedication of those pioneers in the medical and architectural fields, and tells us touching stories. Of particular importance is the modernist architecture advocated by hospital architecture, which is a model of modern architecture. The book

records the works of the British architectural firm Moorhead & Halse, the Hungarian architect L. E. Hudec, the Russian architect Livin Goldenstadt, the British architectural firm Lester, Johnson & Morriss, the German architect Rudolf Hamburger and the French architectural firm Leonard, Veysseyre & Cruze, as well as the hospital architecture works of the famous Chinese architects Zhuang Jun(Tsin Chuang), Dong Dayou, Xi Fuquan(Ede, Fohjien Godfrey), and Messrs. Kwan, Chu & Yang Architects and Engineers. There are more works by architects yet to be verified.

The book introduces Dr. Sun Keji's Woman's Hospital designed by Zhuang Jun as an example of close cooperation between doctors and architects, which is fully functional and shows a simple and practical "international style" by completely abandoning ornamentation, indicating Zhuang's functionalism: "Always seek to be practical". Dong Dayou designed Shanghai Municipal Hospital and the Pathological Research Laboratory, the first public hospital in the Chinese sections of old Shanghai. As the medical center of Shanghai, the hospital integrated three functions: medical care, research and teaching. The original design of the hospital consisted of nine parts, with a simple modern architectural shape. Only the main building out of the nine in the planning scheme was eventually built. Xi Fuquan's Hongqiao Sanatorium was inspired by the Krankenhaus Waiblingen built in 1926 in Germany, which involved space as part of the "medical equipment" in a specific treatment, making space no longer just a function of isolation. The Woman's Hospital is considered one of the most representative modernist buildings in the city. Shanghai Zhongshan Hospital was designed by Messrs. Kwan, Chu & Yang Architects and Engineers as a teaching hospital with an educational function. The overall shape of the building is a five-story, gigantic Western-style modern architecture as the main body of the ward building, topped with a hipped roof of official Chinese architectural style.

Although the hospitals introduced in this book can only be said to be the tip of the iceberg of modern hospital architecture, more hospital buildings have yet to be thoroughly investigated and proven, and due to the evolution of history, there are still plenty of gaps in this puzzle game of researching modern hospital architecture in Shanghai, and many more buildings are coming into view. The study of hospital architecture is an interdisciplinary and comprehensive study of academic disciplines. As time goes by and the study of hospital history deepens, the full picture of modern hospital architecture is bound to become clearer and clearer.

To focus on hospital architecture is also to pay attention to the social development of the city, public services and medical and health care, modern urban life and modern science and technology, the value orientation of the city, and the preservation of historical buildings. This book allows us to broaden our horizon, in which every hospital, every building and every person is a piece of history, and history becomes the collective memory of the past injected into architecture. History guards the hearts and minds of the society. Focusing on history implies a sense of cultural introspection, and it is actually looking back at the past, viewing the present, and looking forward to the future.

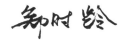

June 17, 2023

前　言

近年席卷全球的新冠疫情，让大众的目光聚焦公共卫生与医疗机构。

1936年9月20日，英文《大陆报》（The China Press）曾出版一期上海医院专刊（hospital supplement），图文并茂地介绍了国立上海医学院、中山医院、红十字会总院、仁济医院、公济医院、上海市立医院、宏恩医院、福民医院、红房子医院等上海医学机构。专刊不仅展示了各大医院的诊疗室、手术室、病房、婴儿室和实验室等，还刊登了医学建筑群规划图、建筑设计图、建筑模型和建筑施工照片。这本医院专刊中的上海医院大都运营至今，院区里还保留着一座座见证医院历史的老建筑。

这些上海医院历史悠久。19世纪中叶，西医随着外国传教士进入上海。根据上海医学史专家陆明的"上海近代西医医院概述"，自1844年到1949年，上海曾有近300家西医院，其发展历程分为两个阶段：1. 创建期（1844—1899），以教会医院和外国人兴办的医院为主；2. 发展期（1900—1949），教会、公立、私立医院三足鼎立，抗战后市立综合性医院和专科医院初具规模。

1844年初，上海第一家西医院、由英国传教医生雒魏林（William Lockhart）创办的仁济医院就开诊了，当时上海才刚开埠。如今，这座医院仍位于外滩附近的旧址，保留着老院名和1931年兴建的"新大楼"。

在创办之初，仁济医院是一间开在民宅里的小诊所。后来陆续开办的上海医院规模也不大，有的仅有一位驻院医师和几十张病床。随着上海城市的发展，这些百年前创办的医院逐渐发展为一家家大型公立医院和专科医院：仁济医院、第一人民医院、瑞金医院、华山医院、中山医院、华东医院、上海市精神卫生中心、长宁区妇幼保健院、红房子妇产医院等。如今，这些现代化的上海医院拥有数百上千张床位和多个院区，以国内领先的医疗技术吸引来自全国各地的病患前来就医。

但百年前设计建造的医院老建筑难以满足快速发展的需要。岁月变迁中，许多上海老医院里的建筑被拆除重建，为一座座大型现代化诊疗大楼腾出空间，接待人数日益增长的病人。

不过，仍有一些深藏于上海医院里的历史建筑保留至今，并延续着昔日的医疗功能。它们好像一颗颗医学人文历史的珍珠，散落在城市的各个角落。这些幸存的医院建筑建于 20 世纪 10 到 40 年代，建筑风格从古典主义到现代主义，较完整地展现了近代上海医学建筑的风貌。

医院建筑是一种功能性强、人流量大、建造预算相对有限的公共建筑类型。很多上海医院里的历史建筑也设计得简洁实用，自然地采用了"形式追随功能"的现代风格。在《X 光建筑》（X-Ray Architecture）一书中，西班牙建筑学者科伦米娜（Beatriz Colomina）提出猜想，认为 20 世纪 20 年代兴起的现代建筑是由当时最困扰人类的疾病肺结核和新诊断技术 X 射线所塑造的，医疗技术和疾病治疗在决定现代建筑的特征方面发挥了重要作用。

梳理设计近代上海医院的建筑师，发现很多知名中外建筑师和事务所: 英商德和洋行 (Lester, Johnson & Morriss)、法商赉安洋行 (Leonard, Veyssyre & Kruze)、斯裔匈籍建筑师邬达克（L. E. Hudec）、德国建筑师汉堡嘉 (Rudolf Hamburger)、俄国建筑师李维（Livin Goldenstadt）、中国建筑师庄俊、董大酉、奚福泉、基泰工程司等。其中，庄俊、董大酉、奚福泉和设计中山医院的基泰工程司建筑师朱彬都是近代中国第一代建筑师中的代表人物。很多上海医院建筑堪称现代建筑的设计典范，既实用经济，又美观亲切，映射了近代上海建筑师们的"匠心"。邬达克设计的宛若度假酒店般的宏恩医院、奚福泉的摩登虹桥疗养院和庄俊的转型之作——孙克基产妇医院，更是列入上海建筑史甚至中国建筑史的佳作。

与宾馆、银行、商店等商业用途的上海历史建筑相比，上海医院里的老建筑简洁朴素，但它们蕴含的历史也许更加迷人。在上海医院建筑里，闪动过一个个动人的身影。

这些上海医学史重要历史人物的事迹非同凡响。德国医生宝隆（Erich Paulun）2岁就成为孤儿却"散发出热力、生命力和阳光"，为中国穷人创办了同济医院。美国纽约女裁缝威廉森夫人（Margaret Williamson）为上海妇儿建"红房子医院"捐出自己菲薄的积蓄。英国富商雷士德（Henry Lester）在去世前为上海捐赠几乎所有财产，用于建造仁济医院新楼、雷士德医学研究

院和作为海员医院使用多年的雷士德工学院。中国红十字会创始人沈敦和的杰出工作让日内瓦国际红十字会议代表"感到惊讶"。创办中山医院和上海医学院的颜福庆认为"医学为民族强弱之根基，人类存在之关键，要以为公众利益的目的去学医，而不是赚钱"。骨科名医牛惠生的遗嘱提到"所用棺木不能超过四百元，金钱应用于有益社会人群之事业"。

这不是一两个人，而是一批来自医学界和支持医疗事业的人，既有中国人也有外国人。他们不仅各有专长，而且人品高尚，富有"仁心"。在百年前动荡的时代，他们克服难以想象的困难，为建设好一座座上海医院付出大量心力，开创了很不一般的医疗事业，为无数人疗愈病痛，也为上海医学事业打下基础，惠及今人。

本书尝试顺着时间脉络，讲述从1844年到1949年，30个幸存至今的上海医学历史建筑的故事，从西人创办的教会医院和民营医院，到中国人创办的公立

医院、私立医院、市立综合性医院和专科医院，最后介绍用于医院功能的历史建筑住宅和医学会、医学研究机构建筑。

这些朴素的上海医院建筑映射了近代建筑师的"匠心"，又蕴藏着近代医者和医学事业支持者的"仁心"。"匠心"与"仁心"交相辉映，是上海医院建筑最独特最大的魅力。

乔争月

2022 年 6 月 1 日

上海武康路月亮书房

Foreword

The Covid-19 pandemic since 2020 has drawn people's attention to public health and medical institutions.

On September 20, 1936, English newspaper "The China Press" published a supplement of Shanghai hospitals, which introduced the National Medical College of Shanghai, Chung Shan Hospital, Chinese Red Cross General Hospital, Renji Hospital, General Hospital, Shanghai Municipal Hospital, Country Hospital, Foo Ming Hospital, Margaret Williamson Memorial Hospital among other Shanghai medical institutions. The supplement displays not only operation rooms, wards, nurseries and laboratories of major local hospitals, but also planning blueprints, architectural drawings, building models and construction photos of these medical buildings. Most Shanghai hospitals introduced in the 1936 supplement are still in operation now till now. A rainbow of historical buildings, the witnesses of Shanghai medical history, have also been well preserved in the hospital compounds.

These Shanghai hospitals have rich histories behind. In the mid-19th century, Western medicine was introduced to Shanghai through foreign missionaries. According to the thesis titled "An Overview of Modern Western Hospitals in Shanghai" by medical historian Lu Ming, around 300 Western hospitals were founded and operated in Shanghai from 1844 to 1949.

The development of local hospitals can be divided into two periods. During the Establishment period (1844-1899), most hospitals were founded by missionary societies or expatriates in China. While during the development period (1900-1949), missionary hospitals, public hospitals and private hospitals all played important parts. After World War II, municipal hospitals and specialized hospitals began to take shape.

In early 1844, Shanghai's first Western hospital, Renji Hospital was founded by British medical missionary William Lockhart. It was a time when Shanghai had just opened its port for a few months. Today, this hospital still perches at the old site near the Bund, retaining its old-time name and a modern ward building built in 1931.

At the beginning, Renji Hospital was only a small clinic opened in a private house in the old town. At that time, all the old Shanghai hospitals were very small. Some hospitals started with only one resident physician and dozens of beds.

With the fast growing of the city over the past century, these old Shanghai hospitals have gradually developed into large public or specialized hospitals: Renji Hospital, General Hospital, St. Marie's Hospital (Ruijin Hospital), Chinese Red Cross General Hospital (Huashan Hospital), Chung Shan Hospital (Zhongshan Hospital), Country Hospital (Huadong Hospital), Shanghai Mercy Hospital (Shanghai Mental Health Center), Woman's Hospital (C. N. Maternity & Infant Health Hospital), Margaret Williamson Hospital (Obstetrics & Bynecology Hospital of Fudan University) etc. Today, these modern hospitals have hundreds of beds and multiple branches. They've attracted patients from all over the country to seek medical treatment with leading medical technologies and services.

However, the old hospital buildings designed and constructed some 100 years ago are not able to meet the needs of rapid development. Over the years, many buildings in old Shanghai hospitals have been demolished or rebuilt to make room for large, modern medical buildings to receive an ever-increasing number of patients.

Fortunately, some historical buildings well hidden in the hospitals have been preserved to this day and still used for medical functions. They are like pearls scattered in every corner of the city. These surviving hospital buildings had been built from the 1910s to 1940s. Their architectural styles range from classicism to modernism, and more completely show the features of modern Shanghai medical architecture.

The genre of hospital buildings features functionality to receive large flow of people, and relatively limited construction budget. Many historical buildings in Shanghai hospitals were designed to be simple and practical, naturally adopting the modern architectural conception of "form follows function".

In the book "X-Ray Architecture", Spanish architectural scholar Beatriz Colomina conjectured that the modern architecture which emerged in the 1920s was caused by the most troubling diseases of the time, tuberculosis and its new diagnostic technology X-rays. Medical technology and treatments have played an important role in determining the character of modern architecture.

After sorting out the architects who designed modern Shanghai hospitals, I found many famous names of Chinese and foreign architects and firms: British firm Lester, Johnson & Morriss, French firm Leonard, Veyssyre & Kruze, Slovakian-Hungarian architect L. E. Hudec, German architect Rudolf Hamburger, Russian architect Livin Goldenstadt, Chinese architects Zhuang Jun, Dong Dayou and Xi Fuquan, and Chinese firm Messrs. Kwan, Chu & Yang Architects and Engineers.

Among them, Zhuang Jun, Dong Dayou, Xi Fuquan, and Zhu Bin of Messrs. Kwan, Chu & Yang Architects and Engineers who designed the Zhongshan Hospital, are all representative figures of the first-generation architects in modern China. In addition, many Shanghai hospital buildings are model designs of modern architecture, which are practical, economical, beautiful and human-friendly, reflecting the ingenuity of architects. The hotel-like Country Hospital designed by L. E. Hudec, the avant-garde Hongqiao Sanatorium by Xi Fuquan and Zhuang Jun's groundbreaking work, Woman's Hospital, are listed as masterpieces in the architectural history of Shanghai and China.

Compared with the historical buildings for commercial purposes such as hotels, banks and shops, the old Shanghai hospital buildings are simple and sober. However, the history they convey may be more significant. A galaxy of legendary people had worked in these buildings.

The achievements made by these important figures in Shanghai medical history are extraordinary. Erich Paulun, a warm-hearted German doctor who was orphaned at the age of 2, founded Tung Chee Hospital with love and care for the poor in China. Margaret Williamson, a New York seamstress, donated her meager savings for the construction of the "Red House Hospital" for women and children in Shanghai. Before his death, British tycoon Henry Lester bequeathed almost all his assets to Shanghai for the construction of the new building of Renji

Hospital, the Lester Institute for Medical Research and the Lester Institute of Technology (later used as a seaman's hospital). The outstanding work of Shen Dunhe, founder of the Red Cross Society of China and Chinese Red Cross General Hospital, surprised delegates to the International Red Cross Conference in Geneva. Medical educator Yan Fuqing, who founded Chung Shan Hospital and National Medical College of Shanghai, believed that "medicine is the foundation of a nation's strength and the key to the existence of human beings. It is necessary to study medicine for the purpose of public interest, not for just making money". Famous orthopedic doctor Niu Huisheng mentioned in his will that his coffin "should not exceed 400 yuan because money needed to be used for the cause of benefiting the society".

They were a group of people including medical professionals and supporters of medical causes, both Chinese and foreigners with different backgrounds. They were gifted with not only professional expertise, but also noble personalities and benevolences. In the turbulent Shanghai a century ago, they overcame unimaginable difficulties, devoted a lot to the founding and operating of Shanghai hospi-

tals, created incredible medical cause, healed countless lives and laid a solid foundation for Shanghai medicine. Their efforts are still benefiting people today.

This book tries to follow the timeline from 1844 to 1949 and tells the stories of 30 surviving medical historical buildings in Shanghai, from the missionary hospitals and private hospitals founded by Westerners to public hospitals, private hospitals, specialized hospitals and municipal hospitals established by Chinese. It also introduces old villas used for hospital functions as well as historical buildings that housed medical societies and research institutions.

These simple Shanghai hospital buildings reflect both the "ingenuity" of modern architects and the "benevolence" of modern medical professionals and supporters. "Ingenuity" and "benevolence" complement each other, which in my opinion is the most unique and biggest charm of Shanghai hospital architecture.

Michelle Qiao
June 1, 2022
Moon Atelier, Wukang Road, Shanghai

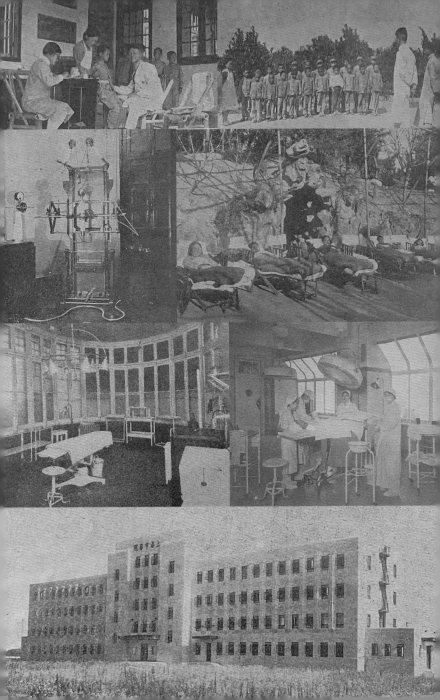

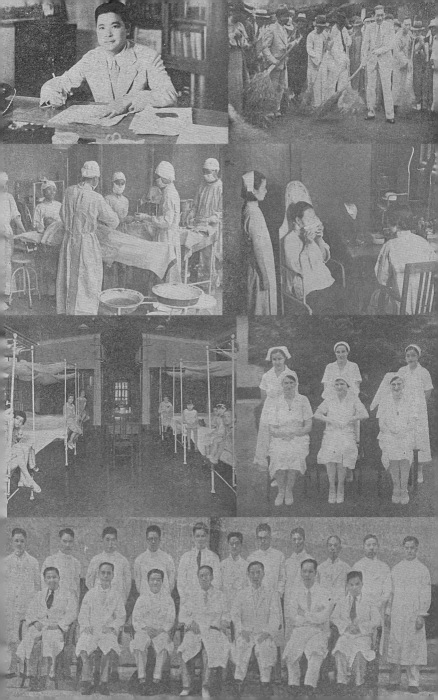

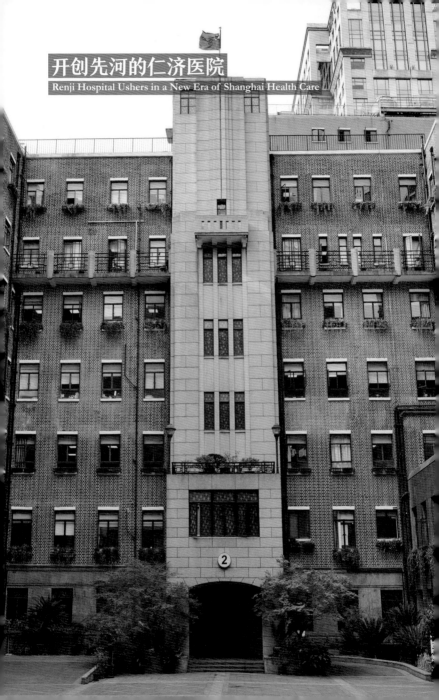

开创先河的仁济医院

Renji Hospital Ushers in a New Era of Shanghai Health Care

1931年12月15日，英文《北华捷报》（The North-China Herald）报道了富商雷士德（Henry Lester）为仁济医院捐建的"新家"。这座"新大楼"位于上海外滩附近的仁济医院西院内，至今仍在使用。仁济医院创办于1844年，是上海的第一家西医院。

1843年11月5日，英国伦敦圣公会（the London Missionary Society）传教士雒魏林（William Lockhart）来到上海，比11月17日上海正式开埠的时间还早。1844年初，他在上海老城南门外租赁民居，创设了一间为华人免费治病的诊所。这间小小的诊所开创了上海近代西医事业的先河，后来发展为仁济医院。

《上海宗教史》记载，建所伊始为吸引中国民众就医，雒魏林以免费为号召，以致该诊所"每日涌来大量的人，急切地，经常是吵吵嚷嚷地要求就诊。病人不仅有来自上海的，还有许多来自苏州、松江及附近其他城镇，甚至远在崇明岛的。"（转

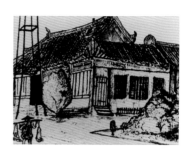

引自雒魏林《在华行医传教二十年》英文版）自1844年5月1日至1845年6月30日，诊所接待病人达10978人次。

仁济医馆历经搬迁。1846年，雒魏林募款在老城外北门附近购地建院，开始时有60个床位，英文名叫"Chinese Hospital"（华人医院），中文名叫"仁济医馆"。1861年，医院又于山东路麦家圈择地建院，英文名改为"Shantung Road Chinese Hospital"（山东路华人医院），中文称为"仁济医院"。

雒魏林年富力强，他不仅医术高超，而且擅长创办与管理组织机构。他联合本地精英成立了董事会，每年召开董事会评估医院发展，同时募集办院资金。

上海图书馆研究员黄薇发

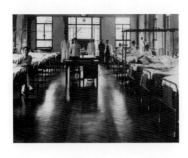

现，仁济医院从创办开始就不同于一般的教会医院。医院虽然由伦敦会传教士雒魏林发起，但实际上是一家由在沪英侨捐款建立、拥有和管理的慈善医院。伦敦会只有派遣医生承办的经营权。仁济医院的主要功能是医疗、救济和传教，资金来源以捐款为主。捐赠者除了英国人，还有华人、美国人、印度人等。

她研究仁济医院早期档案发现，从1844到1856年间，医院治疗了15万病患，接诊人数连年增长。雒魏林后来又创立北京施医院，是北京协和医院的前身。

"雒魏林在中国生活22年，合计医治的病人20万名，其中也有少数人成为基督徒。虽然作为传教士不算非常成功，但是作为医生他的成绩值得重视。传教士医生这个群体，比起像海关医

生、军队医生等来华医生团体，人数最多，影响也最大。雒魏林是其中非常重要的人物，尤其是在上海、北京建立仁济医院和施医院，让更多的中国人接触和认识近代的西方医学。其实，伦敦会后来在中国很多地方建立的医院也都以仁济来命名，可见上海仁济医院的成功和重要性。"黄薇说。

1857年雒魏林回英国后，仁济医院由合信（Benjamin Hobson）主持。这位继任院长写作翻译了《西医略论》、《妇婴新说》和《内科心说》等多部专著，将西方医学介绍到中国。

1863年，仁济医院英国医生韩雅各（James Henderson，1829—1865）又出版了一部《上海卫生》（Shanghai Hygiene），分食物、饮料、运动、衣服、沐浴、排汗等11个章节，介绍在华生活卫生保健的注意事项。当时在上海的外国侨民生活得并不健康，死亡率高。韩雅各在书中提到："我禁不住想，去年在上海死亡的1600个欧洲人，如果得到照顾并且采取适

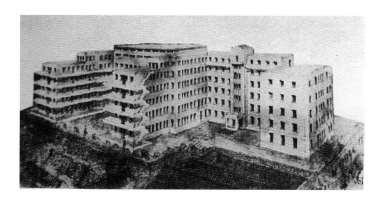

当的预防措施来保健的话，那么至少有1000人本应还活着。"他建议"炎热天气里多喝茶和咖啡吧，少喝烈性酒和啤酒，让法国和德国葡萄酒取而代之"。

1914年，仁济医院创办了上海最早的女子护理学校之一，1927年获得英国富商雷士德遗产捐赠后，更名为Lester Chinese Hospital（雷士德华人医院），亦称德和医院。1932年，用雷士德遗产资金建造"新大楼"落成，仁济医院成为当时上海规模最大的医院。

1840年2月26日，雷士德（Henry Lester）出生于英国南部港口城市南安普敦市。他曾在伦敦接受建筑师和土地勘测师的训练，1863年到上海后受雇于工部局负责公共租界土地测量的工作，后来也为法租界测量土地。这些工作完成后，雷士德回归建筑师的角色。他先与一名建筑师合作，但很快独立创业，沿着黄浦江岸设计建造了许多著名的洋行、码头和仓库。

1913年，雷士德又与强生(George A. Johnson)和马立斯（Gordan Morriss）联合创办德和洋行（Lester, Johnson & Morriss），专营建筑设计、土木工程、测绘检验、房地产抵押放款等业务，后来发展成为近代上海实力最强的设计事务所之一。富有眼光的雷士德很早发现了上海的潜力，大量投资不动产，在上海的运气特别好，无论做什么都能"点石成金"，做成了上海历史上最大的几笔土地交易。

1926年5月14日，雷士德在上海公济医院（General Hospital，今上海第一人民医院）病逝，他在去世前已成为上海最大的土地拥有者之一。虽然拥有当时就价值数百万英镑的巨额财富，雷士德却终身未婚，生活简朴。他留下一份惊人的遗嘱，除了少量遗产赠予个人，将几乎所有遗产留在上海用以成立"雷士德基金会"，发展医疗、教育和慈善事业。

他生前指定用遗产主要资助建造仁济医院新大楼、雷士德医学研究院和雷士德工学院及学校。遗嘱还设立5万两银子的雷士德奖学金，面向在上海就学的所有国籍、无论宗教信仰的14岁以下的男女学生。从这份遗嘱可以看出，雷士德高瞻远瞩，重视医学和教育事业。

1927年，雷士德基金会即按照这份遗嘱开展筹建工作，由德和洋行负责设计。雷士德去世后的十年内，他遗嘱中提到的三大项目都建成了，而仁济医院位于山东路的新大楼是最先投入使用的。

在《仁济医院九十五年1844—1938》（Ninety-Five Years A Shanghai Hospital 1844-1938）一书中，医院董事会秘书埃利斯顿（Eric S. Elliston）提到雷士德与这所为华人提供服务的慈善医院有着深厚渊源。1873年时，雷士德曾负责仁济医院男子病房的设计工作，此后长期为医院提供捐赠。在1924年12月订立的最后一份遗嘱中，雷士德捐赠100万两款项用于建造仁济医院新楼，此外还赠予医院四块地皮。

雷士德的捐赠附有几项条件，除了提出医院需改名为"The Lester Chinese Hospital"，还要求医院为穷苦病人免费治疗。1927年，医院又收到一张数额达64358.99两的支票，款项是来自雷士德赠予土地的收入。埃利斯顿透露，仁济医院新大楼原计划盖5层，因为后来决定让雷士德医学研究院使用其中一层，这座钢筋混凝土结构的大楼加建为6层。

"医院每个方面都很现代：柔和色调的墙壁取代了以前令人不快的刺眼的白墙，手术室富有效率。从过去的记录来看，仁济医院在一年里可以为多达15万名门诊患者提供服务。" 1931年12月15日《北华捷报》的报道写道。

报道还提到，医院的"新家"现代、卫生、功能完善。食物通过服务升降机运送到病房，这样就不需要用托盘或推车了。所有的食物都在一个外间里清洗和准备好，然后才被送入闪亮的大厅。

医院的四楼有四间手术室，漆成柔和的绿色，对疲惫的眼睛有益。病房的三边都有窗户。四楼专供妇女儿童使用。有一间明亮的小房间是为孩子们设计的，浅黄色的墙壁，有关于幼儿教育的图画，可容纳12名婴儿。产科病房在三楼，配有带轮子的婴儿篮，供不愿意让孩子离开自己的妈妈们使用。大厅的下方是育婴室，一排排的婴儿在那里度过了生命中前三周的大部分时光。X光室和其他手术室位于二楼，

此外还有医院的药房、专科门诊、牙科、耳、眼、鼻、皮肤和妇科门诊等。男科位于一楼，急诊室和观察室就在医院入口的对面。

"虽然医院位于市中心，但幸运的是，从病房可以眺望宜人的开阔场地。这座用泡沫混凝土和灰泥制成的建筑的外观为棕褐色和砖色，庄严而令人愉悦，其铺着碎石的道路通向门廊和一棵常青树。建造者有先见之明，将北侧房间用于实验室、手术室和办公室，而病房则保证有令人愉快的阳光。"《北华捷报》报道写道。

报告特别指出，新大楼的五楼主要由雷士德医学研究院临床部使用。雷士德捐建的两家医学机构——仁济医院与雷士德医学研究院在这座新大楼里一起办公，开展良好的密切合作。研究院接办了医院的化验部，帮助其开展细菌学、血清学、临床化学、病理学、临床造影等方面的研究应用。埃利斯顿评价，研究院的医学专家对医院提供了给力的帮助，而供研究院使用的五楼

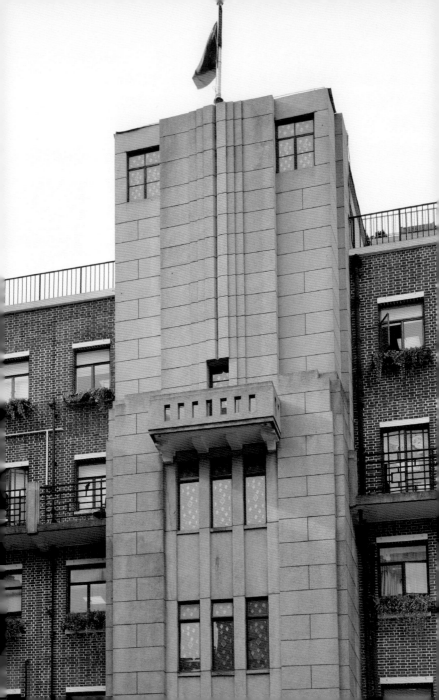

保留了一些病房，以供专家研究临床疾病。基础研究与临床治疗的结合使仁济医院的水准在当时沪上首屈一指，而两家医学机构都为近代中国培养了很多医疗技术人才，为今天上海的医疗卫生事业奠定了一定的基础。

在"新大楼"投入使用的20世纪30年代，更多中国医生参加了仁济医院的工作。抗战后，原南京中央医院泌尿科主任、上海圣约翰大学医学院教授陈邦典担任仁济医院院长，此时医院床位增加至318个。

2014年，雷士德捐建的这座大楼历经修缮重新投入使用，昔日宽敞的大病房和水磨石楼梯犹存。如今，仁济医院已发展为一所集医疗、教学、科研于一体的综合性三级甲等医院，有四个院区，超过2000张床位。昔日的山东路"新大楼"位于西院区。

2019年12月，这家沪上最老的西医医院庆祝建院175周年，开设了院史馆。展品珍贵而丰富，其中就有这座"新大楼"1932年竣工时制作的铜雕模型。

昨天： 仁济医院　**今天：** 仁济医院　**地址：** 山东中路 145 号　**建造年代：** 1932 年
设计师： 德和洋行　**参观指南：** 雷士德捐建的大楼今日犹存，仍旧用作诊疗功能。

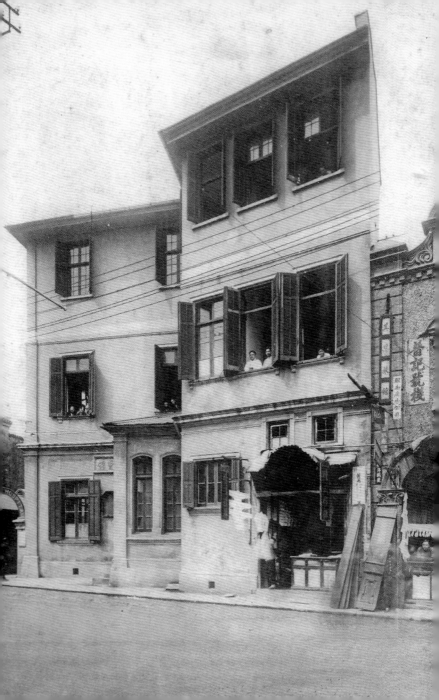

It would be fair to say Western medical practise was still very primitive in mid-19th century China. But, thanks to English medical missionary William Lockhart and several other pioneering philanthropists, medicine, health care and hospitals developed, became more sophisticated and a new era of hospital care was born.

Shanghai's first Western hospital

The North-China Herald introduced the "new home" for the Lester Chinese Hospital on December 15, 1931. This "new building" still stands on the historic Shandong Road site of the hospital, which was Shanghai's first Western hospital and retains its old Chinese name, Renji Hospital. This modern medical building was also one of benevolences left by legendary British billionaire Henry Lester who called himself a Shanghainese.

"Founded in 1844 by English medical missionary William Lockhart, this hospital started the history of Western medicine in Shanghai," says medical historian Lu Ming from Shanghai No. 4 People's Hospital.

Sent by the London Missionary Society, Lockhart was one of the earliest expatriates to come to Shanghai. He arrived in town on November 5, 1843 before the city officially opened its port on November 17, according to Taiwan historian Wang Ermin's book *Modern Shanghai Pioneers of Science and Technology*.

As Walter Henry Medhurst, another missionary from the London society arrived in December, Lockhart discussed with him and then opened a clinic simply called "Chinese Hospital" in a humble house outside the north gate. This small clinic, which treated Chinese patients for free, was seen as Shanghai's first Western hospital and predecessor of today's Renji Hospital.

Though small and simple, the hospital was successful from the beginning and treated some 19,000 patients from 1844 to 1845. After several relocations, Lockhart purchased a site between today's Shandong and Fujian Roads and made it the hospital's permanent address in 1846, with 60 beds. The "Chinese Hospital" was widely called "Shantung Road Chinese Hospital" by expatriates, although the Chinese people called it "Renji Hospital". "Renji" means mercy and relief in Chinese.

Lockhart was not only a high-skilled doctor, but also a brilliant founder of an institution. He formed a committee of trustees joined by local elites, which hosted annual meetings to evaluate the hospital's development, and helped to raise funds.

"From the beginning, Renji Hospital differed from other missionary hospitals. Although London Society missionary initiated it, it was a charitable hospital owned and managed by British residents in Shanghai. The main source of funding was through donations," says Huang Wei, a PhD researcher of Shanghai modern history from the Shanghai Library.

According to her study on Renji Hospital's incomplete early medical records, the number of its patients from 1844 to 1856 reached 150,000 and continued to grow over the years. Lockhart later founded another Chinese hospital named Shi Hospital in Beijing, which developed into the famous "Peking Union Medical College Hospital".

"Lockhart had lived in China for 22 years and treated over 200,000 patients, a few of whom turned Christians. Although not very successful as a missionary, Lockhart's achievements as a doctor was remarkable. Renji Hospital and Shi Hospital founded by him enabled more Chinese to contact and understand modern western medicine, " Huang said.

After Lockhart returned to England, Renji Hospital was managed by his successor, Dr. Benjamin Hobson, who later authored and translated a rainbow of books to introduce Western medicine in China.

"The hospital founded one of Shanghai's first nurse schools in 1914 and saw a period of fast development after 1927. After receiving Henry Lester's benevolence that year, it was renamed Lester Chinese Hospital and built a steel-and-concrete building in 1932, which was the city's largest hospital building of its times, " says medical historian Lu Ming.

Lester's legacy

This steel-and-concrete building built with Lester's legacy was described as a "new home" by the 1931 *North-China Herald* newspaper. According to the hospital's 1927 annual meeting, Lester's legacy to the hospital amounted to 1 million taels in money for the purpose of rebuilding and about 1 million taels in property for endowment.

During the meeting, Judge Peter Grain, chairman of trustees of the hospital, said the late Mr. Lester's legacy allowed them to

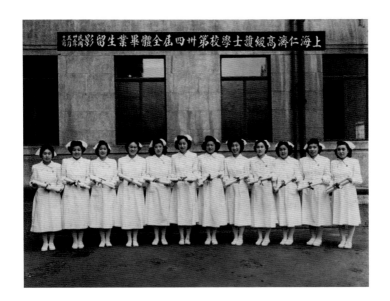

上海仁濟高級護士學校第卅四屆全體畢業生留影 [?]

have the main hospital in its present position at Shantung Road for "one reason to deal with street accidents" which were numerous.

Born in 1840 in Southampton, Lester, who had received training in London as an architect and land surveyor, came to Shanghai in 1863-1864 to survey a Shanghai Municipal Council settlement. After this service was completed, he started his own business. His company, Lester Johnson & Morris, became one of the most well-known architectural firms in town. A man of great foresight, he saw the potential of Shanghai and made large investments in property. Prior to his death, he was one of the largest landowners in Shanghai.

He never married and lived a very simple life. Before he died in May 1926, Lester bequeathed most of his assets to philanthropy, particularly for the building of the Lester Chinese Hospital, the Lester Institute of Medical Research and the Henry Lester School and Institute of Technical Education.

Within a decade after he left this philanthropic will, the three medical and educational projects were completed one after another in the early 1930s. And Renji Hospital's (Lester Chinese Hospital) new building was the first to be put into use.

"Modern in every respect, from the soft-toned walls that have replaced the unpleasantly dazzling white of another era to the efficient operating theatres, the Lester Hospital should service as many as 150,000 outpatients during its first year, judging by past records," *The North-China Herald* reported on December 15, 1931.

According to the report, the "new home" was modern, hygienic and functional. Food was transferred to the ward kitchens throughout the building by service lifts, thus obviating the necessity for trays or carts. All food was cleaned and prepared in an outer room before it is brought into the shining hall.

Four operating rooms were on the fourth floor, painted a soft green, which is believed to do good to tired eyes. The wards, as is the case throughout the building, had windows on three sides.

The fourth floor was reserved for women and children, with the latter—a bright little room with a nursery frieze and buff-colored walls—accommodating 12 infants. The maternity ward was on the third floor, with its baskets on wheels for the infants whose mothers resent having them far away. And down the hall was the nursery, "where rows and rows of babies sleep away the better part of their first three weeks of life (presumably)".

X-ray and other operating rooms were on the second floor, as well as the hospital pharmacy, special clinics, dental, ear, eye, nose, skin and the outpatient department for women. The corresponding section for men was located on the first floor while the emergency rooms and observation ward were just opposite the entrance to the hospital.

"Though in the center of the city, the hospital is fortunate in its pleasant grounds overlooked by the wards. The building, of aerocrete and plaster, in tan and brick-color, is dignified and pleasing, with its sweep of graveled drive to the porte-cochere and its single evergreen tree. With characteristic foresight, the northern rooms are devoted to laboratories, operating theaters and offices, so that the pleasant sunshine is ensured for the wards, " the newspaper describes.

The report specially noted that the fifth floor was largely devoted to the Lester Institute for Medical Research, for clinical as well as laboratory work.

In his book *Ninety-Five Years A Shanghai Hospital 1844-1938*, Eric

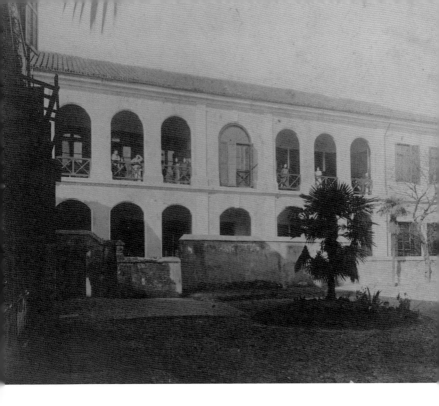

S. Elliston, the then secretary of trustees of the hospital, wrote that Lester had long been connected with the hospital since he was architect for the planning of the new hospital building in 1873. Since those earlier days, he had been a constant supporter of the hospital in many ways, contributing considerable sums from time to time.

He said that the Lester Institute added an extra floor to the original five-storied building plan for special use.

"Later on the Lester Hospital and Lester Institute of Medical Research located on the new building's fifth floor cooperated in an intensive way. The institute not only undertook technical guidance to hospital, but also took over its laboratory department to help carry out various aspects of research and application in bacteriology, serology, and pathology. The combination of basic research and clinical treatment made the hospital's standard second to none in Shanghai," Lu Ming said.

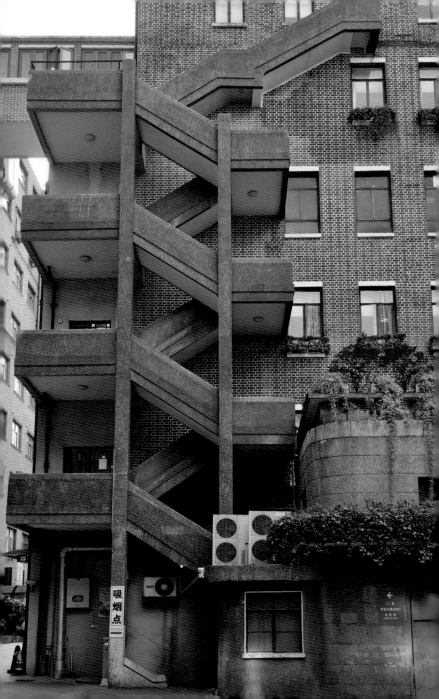

He added that more domestic doctors joined the hospital since the 1930s. After World War II ended, Chinese doctor Chen Bangdian became the director. In 1948, the hospital had up to 318 beds.

During the next 50 years, this oldest Western hospital of Shanghai continued to grow and now has four branch hospitals of more than 2,000 beds across the city plus a medical research institute specialized in tumor. The old hospital on Shandong Road, where the bricked building donated by Henry Lester still stands, is called the Western branch of Renji Hospital.

In December 2019, the hospital celebrated its 175th anniversary by opening a hospital museum.

"Renji Hospital has witnessed the vicissitudes of history, the prosperity of Shanghai, and led to the development of medicine over 175 years. She will continue to be full of vitality, and will continue to strive to reach the peak of medicine," as is written in the museum's preface.

Yesterday: Renji Hospital   **Today:** Renji Hospital   **Address:** 145 Shandong Road M.
Built in: 1932   **Architect:** Lester, Johnson & Morris Co.
Tips: The building donated by Henry Lester is still for medical use.

英国慈善医学先驱去世

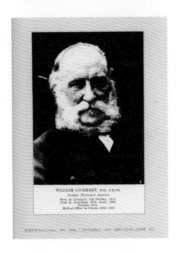

WILLIAM LOCKHART, M.D., F.R.C.S.
(London Missionary Society)
Born at Liverpool, 3rd October, 1811.
Died at Lewisham, 29th April, 1896.
Founder 1844.
Medical Officer in Charge, 1844–1856.

威廉姆·洛克哈特(William Lockhart, 1811—1896),上海仁济医院创始人,1844—1856年为仁济医院院长。提译

　　在远东知名的医疗传教士洛克哈特先生（William Lockhart，又名雒魏林）于 4 月 29 日上午在布莱克希思（Blackheath）的住所去世，享年八十四岁。

　　洛克哈特先生曾在都柏林的盖伊医院（Guy's Hospital）和米斯医院(The Meath Hospital)攻读医学专业，并于 1834 年成为英格兰皇家外科医学院的成员。他先担任利物浦韦恩莱特先生（AS Wainwright ）的助理，并在那里待了三年多。当约翰·威廉姆斯(John Williams)和莫法特博士(Dr. Moffat)传教归来后，他也燃起成为一名医学传教士的愿望，为伦敦会服务。他被派到中国，与麦都斯先生（注：Walter Henry Medhurst, 19世纪来华重要的传教士之一、著名汉学家/出版家）一起从英国启程，在巴达维亚(Batavia)的华人间做传教工作。

　　1839年，洛克哈特先生开始在澳门工作。他从澳门来到舟山，1843年上海刚开埠他就搬到了那个城市，并在那里创办了一家医院。这家医院从一开始就非常成功，中国病人的人数很快在十个月内达到上万人。 1858年他回英国前，将医院置于有效率的监管之下，

并扩展了医院的适用领域。他很满意地了解到那是目前中国最重要的华人医院。

1861年，洛克哈特先生作为英国驻京使馆的医务官返回中国，在两年半的时间里，治疗了3万多名患者。他最终于1864年返回英国，并一直从事工作到1895年。

在职业生涯中，洛克哈特先生反应迅速、操作熟练、耐心对待结果。凭借着敏锐的洞察力，他总是能快速做出诊断。直到生命的最后阶段，他都随时做好准备响应工作的召唤。他充满爱心，仁慈温柔又开朗，深受患者的喜爱。他一直很关照病人，不仅是他们值得信赖的顾问，而且是深受爱戴的朋友。

他收藏了大量珍贵的关于中国的藏书，其多样性和完整性是独一无二的。他最近将这些收藏交给伦敦会，这批藏品经过仔细整理，以便在传教士之家阅览参考，这里也被称为"洛克哈特图书馆"。

洛克哈特先生广受欢迎，直到生病的前一天，他都充满活力、光彩和精力。他在作为医学传教士的职业生涯中所表现出的奉献精神与高尚的克己精神贯穿于他后来的人生中，很难找到一个比他更正直、更高尚的人。在他异常多变的人生最艰难的情况下，他总是表现出最大的毅力，而他的善心让所有认识他的人都喜欢他。

摘自 1896 年 12 月 1 日《教务杂志》

Philanthropic British medical pioneer dies at the age of 84

Known as a medical missionary in the Far East, William Lockhart passed away on the morning of April 29 at his residence at Blackheath at the ripe age of eighty-four years.

Mr. Lockhart pursued his medical studies at Guy's Hospital and at The Meath Hospital, Dublin and became a member of The Royal College of Surgeons of England in 1834. He first began practice as assistant to Mr. AS Wainwright of Liverpool, where he remained for three years, but on the return of John Williams and Dr. Moffat from their missionary journeys he was fired with the desire of becoming a medical missionary and offered his services to the London Missionary Society in that capacity. He was appointed to China and left England with Mr. Medhurst, then engaged as a missionary to the Chinese in Batavia.

Mr. Lockhart began his work at Macau in 1839. From Macau he moved to Chusan, and as soon as Shanghai was opened up in 1843, he moved on to that city and founded a hospital there, which was most successful from the first, with Chinese patients soon reaching 10,000 within ten months. He returned to England in 1858, leaving the hospital under efficient superintendence for the further extension of its sphere of usefulness, and he had the satisfaction of knowing that it is at the present time the most important hospital for Chinese in China.

Mr. Lockhart returned to China as Medical Officer of the British Embassy in Beijing in 1861 and during the two and a half years over 30,000 patients were treated.

He finally returned to England in 1864 and remained in practice until 1895.

In the exercise of his profession he was prompt, skillful and patient of results. Of keen insight, he was always quick at diagnosis and to the very last always prepared for an instant response to the call of duty. His loving kindness and tender cheerfulness endeared him to his patients, amongst whom he was always looked for, not only as the trusted adviser, but as the much-loved friend.

He had collected a large and valuable library of works on China, unique in its variety and comprehensiveness. This he gave quite recently to the London Missionary Society upon certain conditions, which have been carefully carried out, so that it is available for reference at the Mission House, and is known as the "Lockhart

Library" .

Mr. Lockhart was universally beloved; he was full of life, brightness and energy up to the very day before his short illness. The devotion and noble self–denial exhibited during his career as a medical missionary were carried through every relation of later life, and a more thoroughly upright and honorable man in all his dealings it would be very hard to find. In the most trying circumstances of his unusually varied life he always exhibited the utmost fortitude, while his kindness of heart endeared him to all who knew him.

Excerpt from *The Chinese Recorder and Missionary Journal*
on December 1, 1896

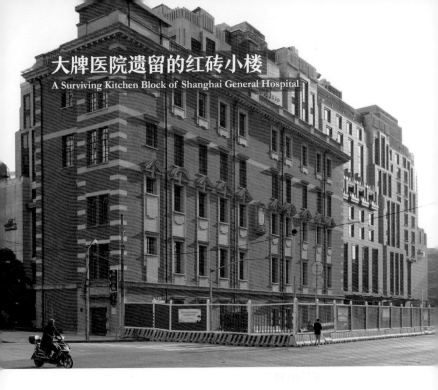

大牌医院遗留的红砖小楼
A Surviving Kitchen Block of Shanghai General Hospital

上海北外滩宝丽嘉酒店的花园里，有一座红砖砌成的古典建筑，是大名鼎鼎的公济医院（Shanghai General Hospital）唯一遗留的小楼。公济医院开办于1864年，曾经是中国规模最大的医院，也是旅沪外侨治疗的首选地。

公济医院院史显示，由于旅沪外侨人数不断增长，1862年时管理旧法租界的公董局委托意大利神父 P. Mannus Desjacoues 筹办一家综合型西医院。神父募集5万两白银资金后，在外滩与高尔朋路（Rue Colbert，今新永安路)转角租下一幢四层楼建筑。如今，这座建筑早已拆除，建造了今天外滩22号大楼。

1864年1月，这家由法国天主教会、法租界公董局和公共租界工部局共同出资的医院正式开业，开始规模不大，仅有17个病房，35张床位，主要收治英国、法国和美国病人，治疗风湿病、梅毒等疾病。医院仅有一位由七人董事会任命的住院医师，但病人可以外请其他医院的医生前来诊疗。医护人员是法国天主教仁爱会的修女，她们不仅负责护理工作，也要管理医院的运营。

根据《上海宗教史》记载，1877年医院迁至苏州河北岸，取名公济医院。公济医院在新址附近不断购地扩建，就是红砖小楼的所在地。1914年英文《北华捷报》(*The North - China Herald*)报道显示，这座幸存的小楼位于院区的东北角，是当时两座新建的建筑之一。

"这两座新楼的设计完全是为了满足医院管理的需要，一座为天主教修女提供急需的住宿，另一座被称为'厨房楼'(kitchen block)，专门安排用于医院后勤工作。建筑均由来自德和洋行(Lester, Johnson & Morriss)的乔治·约翰逊先生(George A. Johnson)设计。建造工作的每个阶段都受到非常仔细的监督，因此在不影响工艺或所用材料质量的情况下，显著地节省了预估成本。很快，这座建筑将展现值得称赞的规划设计和高效经济的施工。它提供的住宿条件充足而舒适，但风格朴素。建筑外部是红砖，有裸露的石材饰面。"这篇1914年12月5日的报道提到。

报道中提到的修女宿舍占地613平方米，高达四层，设有办公室、社区活动室、客厅、储藏室、修女病房和小教堂，很可惜已被拆除。酒店花园中幸存的红砖小楼是同期建造的厨房后勤楼，面积略小，占地约502平方米。

1914年的报道提到，厨房楼的一层是华人工作人员的宿舍，二层为日本护士的房间和梳妆室。小楼配备有储藏室和洗衣房，干衣室配有特殊的蒸汽加热设备。

如今，小楼仍保留着简洁美丽的红砖立面，装饰有石质檐口、券窗和精美石雕。虽然风格简洁，但这两座小楼都是设备齐全的功能性医院建筑，而且似乎"非常适合它们的特殊用途"。

"蒸汽散热器供暖和卫浴安装均由上海自来水公司

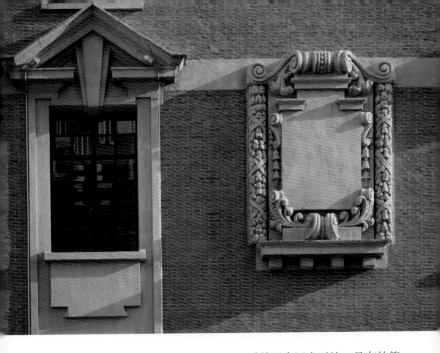

（Shanghai Water Works Company）负责，电线则来自上海电气石棉公司（Shanghai Electric and Asbestos Company）。两座小楼甚至配备了电梯，由Messrs. Smith, Major & Stevens制造。建筑使用大量的钢筋混凝土建造，以便尽可能地防火，也提供消防逃生楼梯以应付紧急情况。"报道写道。

上海市档案馆研究员彭晓亮查阅馆藏的《上海公济医院纪念刊》（1948年）发现，公济医院不对普通中国人开放，具有外籍的华人才能入住。外籍病人不限国籍，有近50个免费床位为无国籍的外侨准备。

"因为医生和病人都来自不同国家，讲各种语言，所以不同国籍的修女对医院工作很有裨益。医院为英国、美国、意大利等国的水手特设病房，商号、海关、捕房人员也享受同样待遇。另外医院还设有婴儿病房、男孩病房和女孩病房，锡克族印度人也尽可能住在同一病房。"他在《苏州河畔的公济医院》一文中

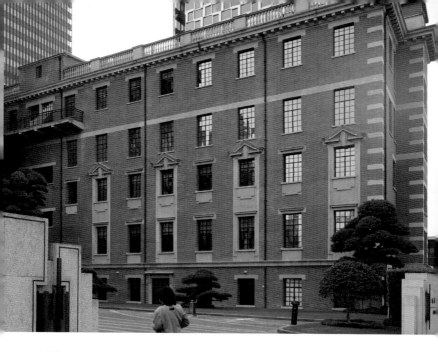

写道。

根据他的研究统计，截至1935年9月，公济医院共有病床270个，住院病人最高达150人。医务人员仅院长1人，住院医师1至2人，修女30名，护士20名。1937年，公济医院开始录用上海震旦大学附设护士学校毕业的中国护士，在修女领导下工作。1937年"八·一三"抗战爆发后，公济医院历经一段动荡坎坷的岁月，医护人员和70名重病患者辗转迁移，后来暂住在爱文义路（Avenue Road，今北京西路）雷士德医学研究院。此后医院遭受两次炮击轰炸，幸未造成人员伤亡。

值得一提的是，捐建雷士德医学研究院的英侨富商雷士德（Henry Lester）也曾经在公济医院治疗，1926年在医院去世前留下遗嘱将几乎全部财产捐给上海的慈善事业。在老上海英文报纸的讣告栏里，公济医院是经常出现的名字，大多数外国侨民在这家医院走完人生旅程。

1940年，公济医院被日军作为病囚集中地，收治来自龙华、

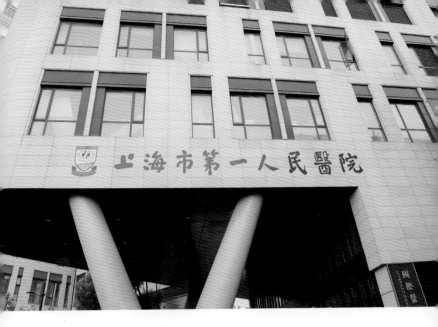

闸北等全市各地集中营的病人，后来又一度被日本海军征用。

"1945年8月15日，抗战胜利的消息传来，公济医院一片欢腾。中国军方派代表前来祝贺，并向病人敬献鲜花。被长期拘禁于此的病囚及其亲友们劫后余生，分外兴奋。当天下午，不同国籍的人们齐集修女院中，高唱赞美诗，庆祝抗战胜利。"彭晓亮写道。

二战结束后，朱仰高接任公济医院院长。他为医院邀请名医，创设为乡民看病的卡车"流动医院"，为公济医院赢得新的声誉。

"公济医院的规模很大，有200多名医护人员，从设备和技术的先进程度上来讲，当时的宝隆医院(今长征医院)是最强的，但公济医院的条件、服务却是上海最好的。除了三、四等病房以外，每一个病房区至少有两个修女和一个护士负责，而且每间病房都有独立的卫浴设备，所以公济医院实质上还是一个贵族医院。"1947年到公济医院工作、后来担任副院长的唐孝均曾在一次访谈中回忆。

1949年后，公济医院由上海

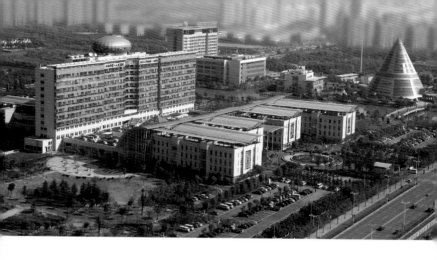

市人民政府接管，1953年改名上海市立第一人民医院，从"贵族医院"转变为"人民医院"，1966年改名为上海市第一人民医院。历经搬迁和扩建后，医院如今坐落于虹口区武进路的现代化院区，在松江也有院区。医院获得包括"中国百家医院"在内的许多国家级奖项，2002年成为上海交通大学附属第一人民医院。2022年成为上海交通大学医学院附属第一人民医院。

昔日公济医院的历史建筑大多不存，仅剩下酒店花园里这座红砖小楼。不过，第一人民医院仍沿用了源自19世纪的英文院名——"Shanghai General Hospital"。漫步医院，有心人会发现很多地方标记着"1864"这个建院的年份，如电梯上方的装饰和门口巨石上的医院标志。

2020年，上海市第一人民医院历经数年终于完成了院志的编纂，有875页之多。这座苏州河边的医院，也是一本厚厚的大书。

昨天： 公济医院　**今天：** 上海市第一人民医院　　**地址：** 北苏州路 190 号　　**建造年代：** 1914
建筑风格： 新古典主义　　**建筑师：** 乔治·约翰逊（George A. Johnson）
参观指南： 可以在天潼路（近北苏州路）欣赏百年医院小楼精美的红砖立面。

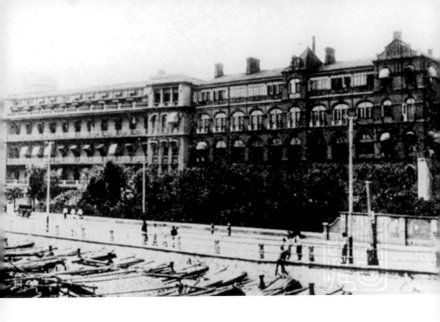

In the stylish garden of Shanghai Bellagio Hotel stands a classic red-brick building which is the only surviving architecture of the once largest hospital in China, Shanghai General Hospital. The hospital, often the first choice for expatriates living in old Shanghai, has operated since 1864.

"Founded by French Catholic medical missionaries in the former French section of the Bund, Shanghai General Hospital treated expatriates only and served also as a sanatorium," says Lu Ming, a medical historian from Shanghai No. 4 People's Hospital.

According to the annals of Shanghai General Hospital, the municipal council of the former Shanghai French Concession planned to establish a comprehensive hospital for the city's growing number of expatriates in 1862. Italian father P. Mannus Desjacoues, who was commissioned for the job, raised 50,000 taels of silver and rented a four-story building at the crossing of the Bund and Rue Colbert (today's Xinyong'an Road) to open the hospital. The site is the present "Bund 22", a life-style complex on 22 Zhongshan Road E2.

The hospital opened officially in 1864 and was funded by the Catholic church, as well as municipal councils from both the French Concession and the International Settlement.

At the beginning, the hospital was small with only 17 wards and 35 beds. It received British, French and American patients and treated dozens of diseases like rheumatism, syphilis and chest problems. With only a resident doctor designated by the hospital's committee of seven council members, doctors from other hospitals were often invited by patients for medical treatment. The nurses were 10 Catholic sisters, who were responsible for medical care and administration work.

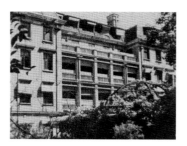

The General Hospital was developed and expanded after moving to an 18-mu site (around 12,006 square meters) purchased along the bank of Suzhou River where the red building of Bellagio Hotel now stands.

A surviving building

According to a 1914 report on *the North-China Herald*, this surviving building is one of the two newly completed extension blocks situated on the northeast corner of the hospital compound.

"The two extensive blocks of new buildings, which are designed entirely to meet the needs of the hospital administration, one providing much needed accommodation for the Catholic sisters, and the other, known as the kitchen block, being exclusively arranged for the domestic work of the hospital. The buildings have been designed by Mr. George A. Johnson (of the firm of Lester, Johnson & Morriss), and the contractor is Koo Lan-chow. Every stage of the work has been very carefully supervised, with the result that an appreciable saving on the estimated cost has been effected, without impairing workmanship or the quality of the materials used. The building will at once be seen to the admirably planned and efficiently and economically constructed, the accommodation being adequate and comfortable, but plain in style. The exterior is of red brick with patent stone facing," the report said on December 5, 1914.

Covering an area of 613 square meters, the four-story building for the Catholic sisters housed offices, community room, a parlor, store rooms, sick wards for the sisters and a chapel. It's a real pity that this building had been demolished. The surviving building in the hotel garden was the five-story kitchen block that covered an area of 502 square meters.

"On the first floor there are quarters for the Chinese attendants and on the second, rooms for the Japanese nurses and dressers. The building is completely equipped with store rooms and a laundry, with special steam-heating apparatus in the drying room," the newspaper said.

Today, the building retains the simple-cut, red-brick façade graced by stone cornice, arched windows and an exquisite stone carving as the centerpiece. Though simple in style, both blocks were well-equipped functional hospital buildings which appeared "to be excellently adapted to their special purposes".

Both the heating by steam radiators and the general sanitary installation were carried out by the Shanghai Water Works Company, while the electric wiring was done by the Shanghai Electric and Asbestos Company. The two buildings were even equipped with electric lifts, which were manufactured by Messrs. Smith, Major & Stevens. A good deal of reinforced concrete was put into the buildings, rendering them as nearly fireproof as possible. Fire escape staircases were provided to meet emergencies.

According to the research of expert Peng Xiaoliang from the Shanghai Archives Bureau, the hospital was not open to Chinese, but foreign patients were not limited to their nationalities. There were 50 free beds prepared for stateless aliens.

"Because doctors and patients of the hospital came from different countries and spoke various languages, nuns of different nationalities were very helpful. There were special wards for foreign sailors, a baby ward, a boy ward and a girl ward. Sikh Indians were arranged to live in the same ward as much as possible," Peng said of his research on a Shanghai General Hospital memorial booklet, which was published in 1948 and preserved in the Shanghai Archives Bureau.

According to Peng's research, the hospital grew to have 270 beds and housed up to 150 inpatients by September 1935. There was one medical superintendent, one to two resident doctors, 30 nuns and 20 nurses. In 1937, the hospital began recruiting Chinese students who graduated from the Aurora University School of Nursing in Shanghai as nursing assistants.

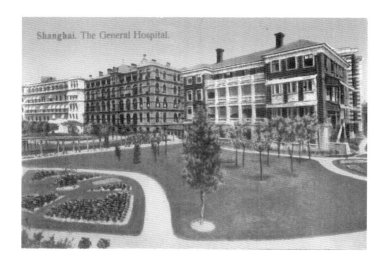

Shanghai. The General Hospital.

After World War II broke out, the hospital underwent a turbulent period. Between September and November 1937, the hospital was bombed twice, but fortunately no one was hurt.

The hospital staff had to transfer more than 70 seriously ill patients to the Lester Institute of Medical Research on today's Beijing Road W.. The institute was built with assets donated by British tycoon Henry Lester shortly before he died of disease in the general hospital in 1926.

In the obituary columns of old Shanghai English newspapers, the general hospital was frequently mentioned as a place where many expatriates passed away in Shanghai.

During World War II the hospital turned into a concentration hospital by Japanese military force. A number of the 160 sick prisoners from Japanese camps were sent to the hospital for medical treatment, some of whom were critically ill, in poor nutritional condition or even dying.

"On August 15, 1945, when the news of the victory of the war against Japanese invaders came, Shanghai General Hospital was full of joy. The Chinese military sent representatives to congratulate and present flowers to the patients. The sick prisoners and their relatives and friends who were detained there for a long time were all very excited. In the afternoon of the same day, people

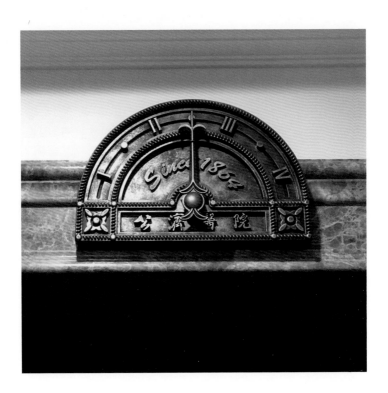

of different nationalities gathered in the sisters' building and sang hymns to celebrate the victory," Peng adds.

After World War II, Chinese doctor Zhu Yanggao became the new director and did much work to boost the hospital's reputation, such as the well-received "mobile hospital" project. The director renovated a truck into a medical vehicle and sent service to people in the countryside.

"The scale of the hospital was very large with more than 200 medical staffs when I joined as an intern doctor in 1947," said Tang Xiaojun, former deputy director of the hospital, in an earlier interview.

"In terms of equipment and technology, the then Paulun Hospital (today's Changzheng Hospital) was the best in Shanghai. But the General Hospital provided the best conditions and services. Except for the third and fourth-class wards, each ward area had at least two nuns and a nurse on service. The wards were equipped with private bathroom facilities. It was essentially a noble hospital," Tang said.

After 1949, the hospital was taken over by the Shanghai government. Its Chinese name, Gongji Hospital, was changed to Shanghai First People's Hospital on January 1, 1953. After relocation and expansion, the hospital moved to the present site on Wujin Road and grew to be a modern comprehensive hospital. Having won many national awards including "China's Top 100 Hospitals", it became the First People's Hospital affiliated to Shanghai Jiao Tong University School of Medicine in 2002. Now the hospital has a branch in Songjiang District.

Today, most historical buildings in the old hospital compound have been demolished, except for the red-brick building in the hotel garden. But the hospital still kept its old English name, Shanghai General Hospital. The founding year, 1864, is seen everywhere, from above the elevators to its logo gracing a big stone fronting the hospital.

In 2020, Shanghai General Hospital completed the compiling work of its newest hospital annals, which is a large book of 875 pages. And this river-side hospital is also like a big, heavy book.

Shanghai General Hospital was another health care hospice at the forefront of medicine and it provided hospitals that followed a blueprint for future medical care.

Yesterday: Shanghai General hospital
Today: Shanghai General Hospital (Shanghai First People's Hospital)
Address: 190 Suzhou Road N.   **Built in:** 1914
Architectural style: Neo-classic   **Architect:** George A. Johnson
Tips: The façade of the century-old surviving building graced by arched windows and a stone carving can be appreciated from Tiantong Road (across Suzhou Road N.).

"铁肺"人到公济医院

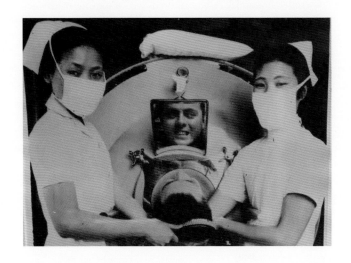

　　"铁肺人"弗雷德里克·斯奈特（Frederick B. Snite）成功完成他回家之旅的第一站，这趟从北京到芝加哥的万里旅程将创造历史。今天凌晨3点15分，他从北平乘坐专列抵达上海北站。"医院"快车在车站8号站台短暂停留后，被转到宝山路一个站台附近，以便将呼吸装置（注：斯奈特使用的是"铁肺"——一个连接泵的密封铁盒子，可以代替肺的功能帮助脊髓灰质炎患者呼吸）转移到救护车上。据透露，这名患者情况良好。

　　"铁肺"中的26岁美国青年斯奈特于今天凌晨3点左右从北平乘坐专列抵达上海北站。昨晚，一位《大陆报》（The China Press）驻南京的记者报道说，在过去 14 个月里一直戴着呼吸器生活的年轻的斯奈特，带着 18 人的随从展开他史诗般的跨越半个地球的旅程。他看上去状态很好也很开朗，于昨天下午 5 点 10 分抵达浦口。

　　晚上7点，斯奈特的火车渡过长江后开往上海。到达这里后，斯奈特带着他的重型"铁肺"人工呼吸器，将被放在一辆特殊的救护车上，然后加速前往公济医院，直到他登上周日前往旧金山的柯立芝总统号为止。

昨晚上海一切准备就绪，将瘫痪病人从北站快速运送到北苏州路总医院。

大上海特别市的警察与和平保护总队将随时准备清理从铁路车站到租界边界的交通。当斯奈特的救护车开进租界时，上海市巡捕房要派摩托车护送。

老斯奈特先生（Frederick B. Snite, Sr.）是芝加哥的富商，也是这位患病青年的父亲，他告诉记者，他的儿子很开朗，吃得很好，在旅途中表现得非常令人满意。

在公济医院，年轻的斯奈特将在那里待近 48 小时，所有工作人员，甚至是苦力，都被告知他的到来。

摘自 1937 年 6 月 4 日《大陆报》

Man in "Iron Lung" Transferred to General Hospital

Successfully completing the first leg of his history-making 10,000-mile trip to his home in Chicago, Frederick B. Snite, "the man in the iron lung" arrived at the North Station in a special train from Peiping at 3:15 o'clock this morning. The "hospital" express, after stopping briefly at platform No. 8 of the station, was shunted near a platform on Paoshan Road, in order to enable the respirator to be moved to the ambulance. The patient, it was revealed, was doing well.

Frederick B. Snite, 26-year-old American youth in the "iron lung" was due at the Shanghai North Station in a special train from Peiping at around 3 o'clock this morning.

Traveling with a retinue of 18 people on his epic journey half way around the world, young Snite, who has been living in his respirator for the past 14 months, was reported last night by a China Press correspondent in Nanking as looking well and cheerful when he arrived at Pukow at 5:10 o'clock yesterday afternoon.

The Snite train, after being ferried across the Yangtse, left for Shanghai at 7pm. Shanghai railway officials stated last night that the special was due at the North Station at about 3:15 o'clock according to the pre-arranged schedule.

On his arrival here, Snite, in his heavy iron artificial respirator, was to be placed in a special ambulance and sped to the General Hospital where he will stay until he boards the President Coolidge which sails Sunday for San Francisco.

Everything in Shanghai was ready last night for the speedy transportation of the paralysis patient from the North Station to the General Hospital on North Soochow Road.

The Greater Shanghai Police and Peace Preservation Corps would be on hand to clear the traffic from the railway depot to the boundary of the Settlement. When Snite's ambulance entered the Settlement Road, a motorcycle escort was to be furnished by the Shanghai Municipal Police.

Mr. Frederick B. Snite, Sr., wealthy Chicago merchant and father of the stricken youth, told pressmen that his son was cheerful, eating well, and standing the trip in a most satisfactory manner.

At the General Hospital, where young Snite will remain for nearly 48 hours, the entire staff, even down to the coolies, were apprised of his coming and everyone who may be even remotely connected with his visit was drilled in correct procedure.

Excerpt from *The China Press* on June 4, 1937

公济医院回家

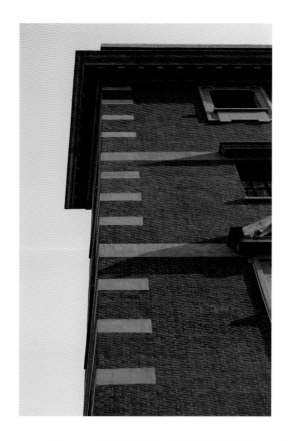

    1 月 14 日，公济医院收复了位于北苏州路的院区。白天，患者和设备从爱文义路1320 号雷士德医学研究院分别转移到消防救护车和卡车上。三辆救护车将30名男女老幼从临时病房运送到虹口，到中午时分全部安全转移。

    公济医院的收治量为220张床位，但目前只有很少的数量可用。

医疗主管钱伯斯医生（Dr. G. Chambers）、财务主管麦尔科先生（J. E. Melchior）和由玛丽亚方济各传教女修会组成的大量护理人员现已全部安置在医院。

总的来说，这座建筑在最近的战争中受到了一些影响。被炮弹击中的手术室已部分修复。花园里，就在北苏州路的围墙内，有两个相当大的弹孔，导弹显然是在炮击过程中从西北方向上空掠过建筑。一枚炮弹在男孩宿舍爆炸，造成了损坏。

为了给患者和工作人员返院做好准备，这里已经热火朝天地忙了一周。

早上，厨房的烟囱里冒出炊烟。医院大门附近的一棵树上挂着一个鸟笼（带鸟），为回归增添了一丝中国风。

这次"回家"结束了始于去年 8 月 16 日的流亡岁月，那时战争才刚刚开始。医院搬迁到南京路新的大通银行大楼（Chase Bank Building），后来它被转移到雷士德医学研究院。

摘自 1938 年 1 月 19 日《北华捷报》

General Hospital is reoccupied

The General Hospital reoccupied its permanent quarters in North Soochow Road on January 14. Patients and equipment being shifted during the day from the Henry Lester Institute of Medical Research, 1320 Avenue Road, in fire brigade ambulances and lorries respectively. Three ambulances were used to convey 30 men, women and children from the temporary wards to Hongkow and all had been safely transferred by noon.

The capacity of the General Hospital is 220 beds, but for the time being only a much smaller number will be available. Dr. G. Chambers, medical superintendent, Mr. J. E. Melchior, treasurer and the large nursing staff composed of Franciscan Missionaries of Mary are now all installed in the hospital.

Generally speaking, the building suffered a little during the recent hostilities. The damage to the operating theatre, which was struck by a shell, has been partly repaired. In the garden, just inside the wall in North Soochow Road, are two sizable shell-holes, the missiles having apparently come over the building from the northwest in the course of Chinese shelling. One projectile exploded in the "boys" quarters, which were damaged.

The heat has been on in the large structure for a week in preparation for the return of patients and staff.

In the morning smoke was pouring from the kitchen chimney. From a tree near the main entrance a bird-cage (with bird) was suspended, lending a Chinese touch to the return.

The homecoming ended an exile which began on August 16, last year, when the hostilities had just started. At that time the hospital removed to the new Chase Bank Building in Nanking Road. It was later transferred to the Henry Lester Institute.

Excerpt from *The North-China Herald* on January 19, 1938

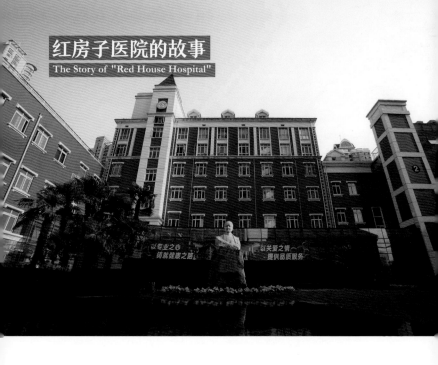

红房子医院的故事
The Story of "Red House Hospital"

　　1885年，西门妇孺医院（Margaret Williamson Memorial Hospital）位于方斜路的新院舍落成。屋顶与外墙覆盖红砖瓦，非常醒目，被人们称为"红房子医院"。

　　这家医院在百年前的院址开设至今，如今是复旦大学附属妇产科医院，但上海市民仍亲切地叫她"红房子医院"。

　　"我们医院是中国近代以来第三个专为妇女和儿童设立的医院，也是上海首家妇儿专科医院。"复旦大学附属妇产科医院王珏副书记说。

　　"红房子医院"源起于1882年，当时美国基督教女公会成员玛格利特·威廉逊夫人（Margaret Williamson）捐款5000美元，用于在上海建造一座妇儿医院。值得一提的是，这位玛格利特·威廉逊夫人是一位纽约的女裁缝，并非富豪。但她不仅慷慨捐出这笔5000美元积蓄，

1883年去世前还留下遗嘱，将财产皆用于建院之需。

善良大方的"玛格利特"未能亲眼看到上海妇儿医院建成，但两位相当能干的"伊丽莎白"很快实现了她的心愿。玛格利特·威廉逊夫人去世这一年，女公会传教医师伊丽莎白·罗夫施奈德（Elizabeth Reifsnyder）抵沪，于老城西门外方斜路租房两间，开办诊所，筹建医院。次年4月，首位来华的基督教传教护士伊丽莎白·麦基奇尼（Elizabeth McKechnie）也参与其中。两人齐心合力建院，在美国基督教女公会等各方支持下，一幢二层建筑在旧法租界与老西门之间落成，于1885年6月3日正式开张，有床位20张。

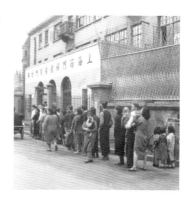

1885年6月5日的英文《北华捷报》（*The North-China Herald*）报道了开幕仪式，介绍这家由简陋诊所发展起来的"优秀机构"。医院命名为"玛格利特·威廉逊纪念医院"（Margaret Williamson Memorial Hospital），以纪念怀着同情心与慈善热情捐出微博积蓄的威廉逊夫人，中文名为"西门妇孺医院"。在医院一楼用作接待和礼拜堂的大房间里，悬挂着这位夫人的肖像。罗夫施奈德医生担任主治医师，文恒理（注：H.W. Boone，著名医生/医学教育家，美国圣公会首任驻华主教文惠廉之子，曾担任同仁医院院长）任兼职医师，麦基奇尼小姐被任命为护士长。

在"红房子医院"建院初期，中国因为贫穷落后，医药卫生状况落后，不科学的旧式接生法造成的产妇死亡率和婴儿死亡率相当高。因此，作为沪上最早的妇儿专科医院，西门妇孺医院比其他教会医院更受社会欢迎。根据《上海宗教史》，开业翌年，西门妇孺医院诊治人数已

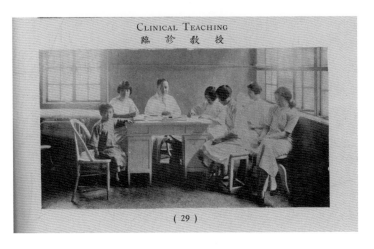

CLINICAL TEACHING
臨 診 教 授

（29）

达16138人，其中初诊病人9361人，到1887年增至18062人，初诊占11448人。

"早期的教会医院大多规模小，且无明确的科别之分。随着人员设施的日渐完备，教会医院皆由专科性向综合性发展。西门妇孺医院初以妇产科为主，到20世纪20年代已是一所拥有门诊部、公共卫生部、内科、外科、妇产科、耳鼻喉科、眼科等颇具规模的综合性医院。"《上海宗教史》记载。

1926年夏天，斯裔匈籍建筑师邬达克（L.E. Hudec）撰写了一份简历，介绍1925年1月创办事务所后设计的项目，其中包括三个医院项目：宝隆医院（Paulun Hospital，今长征医院）、当时刚开业的宏恩医院（Country Hospital，今华东医院）和西门妇孺医院宿舍楼。

邬达克毕业于布达佩斯的匈牙利皇家约瑟夫技术大学建筑系，1914年应征入伍参加一战，1916年不幸被俘。一战后奥匈帝国解体，在遣返途中的他于1918年逃至上海。当时他身无分文且有腿伤，但这个受过专业建筑教育的年轻人正是当时上海需要的人才。

他先在美国建筑师罗兰·克利（Rowland Curry）的克利洋行找到绘图员的工作，后自立门户，至1947年离开上海时，他设计建成了包括远东第一高楼——国际饭店、远东第一影院——大光明大戏院、远东第一豪宅——吴同文住宅、远东最豪华医院——宏恩医院、中国知名学府上海交通大学的扩建规划及其工程馆、中国最大的啤酒厂——联合啤酒厂等54个项目，近百个单体建筑。

邬达克在上海最后一件力作"吴同文住宅"因为通体覆盖绿色釉面砖，又被称作"绿房子"。很少有人知道邬达克还为"红房子"设计过新的医院建筑。

1921年，"红房子医院"附设"上海协和高级护士学校"（Shanghai Union School of Nursing），1924年又与迁沪的苏州女子医学院共同创办"上海女子医学院"（Shanghai Woman's Christian Medical College），是当时上海唯一的女子医学院。

王莉娟和苏智良在《上海西门妇孺医院研究（1884—1952）》一文中评价，1921年是西门妇孺医院发展史上的第一个转折点，"它从一所普通的医院转变为一所与医学教育相结合的医学院，为当时的医学界培养了一批优秀的医务护理人才"。

《上海宗教史》一书提到，上海女子医学院开设解剖、生化、生理、药理、细菌、外科、产科、妇科、神经、精神等14个专业。医学院在美国哥伦比亚特区立案，得授医学博士学位。医学院的开设，使西门妇孺医院在人员、技术上获得充分保障。

医院通过创办卫校和医学院，解决了医护人才不足的难题，同时也不断扩建院区。1924年，一座占地24亩、临床与教学相结合的建筑竣工，内设普通病房、产科室、办公室、医生休息室等。1931年又建成一座产科楼，X光机和其他电子仪器配置齐全，诊治能力显著提高。

1931年6月13日，《大陆报》报道说，"新的西门妇孺医院"将在旧址上建造一个由三个建筑单元组成的院区，造价超过5万美元。其中第一个建筑，梁氏产科大楼将于夏季启用，建筑

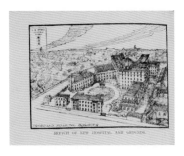

师是邬达克先生。

报道提到，西门妇孺医院产科每月出生的婴儿比上海任何一家医院都多，平均每个月有120到130个，是中国最大的产科诊所。新大楼将有200张床位，会特别关注私人病房的需求。

"参观这座隐藏在老城墙后面的院区，它位于上海老城东门附近的一条狭窄通道上，是一种趣味盎然、充满启发的体验。有45年历史的花园很幽静，周围是老行政楼、老产科楼、贝内特纪念实验室（Bennett Memorial Laboratories）和门诊部、医学院学生宿舍、医生宿舍和新式厨房，还有基本完工的产科大楼。在该地区拥挤、恶臭的生活区的中心，这是一个奇迹。"1931年的报告描述道。

记者的笔触生动介绍了产科

病房里"面容清新、魅力十足的护士们"，有着闪亮的黑发，"长长的白色围裙穿在东方化的蓝色制服上"。

"病人在病房里看起来如此舒服，让你不禁怀疑临时护理是她们在日常生活中体会不到的舒适时光，她们正在为遭受的痛苦而得到补偿。"报道写到。

抗战期间，西门妇孺医院组成了医疗救护队，救治孕妇、新生儿和受伤的妇女。但医院因处南市战区而损失惨重，房舍不是毁于战火，就是被日伪侵占。医院临时迁到徐家汇路，在延安中路另设门诊部和妇科。1942年后，医院由中国人主持，邝翠娥任院长。

1948年，医院把大部分设备搬回方斜路419号原址，恢复原来各科室，将徐家汇路850号作为分院，举行盛大的复院庆典。1952年，著名妇产科专家王淑贞任院长。

一百多年来，"红房子医院"从一个仅有20张床位的小医院发展为有两家分院、800多张床位、集医疗、教学、科研于一体的知名专科医院，年门诊量高达170万人次。

《上海邬达克建筑》一书提到，根据邬达克设计的原始图纸，该医院的建筑设计风格属法国学院派的古典主义风格。水平及垂直三段式构图，双坡屋面庄重平和，南侧东西两端的门廊入口带有西班牙式的三联拱券式列柱门廊，使整个立面设计活泼生动。这种寓变化与统一的设计特点，是邬达克设计作品中常用的神来之笔。而现存的建筑不同于上述的风格。

意大利建筑史专家卢卡·彭切里尼（Luca Poncellini）在《邬达克》（Laszlo Hudec）一书中提到，邬达克替西门妇孺医院"设计了一个新的总规划，替换掉几处废弃已久而无法使用的危房"。但由于保存下来关于这个项目的档案很少且无连贯性，无法判断哪些部分是邬达克设计并建造的，哪些部分是后期以同种风格而建造的。

黄浦区文物档案显示，医院现存的历史建筑（现7号楼办公用房）为二层砖木结构建筑，占地面积461平方米，用红砖、红瓦砌成，高二层，坡顶、门窗为拱形。

"这栋7号楼应该是管理大楼。邬达克的总平面图上也是这么写的。邬达克设计的主要是梁氏产科大楼和护士学校宿舍。"《上海邬达克建筑地图》作者、同济大学华霞虹教授说。

医院精心布置了院史馆，在展览入口处挂着威廉逊夫人和罗夫施奈德医生的肖像。一件件展品和史料，生动讲述着这家由女性捐赠、创办、管理、运营，以疗愈女性病痛为使命的医院的非凡故事。

2003年，复旦大学附属妇产科医院正式使用"上海市红房子妇产科医院"为第二冠名。"红房子"的故事，还在这里续写着。

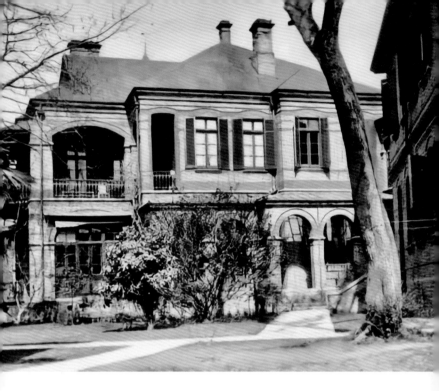

Margaret Williamson Memorial Hospital was nicknamed "Red House Hospital" in old Shanghai for its new building in 1885 covered by eye-catching red bricks and tiles. Operated on the original site until today, the institution is still called "Red House Hospital" by local people.

"This hospital is the third hospital dedicated to women and children in modern China, and the first hospital of its kind in Shanghai," says Wang Yu, deputy party-secretary of the institution, now named Obstetrics & Gyne-cology Hospital of Fudan University.

The humble beginning of the "Red House Hospital" dated to 1882, when Margaret Woodworth Williamson, a New York seam dresser and a charter member of the Woman's Union Missionary Society, gave a sum of $5,000 for the building of a hospital for women and children in Shanghai.

Though she died in 1883, two women of medical background, Dr. Elizabeth Reifsnyder and Miss Elizabeth Mckechnie, the first foreign nurse to China, worked together to start a clinic for treating Chinese women and children in a two-room native house at the former West Gate of Shanghai old town.

According to a report on *the North-China Herald* on June 5, 1885, "the excellent institution" developed from the humble clinic was formerly opened on June 3, 1885. It was called "Margaret Williamson Memorial Hospital for Women and Children" to memorize the woman who donated her meager savings with sympathies and enthusiasms. A portrait of Mrs Margaret Williamson was hanged in a large room used as a reception room/chapel on the ground floor of the hospital building. Dr. Reifsnyder served as the physician, Dr. H. W. Boone was the visiting physician and Miss McKechnie was appointed the head nurse.

Since the opening day, the hospital saw a steady development. It was an era that the maternal and infant mortality rates were very high in China due to old-fashioned delivery methods. In 1936, the Chinese Medical Journal estimated infant mortality rate in China to be around 200 per 1,000 babies.

According to the 1991 book *Shanghai Religious History*, the "Red

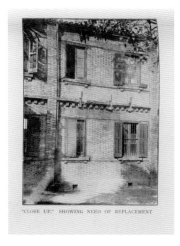

"CLOSE UP." SHOWING NEED OF REPLACEMENT

House" as the city's earliest hospital for women and children, enjoyed more popularity than other hospitals founded by missionary societies. In the year following its opening, the number of patients diagnosed and treated in the hospital reached 16,138, including 9,361 first-visit patients. The number further increased to 18,062 in 1887, 11,448 of whom were new patients.

"Most missionary hospitals were small in scale and had no clear divisions at first. With the improvement of medical staffs and facilities, missionary hospitals all developed from specialized to comprehensive hospitals. The Margaret Williamson Hospital initially focused on obstetrics and gynecology. By the 1920s, it had become a large-scale general hospital with a variety of departments including outpatient, public health, internal medicine, surgery, obstetrics and gynecology, ENT, and ophthalmology," the book notes.

In the summer of 1926, Slovakian-Hungarian architect Laszlo Hudec wrote a curriculum vitae to introduce projects he designed after opening his own offices in January 1925. The projects included three hospitals, the Paulun Hospital (today's Changzheng Hospital), the Dormitory Building of the Margaret Williamson Hospital and the then newly opened Country Hospital (Huadong Hospital).

Born in Besztercebanya (now Banska Bistrica in Slovakia) in the Austro-Hungarian Empire in 1893, Hudec, an architectural graduate student and a World War I soldier, escaped from a Siberian prison to Shanghai in 1918. He became a successful architect in Shanghai and was involved in 54 architectural projects (nearly 100 buildings), including the Park Hotel and the Grand Theatre, during his 29 years in the city.

In 2014 he was voted as a "Shanghai Symbol" by millions of Chinese in an online poll, the only foreigner in a galaxy of Chinese celebrities. One of his master-pieces was D. V. Woo's residence nicknamed "the Green House" on Tongren Road. It's rarely known that he also designed for "the Red House" during a new phase of this history-rich hospital.

In the co-authored paper titled "The Study of Shanghai Margaret Williamson Memorial Hospital (1884—1952)", researcher Wang Lijuan and professor Su Zhiliang discovered that the year 1921 was a transition for "the Red House Hospital" when it turned from an ordinary hospital to an institution combining hospital and education.

In 1921, the hospital founded Shanghai Union School of Nursing to train more Chinese women nurses. In 1924, it established Shanghai Woman's Christian Medical College in cooperation with a women's medical college from Suzhou.

According to "Shanghai Religious History", the Shanghai Woman's Christian Medical College had 14 majors in anatomy, biochemistry, physiology, pharmacology, bacteria, surgery, obstetrics, gynecology, neurology and mental health. The college was incorporated under the laws of the District of Columbia in the U. S. and the charter provided for the granting of the degree of Doctor of Medicine. The nursing school and the medical college supplied the hospital with adequate medical workers and technologies.

The founding of the school and the college also led to building expansions of the "Red House Hospital" from the 1920s until 1930s.

On June 13, 1931, *The China Press* reported that "the new Margaret Williamson Memorial", a three-unit hospital plant, would be constructed on site of old buildings. The plans called for a group of buildings which would cost an excess of $50,000. The first unit, the Laing Memorial Hospital, would be opened that summer. The architect was Mr. L. E. Hudec.

According to the report, more babies were born in the maternity ward here each month than in any other hospital in Shanghai, the average ranging between 120 and 130 each month, constituting the largest obstetrical practice in China. There would be 200 beds in the new building and special attention would be directed to the need of more private rooms.

"A tour of the compound, which is concealed adroitly behind an old wall in a narrow thoroughfare in the native section of Shanghai near East Gate, is a stimulating and enlightening experience. The seclusion of the

45-year-old garden around which are grouped the old administration building, the old maternity home, the Bennett Memorial Laboratories and Outpatient Department, the residence of the medical students, the doctors' residence, and the new model kitchen, in addition to the almost-completed Maternity Hospital, is a miracle in the heart of crowded, fetid living quarters of the district," the 1931 report describes.

The journalist gave a vivid narration of "fresh-faced, utterly attractive nurses" in the maternity ward, whose "long, white aprons worn over the Orientalized blue uniform, but with the conventional cubicle of white on their shiny black hair".

"So comfortable do the patients appear to be in their ward beds, that you suspect that the interim of care is an episode of comfort unknown in the ordinary routines of their lives, and that they are being for the few moments compensated for their suffering," the report wrote.

During the Chinese War against Japanese Aggression, the "Red House Hospital" suffered heavy losses. The premises were either destroyed or occupied by the Japanese army. The hospital moved to Xujiahui Road but set

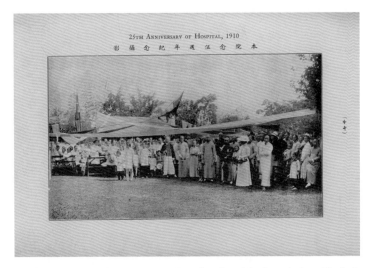

up the outpatient department and the gynecology department on Yan'an Road M.

In 1948, the hospital resumed operations at the original site and converted the Xujiahui Road site as branch. In 1952, famous doctor Wang Shuzhen was appointed the superintendent. Awarded "Baby Friendly Hospital" by World Health Organization, the hospital has grown from the 20-bed humble clinic to a big hospital with two branches, more than 800 beds and a galaxy of medical experts and workers.

Today, the hospital still preserves a historical house, Building No. 7 used for administration.

The book *Hudec's Architecture in Shanghai* notes the architectur-

al style of the hospital on Hudec's original blueprint had been neoclassical. Along with the balanced composition of horizontal and vertical triadic divisions and a superb gable roof, the Spanish porch of triplet arched columns made the façade vivid. It was a common stroke of genius in Hudec's design to intertwine a variety of elements into a new unity. However the existing buildings are different from the above-mentioned styles.

Shanghai Huangpu District Cultural Relics Archives showed that the existing Building No. 7 was a two-story brick-and-wood structure covering an area of 461 square meters. It had steep roof, arched doors and windows and was covered by red bricks and tiles.

"It was most likely the former administration building. Hudec designed a dormitory building and the Laing Maternity Hospital Building," said Tongji University professor Hua Xiahong, deputy editor-in-chief of the book *Shanghai Hudec Architecture*.

Today the hospital has built an informative museum to tell its extraordinary history of how women donated, founded and operated a hospital to alleviate the pains of women, and how women trained women to be doctors and nurses. At the entrance of the museum hang portraits of doner Margaret Williamson and founder Dr. Elizabeth Reifsnyder attired in

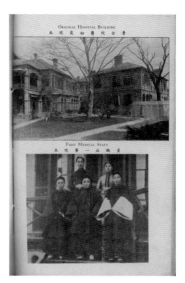

19th-century dress. The story of "Red House Hospital" continues in the city.

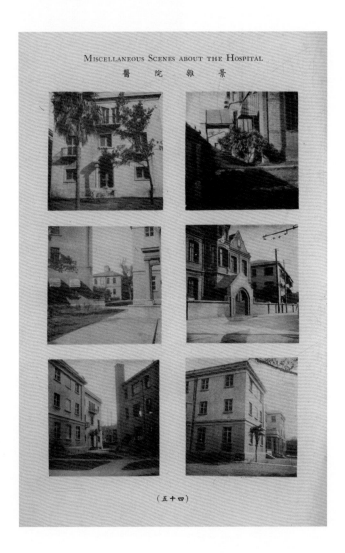

MISCELLANEOUS SCENES ABOUT THE HOSPITAL

醫 院 雜 景

（五十四）

五十岁生日在中国是非常重要的日子，但很少有机构能庆祝为中国公众服务50周年。

位于西门区的西门妇孺医院将于5月11日庆祝成立50周年和成功提供医疗服务50周年。周六下午已安排了精心策划的庆祝活动。

在开办的50年岁月里，医院已经发展到两个院区，有很多大型且设备齐全的建筑。除了可容纳200人的医院外，还有一所护士培训学校和一所医学院。门诊部每年接待3万名患者。

医院扩建

1886年医院成立一周年时，美国的两姐妹每人为医院每年捐100元金币。医院就这样发展壮大了，除了上述各项资金，还有海内外朋友的馈赠，以及来自感谢医院服务的有钱病人和宗教团体的支持。

包括儿童和婴儿诊所在内的门诊部经常只收患者低至六个铜板的治疗费用。

护士培训学校已经招收了70名高中学历的年轻女性。

医院的成长和学校的发展，从以下记录可以一目了然。药房成立于1883年，医院、病房和行政楼建于1885年，1910年25周年庆时增加了妇产大楼，1921年开办护士学校，1922年建造护士宿舍，1924年创办医学院，1925年建实验室，1926年医学生宿舍竣工，1929年建造医生宿舍，1931年改建医院的第一建筑单元竣工，1935年建院50周年。

摘自 1935 年 5 月 9 日《大陆报》

50 Years' Anniversary

Fiftieth birthdays are very important occasions in China, but celebration of 50 years of service to the public in China is something few institutions can boast.

The Margaret Williamson Hospital, situated in the West Gate district, will celebrate the 50th anniversary of its founding and 50 successful years of medical service on May 11. Arrangements for an elaborate celebration program have been made for Saturday afternoon.

In the 50 yeas of its existence, the hospital has grown to include large and well-equipped buildings in two compounds. In addition to a hospital which can accommodate 200 persons, there is a training school for nurses and a medical school for doctors. The out-patients department takes care of 30,000 patients yearly.

Hospital expands

When the hospital had its first anniversary in 1886, two sisters in the United States gave $100 gold each for each year of the life of the hospital. Thus the hospital has grown, supported by various funds beside those mentioned above, gifts from friends in Shanghai and abroad, and from rich patients who are thankful for the hospital's service. Missionary societies supported.

The outpatients department which includes clinics for children and babies, often treats patients for as little as six coppers.

The nurses' training school has an enrollment of 70 young women possessing high school educations.

The growth of the hospital and development of schools may be noted in a glance at the following record. The dispensary was founded in 1883; hospital, ward and administration building in 1885; addition of maternity building in 1910 when the 25th anniversary was celebrated; establishment of a nursing school in 1921; building of the nurses' dormitory in

1922; establishment of the medical school in 1924; building of laboratories in 1925; completion of the residence for medical students in 1926; erection of the doctors' residence in 1929; completion of the first unit of the rebuilt hospital in 1931, and 50th anniversary in 1935.

Excerpt from *The China Press* on May 9, 1935

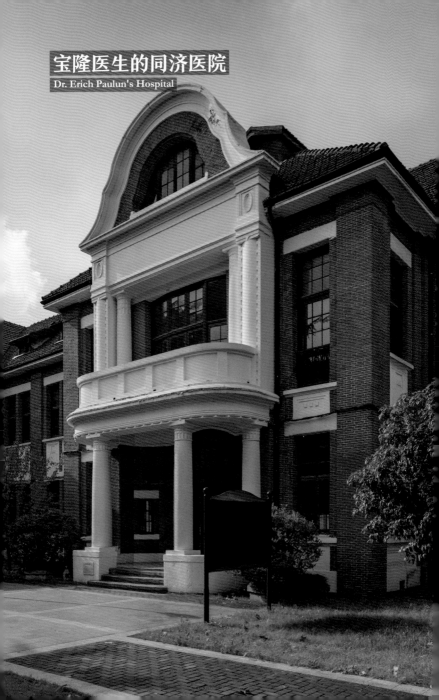

宝隆医生的同济医院

Dr. Erich Paulun's Hospital

2020年武汉新冠疫情爆发后，负责收治重症患者的武汉同济医院频频出现在新闻中。医院的官网写着"长江之滨，黄鹤楼下，有一所海内外闻名遐迩的医院……同济医院1900年由德国医师埃里希·宝隆创建于上海，1955年迁至武汉"。官网还配了一张这位大胡子德国医生的照片。

这位曾被上海人昵称为"大宝医生"的宝隆（Erich Paulun）1862年3月4日出生于德国，2岁时父母患肺结核双双去世，他不幸成为孤儿。由亲戚抚养长大的宝隆选择参军，1882年在基尔的皇家弗里德里希·威廉外科医学学院学习，后成为一名德国海军的上尉随舰医生。

1891年，他在德国海军服役期间随军舰第一次到访上海，亲眼见到老城里卫生条件不佳，流行病和瘟疫肆虐，穷人缺医少药深受疾病之苦。宝隆深受触动，想用自己所学改变这些悲剧。他后来写信给常驻上海的德国医生策德里乌斯（Carl Zedelius），表达了自己的强烈愿望：希望用自己所有的力量和知识为中国的穷人办一家医院。这位精力充沛的德国医生是个行动主义者。为了实现自己的想法，他开始认真地做准备工作，先回国进修学习，到两家医院工作提升外科医术，并继续到大学进修，同时也为筹建医院积攒资金。

19世纪90年代初，宝隆再次来到上海，先担任策德里乌斯的助理。1899年，策德里乌斯去世后，宝隆接替了他的工作。同年，他与另一位德国医生冯沙伯（Oscar von Schab）成立了上海德医公会，起初在德国驻沪领事馆行医，随后在后来的白克路、静安寺路（今凤阳路、南京西路）买了一块地，终于开办了收治中国穷人的"同济医院"（Tung Chi Hospital），并担任院长。"同济"二字从德语"Deutsche"（德意志）在上海话的谐音而来，也有"同舟共济"的寓意。根据1909年4月3日英文《北华捷报》（The North-China Herald）报道，这家成立于1900年的医院开始仅有几座从德国军方购买来的白

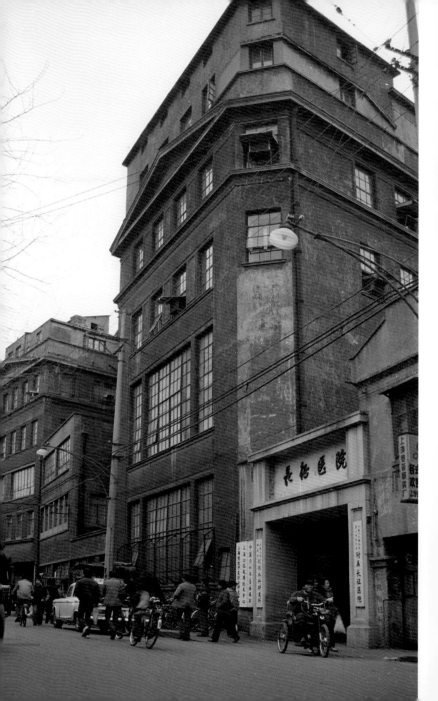

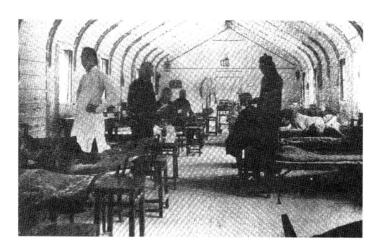

铁皮房子，只有20张床位，十分简陋。同年，宝隆和策德里乌斯的女儿结婚，在上海正式安家落户。

到了1901年，医院用来自中德人士的捐款在原址建起一座红砖建筑。

一份1909年关于医院的新闻报道写道："一楼有一间药房、几个储藏室、门诊室、仪器室和手术室。主要的手术室有三张手术台，并配有消毒器、器械箱、洗手池，实际上配备了现代无菌手术所需的所有条件。手术室外面有一个设备充沛的仪器室，外面是一个装有电灯浴的小房间，用于治疗风湿病人。此外，还有其他电气设备。大楼另一端的主药房与门诊室相连，德国医生每晚在这里慈善义诊50到70位病人。楼上有12间供中国付费病人使用的房间，男女病人各6间。"

同济医院对病人"区别对待"——穷苦华人可享受免费治疗，而德国公司的中方雇员看病需要支付费用。医院得到时任德国总领事克奈佩（Wilhelm Knappe）、上海道台和一些华商的捐助，包括沪上工商界领袖人物叶澄衷、朱葆三和虞洽卿。

在生命的最后几年，宝隆医生深感医务力量不足。在中德两国政府和各界人士的支持下，他在白克路同济医院对面租房创办了一所专门培养中国医生的医科学校。1907年10月1日，这所名为"德文医学堂"的学校举行隆重的开学典礼，医学堂由董事会管理，宝隆任董事会总监督（董事长）兼学堂首任总理（校长）。1908年，学校改名为"同济德文医学堂"。

1908年到1916年间，德国工程技术学院（Deutsche Ingenieur Schule）在今复兴中路陕西路口先后建起宿舍楼、教学楼、机电楼和后勤楼等，由德国建筑师倍克（Carl Baedecker）设计。同济德文医学堂与工学院同在这所校园内，合并为"同济医工学堂"。在接下来的动荡岁月中，学校历经沧桑，最终发展成为一所工科综合性大学，就是同济大学。

德国学者华纳（Torsten Warner）在《德国建筑艺术在中国》一书提到，倍克设计的这座校园布局以普鲁士皇家机械学校的设计方案为蓝本。华纳引用1914年德文报纸"The Shanghai Nachrichten"（上海新闻）对建筑群的描述："步入校园，首先看到的是工程技术学院雄伟的教学大楼，在教学楼对面是机电楼，楼内设有各种实验室、电机房、学徒实习车间、铸造车间、锻工场和木工房，走过位于校门两侧的教学楼与机电楼便是设有教师阅览室的语言学校和两座在同济德文医学堂创办初期盖的学生宿舍。在整个建筑群的中间是一幢造型典雅的建筑，其两边分别写着'生理学''解剖学'的字样。在这约三万平方米的校园南端，坐落着宽敞的健身房和在所有建筑物中规模最大的新宿舍楼，这幢宿舍楼可容纳两百名学生。新造的楼房均为砖块砌筑的清水墙面，其周围是绿色的草坪。"

不过世事难料，1909年3月5日，宝隆医生英年早逝，年仅47岁。

宝隆医生去世后，"同济医院"改名为"宝隆医院"，以示纪念。1926年，国际饭店设计师邬达克曾负责医院新楼的设计。意大利建筑史专家卢卡·彭切里尼（Luca Poncellini）在《邬达克》（*Laszlo Hudec*）一书中写道，除了宏恩医院，1926年时邬达克还指导建造了另外两个医疗设施项目：宝隆医院和西门妇孺医院。在第一个项目中，"邬达克在原白克路医院的基础上，设计了大型的加建"。

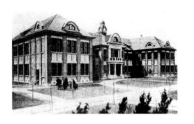

邬达克设计的建筑之一就位于现在长征医院骨科大楼的位置。据长征骨科丰健民教授回忆，他1980年大学毕业到长征医院工作，骨科大楼就是历史照片的样子，后来因为加固工程，大楼被包上现在的外观。

巧合的是，在接手宝隆医院一年前的1926年，邬达克在上海设计了另一家外侨捐建的医院：宏恩医院（The Country Hospital，今华东医院一号楼）。在落成时，匿名出资的美国富商用两名外国医生的名字为宏恩医院的两间病房命名，以表达他"最崇高的敬意"，其中一位就是宝隆。

1946年抗战胜利后，宝隆医院更名为中美医院，1951年又更名为同济大学附属同济医院。1951年到1955年，同济医院分批迁往湖北武汉，更名为"武汉医学院附属第二医院"。1955年10月1日，国防部颁发执行"中国人民解放军第二军医大学外科急症医院编制表"，经上海市批准，院址在黄浦区汉口路515号。1958年，医院被命名为"第二军医大学第二附属医院"，1959年，急症外科医院与长海医院部分人员以及原同济医院少量留用人员合并扩建为综合性教学医院，并于9月迁至凤阳路415号新院址，对外称上海同济医院，后更名为上海长征医院。凤阳路上留下的院址，成为今天长征医院所在地。如今，长征医院在院史中也专门介绍宝隆和同济医院的悠久历史。

迁往武汉的同济医学院和同济医院发展为华中科技大学同济医学院和其附属同济医院，医院的院训是"与国家同舟，与人民共济"。2020年新冠疫情爆发

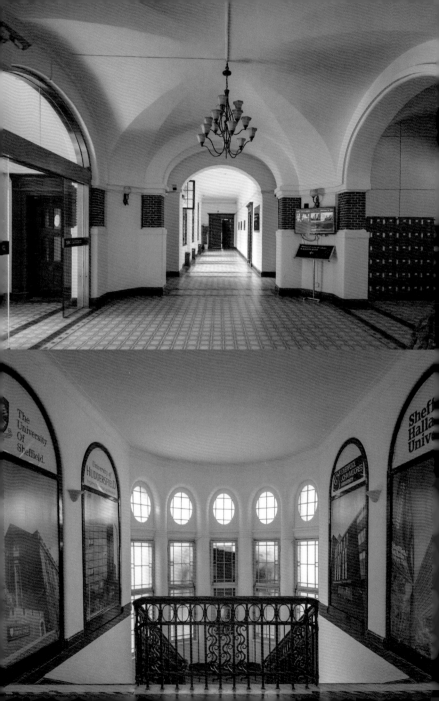

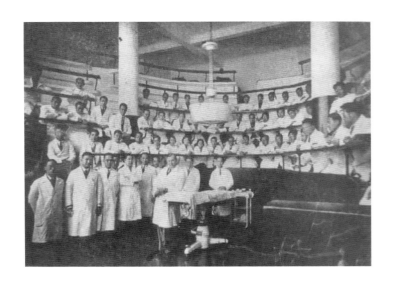

后，武汉同济医院成为收治新冠肺炎重症患者最多的医院之一。全国医务人员驰援武汉，其中也有来自同济医院创办地上海的医疗队，他们与武汉同济医生一起真正地"同舟共济"，并肩作战。

在宝隆创办的同济德文医学堂复兴路校区，由德国建筑师设计的百年校园建筑大部分保留至今，如今由上海理工大学使用。古典风格的红砖建筑设计精致，校园里有偌大的绿色草坪，虽然位于市中心繁华地段，却有一份独特的沉静之美。校门口的陕西南路一度被命名为宝隆路。

2000年，同济大学合并上海铁道大学，将铁道大学附属甘泉医院更名为同济大学附属同济医院。

而在位于四平路同济大学校园内的校史馆里，宝隆医生的雕像就在入口处，仿佛仍在散发着他的热力、生命力和阳光……

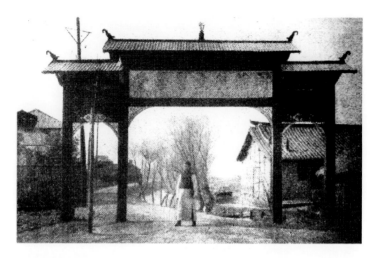

German doctor Erich Paulun was orphaned at the age of 2 but he had a loving heart of determinations. Today, both Shanghai Changzheng Hospital and Tongji University originated from the charitable "Tung Chee Hospital" Paulun founded in the heart of Shanghai for poor Chinese patients.

The name "Tung Chee" or "Tong Ji" represents the transcription of the word "German" or "deutsche" pronounced in Shanghai dialect. This name not only indicated the charitable hospital for Chinese was initiated by Germans, but also referred to the Chinese idiom "tong zhou gong ji" meaning "on the same boat".

Born in Pasewalk of Germany in 1862, Paulun had studied in the Friedrich Wilhelm University in Berlin, an army medical institution, and served on Germany navy ships S. M. S. Wolf and Iltis in Asia in the late 1880s and early 1890s.

In a letter to a Shanghai-based German doctor Carl Zedelius, whom he knew during navy times, Paulun shared his idea to found a charitable hospital for poor Chinese patients who were suffering from illness and without access to medicine in old Shanghai.

To realize this hospital dream, he left the navy, worked in two hospitals in Germany to improve his surgeon skills and began raising funds. In 1895 he returned to Shanghai to work as assistant to Zedelius and became his successor after he died in 1899.

In the same year Paulun and German doctor Oscar von Schab founded the Shanghai German doctors' guild and purchased a land in Burkill Road (today's Fengyang Road) across Bubbling Well Road (today's Nanjing Road W.) to build the Tung Chee Hospital.

According to *The North-China Herald* on April 3, 1909, the hospital founded in 1900 "at first consisted only of a few corrugated iron buildings purchased from the German military authorities". In 1901 a brick building was erected by funds contributed by both German and Chinese residents.

"On the ground floor there are a dispensary, store-rooms, out-patients' rooms, instrument rooms and operating theatres," the 1909 news report documents.

According to the newspaper, the main operating theatre had three tables and was equipped with sterilizers, instrument cases, washbasins and in fact with every requisite for a modern aseptic surgery. A well-stocked instrument-room opened out of this theatre, and beyond was a small chamber fitted with a Sanitas electric light bath for rheumatic patients and other electrical apparatus. The main dispensary, at the other end of the building,

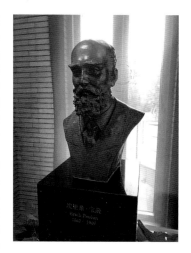

connected with the out-patients' room, where the German doctors see between 50 and 70 charity patients every evening. Upstairs were 12 rooms for Chinese paying patients — six for men and the same number for women.

The hospital treated two kinds of patients — poor Chinese in the International Settlement were treated for free while Chinese employees working for German firms were charged fees.

The hospital was founded with the support of the then German Consul General Wilhelm Knappe who wanted to increase German influence in China through education and medical services. The hospital also received funds from Shanghai Taotai (the circuit intendant for foreign affairs in Qing

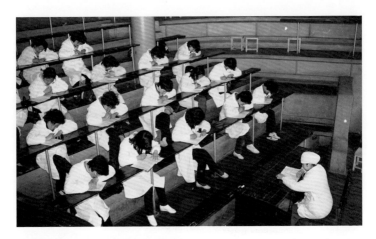

Dynasty) and prominent Chinese merchants including Ye Chengzhong, Zhu Baosan and Yu Yaqing.

The hospital was renamed Paulun Hospital after the German doctor died of disease a day after his 47th birthday in 1909. In the news story regarding the change of hospital name, *The North-China Herald* says a few foreign residents, besides Germans, knew of the existence of the hospital which had become well-known to the Chinese.

"No more fitting memorial could be found to the name of one who gave up so much for others than to establish the institute for ever as the Paulun Hospital," *The North-China Herald* reported.

Unfortunately the old buildings of the Paulun Hospital do not remain today. It's possible that the huge extension part, designed in 1927 by Park Hotel architect Laszlo Hudec, is wrapped inside a modern surface added during a 1980s renovation.

When Hudec's other hospital, the Country Hospital (the No.1 building of today's Huadong Hospital), was unveiled in 1926, the anonymous donor endowed two wards each in memory of Shanghai's departed philanthropists—the late Dr. MeLeod and the late Dr. Paulun "for whom the donor had the greatest respect", according to a report in *The China Press* on June 9, 1926.

In the 1950s Tongji Hospital was moved to Wuhan of Hubei Province and the site since then has been used by the Shanghai Changzheng Hospital which was attached to the Second Military Medical University.

During the last few years of his life, Dr. Paulun founded Tongji German Medical School in Burkill Road hospital with support from both German and Chinese governments. The school hosted a grand opening ceremony on October 1, 1907, which was attended by representatives of German consulates and Shanghai Taotai.

From 1908 to 1916, German school "Deutsche Ingenieur Schule" commissioned German architect Carl Baedecker to design a new campus today's Fuxing Road M. Tongji German Medical School was also located in the spacious campus featuring dormitories, teaching buildings, laboratories and workshops. The two schools were merged and got its new name as Tongji Medical and Engineering School. In the following turbulent years, the school endured many changes and moves and eventually grew to be a comprehensive university specializing in engineering which is today's Tongji University.

In 1978, the then Tongji University president Li Guohao re-

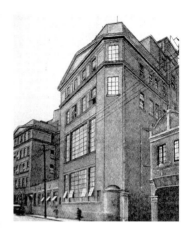

stored the university's relationship with Germany.

Though the Paulun Hospital buildings have been demolished, Changzheng Hospital introduces history and heritage left by this pioneering hospital in its own hospital history today.

At the Fuxing Road campus, red-brick buildings designed by German architect are largely preserved and used by the University of Shanghai for Science and Technology.

In the Tongji University History Museum situated in a quiet corner of its Siping Road campus, a statue of Dr. Paulun welcomes visitors at the entrance.

Yesterday: Paulun Hospital   **Today:** Shanghai Changzheng Hospital
Address: 415 Fengyang Road   **Architect:** L. E. Hudec

宝隆医生逝世

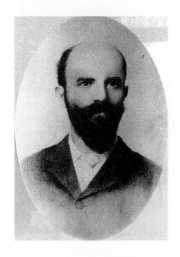

　　"大家都非常遗憾地得知宝隆医生去世的消息。他几天前因感染伤寒被送医，因为肾脏并发症，他于昨天凌晨4点死于尿毒症。几年前，他创立了一家面向中国人的慈善医院，后来又创办位于白克路（今凤阳路）的德文医学院。对于上海这座城市来说，他首先是一名外科医生。众所周知，宝隆医生的昵称'大宝医生'是对他的医术和勇气的称赞。宝隆医生的敏捷和决断力挽救了很多人的生命。无论天气好坏，无论白天黑夜，他总是为了病人而随时待命，对待免费病人和有钱病人一视同仁。许多他的穷苦病人都能说出宝隆医生所做的善事，他会为病人急需的假期资助费用，对病人耐心照顾。就在他去世前不久，宝隆医生还说希望再活20年，以便继续从事他所奉献的职业。"

摘自 1909 年 3 月 6 日《北华捷报》

Shanghai in mourning after philanthropic doctor dies

The news of the death of Dr. E. H. Paulun will be learnt with extreme regret by the whole community. Dr. Paulun was taken to the General Hospital only a few days ago, suffering from typhoid fever. Kidney complications set in, and he died at 4 o'clock yesterday morning from uremia.

Dr. Paulun was one of the best known Germans in Shanghai, not only to his fellow-countrymen, but throughout the entire community.

He founded a charitable hospital for Chinese, the natural corollary to which was the German Medical School for Chinese in Burkill Road. He was a Governor of the General Hospital, member of the German School committee and a committee member of the Club Concordia, in which capacity he rendered invaluable service with his suggestions regarding hygiene in the new building.

To all Shanghai, however, he was, first and foremost, a surgeon. The nickname by which he was familiarly known was a compliment alike to his skill and nerve. Many persons owe their lives to his promptness and decision.

In good or bad weather, at any hour of the day or night, he was always at the disposal of his patients, and he treats those from whom he knew he could receive no fee with the same consideration as the wealthy. Many of his poor patients can tell of kindly acts, of money unostentatiously given them for a much needed holiday, of his care and patience during their illnesses.

Only a short time before his death Dr. Paulun said that he would have liked to live for another 20 years to carry on the profession of which he was so devoted an exponent. Though honors fell thick upon him during his career the most lasting monument of his work will be tender regard in which his memory will be held by many who had every reason to appreciate his services.

— Excerpt from *the North-China Herald* on March 6, 1909

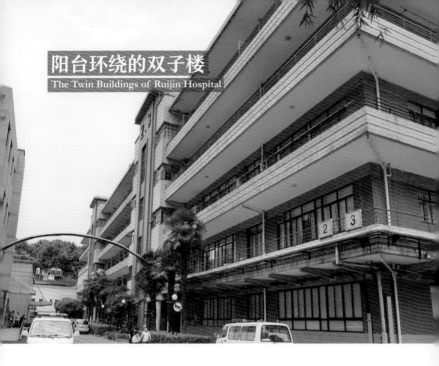

阳台环绕的双子楼
The Twin Buildings of Ruijin Hospital

　　上海瑞金医院美丽院区的一角，坐落着一对外观朴素的双子楼。两座大楼简洁现代，墙面斑驳，只有贯通的大阳台引人注目。常有穿病号服的病人到大阳台上透透气。在20世纪三四十年代，双子楼是上海最现代化的病房大楼之一，由著名的法商赉安洋行（Leonard，Veysseyre & Kruze）设计，后来还成为瑞金医院"内科的摇篮"。

　　研究瑞金医院院史的许善华老师介绍，这两座双子楼虽然外观普通，却是瑞金医院著名的"2号楼"和"3号楼"，包括五位中科院院士在内的很多著名内科医生都在此工作过。

　　两座病房大楼的建造计划始于1932年，这一年正好是瑞金医院前身广慈医院（Ste. Marie's Hospital）成立25周年纪念。

　　瑞金医院院志记载，1900—1904年期间，天主教江南代牧区主教姚宗李（Prosper Paris，1846—1931）与旧法租界公董局合作，在金神父路（Route Pere

Robert，今瑞金二路）购地10.6公顷创办医院。1907年10月13日，医院举行开业典礼，院名为"Ste. Marie's Hospital"（圣母医院），取意"广为慈善"，故中文名为广慈医院。

1932年医院举小建院25周年庆典时，法国驻沪总领事梅耶尔先生（M. Meyrier）在致辞时提到广慈医院创办伊始规模小，病床少，设备也很匮乏。

"广慈医院在过去的25年里稳步发展，如今已成为一所现代化的、设备齐全的医疗机构。仅在1931—1932年间，医院就治疗了7080名患者，产科接生560例，手术1124例，其中大手术756例，共有2240名患者在放射科接受检查或治疗。总而言之，在医院第一个25年里，近10万名患者在此得到了治疗。"1932年10月26日英文《北华捷报》（the North-China Herald）刊登的总领事致辞提到。

由于入院病人不断增加，医院决定建造新楼。1933年，广慈医院拆除用作贫苦男子病

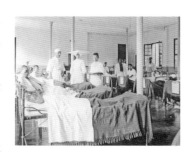

房的圣味增爵楼（St. Vincent Pavilion），新建2幢病房大楼，分别于1935年和1940年投入使用，就是今天的"2号楼"和"3号楼"。

1935年，法国总领事梅耶尔先生为新圣味增爵楼主持了隆重的竣工典礼，200余位中、法、美、英等国代表在这座新楼里的一个大房间出席了活动。

新圣味增爵楼设施完备，有300个床位，主要用于收治贫苦的华人男病人。1935年1月5日英文《大陆报》（The China Press）的报道透露，大楼面宽超过200英尺，高达4层。底层分配给眼科和儿科，内科外科和综合办公室则位于二三四层。这座"优雅而素淡的建筑"由赉安洋行设计。

"宽敞的阳台环绕着新大楼

的四面八方，将为患者提供最多的空气和阳光。内部住宿是与上海最好的专家——广慈医院的医生和震旦大学医学系的教授，合作设计的。眼科诊所的安排是由越南中国眼科诊所主任莫塔尔斯博士（Dr. Motals）做出的。"《大陆报》报道说。

广慈医院自从1912年起，就是震旦大学最主要的教学医院。医科学生有三分之一的时间在广慈医院和安当医院（现瑞金医院卢湾分院）进行临床见习和实习，优秀毕业生经选拔后可留任广慈医院担任住院医师。

负责新大楼设计的赉安洋行由三位酷帅的法国建筑师赉安（Alexandra Leonard）、韦西埃（Paul Veyssyre）和克鲁泽（Arthur Kruze）合伙经营，他们三人的名字组成了洋行的英文名"Leonard, Veyssyre & Kruze"。赉安洋行对许多人来说是一个陌生的名字，但洋行的建筑作品，如白色经典的上海花园饭店（原法国球场总会，Cercle Sportif Francais）和巧克力色的上海市妇女用品商店（原培文公寓，Bearn Apartments），都是很眼熟的地标建筑。

成立于20世纪20年代的赉安洋行是一家既高产又注重设计品质的事务所，1925年因为法国球场总会一炮走红。

同济大学郑时龄院士在新版《上海近代建筑风格》中评价，这家法国建筑师事务所对上海的现代建筑和高层公寓建筑设计做出了重要的贡献，其设计和建造活动始于1920年代初，一直持续到1940年代初，是旧法租界、也是上海最活跃和最重要的建筑师事务所，已知保留的作品60多件。

他提到，赉安洋行还承担了法租界的许多公共服务设施的设计，作品涵盖多种建筑类型和建筑风格，包括住宅、公寓、办公楼、教堂、修道院、学校、医院、警察局、俱乐部、博物馆等。他们的作品体现出法国的文化品位，对上海城市空间的形成影响非常大，在近代上海建筑发展进程中也起了相当大的作用。

研究旧法租界城市空间和建

筑的同济大学建筑学院刘刚教授指出，创办赉安洋行的赉安（Alexandra Leonard）是一个很有趣的人，也是一个真正的国际主义者。"他很有天赋，自由奔放。我相信赉安是公司的灵魂人物。"他说。

1934年的《北华捷报》报道透露，就在这座优雅素淡的病房大楼落成前夕，赉安的妻子伊丽莎白在广慈医院不幸病逝，年仅35岁。这位法国建筑师后来再婚，1946年在上海神秘失踪，他的最终下落至今仍是谜团。赉安洋行的第二位合伙人韦西埃（Paul Veysseyre）于1937年前往越南工作，在那里他大展身手，设计了许多与赉安洋行上海作品风格相似的摩登建筑，如越南末代皇帝保大的夏宫。第三位合伙人克鲁兹据说去了越南河内。

1935年，新圣味增爵楼竣工后，广慈医院的床位增加到700张床位，"位居上海各大医院之首"，成为"远东地区最重要的医疗机构之一"。1940年，为贫苦华人女病人而建的圣路依士楼（St. Louise Pavilion）也落成了，就是今天的"3号楼"。

许善华指出，两座平民病房大楼虽然建造年代相距5年，但建筑师聪明地将它们设计为一体，两座楼之间有一条不容易看出来的裂缝。

1951年，上海市政府接管了医院。广慈医院历经几次更名后，2005年正式更名为上海交通大学医学院附属瑞金医院。

院史档案显示，1952年两座病房大楼的五楼打通后由医院的内科使用，迎来"高光时刻"。

瑞金医院内科奠基人、时任内科主任的邝安堃教授在这里孕育了5大专业和无数人才，从这两座昔日的"平民病房"里走出了五位院士：王振义、陈竺、陈赛娟、陈国强和宁光。这两座阳台环绕的大楼也因此被称为瑞金医院"内科的摇篮"。

如今，瑞金医院园林般的院区里散落着几座广慈医院不同时期的历史建筑，如建于1922年的8号楼行政楼（原产科大楼）和1907年建院至今唯一留存的建筑——9号楼院史馆。

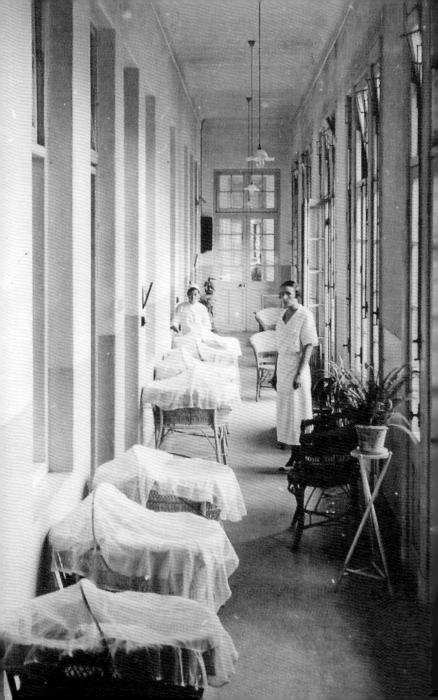

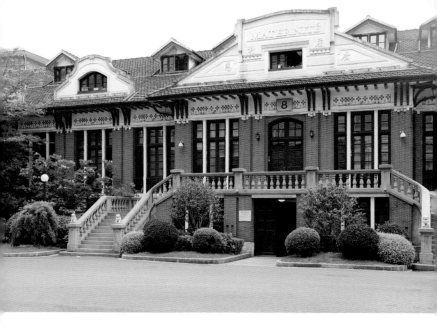

今天的瑞金医院已经发展为一所集医疗、教学、科研为一体的三级甲等综合性医院，占地面积11万平方米，有4000多名员工，1893张床位。办院精神"广博慈爱，追求卓越"源自百年前的名字——"广慈"。

位于院区西北角的双子楼，虽然斑驳沧桑，仍然作为内科大楼使用。这两座优雅素淡的建筑见证着医院广博慈爱的新时代。

昨天: 广慈医院 Ste. Marie's Hospital　**今天:** 瑞金医院　**地址:** 瑞金二路 197 号
建筑风格: 现代风格　**设计师:** 赉安洋行（Leonard, Veysseyre & Kruze）
参观指南: 可以欣赏 2 号楼和 3 号楼的建筑立面和超长阳台。

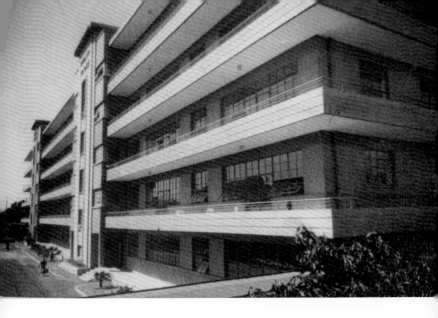

Perched in a corner of the garden-style Ruijin Hospital, a pair of worn-out twin buildings with mottled facades look out over the metropolis.

Back in the 1930s, they were the city's most advanced medical buildings and at the cutting edge of international health care. Designed by the famous French architectural firm Leonard, Veysseyre & Kruze, the buildings later became known as the cradle of internal medicine.

"The twin buildings may look plain today, but they are the famous 'Building 2' and 'Building 3' of our hospital. A galaxy of China's top medical masters, including five academicians of Chi-

na's Academy of Sciences, have worked here," says Xu Shan-hua, a researcher from the office of Ruijin Hospital Record, who has worked in the twin buildings since the 1970s.

According to the hospital archives, the planning of the twin buildings started in 1932 when the predecessor of Ruijin Hospital, a French Catholic hospital named Ste. Marie's, celebrated its 25th anniversary.

The hospital was built on a 106,720-square-meter site purchased by French father Le. T. R. Pere Robert, with support from the French municipal council. In 1906, today's Ruijin Road 2, fronting the hospital gate, was named

Route Pere Robert to honor the work of the French father, who later left Shanghai. His job was taken over by Father Prosper Paris, who opened St. Marie's Hospital on October 13, 1907. The hospital's Chinese name "Guang Ci" means "extensive charity and love".

During its 25th anniversary in 1932, French consul general M. Meyrier said that the hospital started from four modest buildings with a limited number of beds and a scarcity of equipment.

"The hospital has grown steadily during the past quarter of a century to its present splendid position of a modern and well-equipped institution. During the year 1931—1932 alone, St. Mary's Hospital treated 7,080 patients. There were 560 births in the maternity department and 1,124 operations were performed, of which 756 were major operations. And finally, 2,240 patients were examined or treated in the Department of Radiology. All in all, in the first quarter of a century of its existence, nearly 100,000 patients had been cared for at St. Mary's," the consul general said in his speech reported by *the North-China Herald* on October 26, 1932.

Elegant, sober architecture

To accept a growing number of patients, it was then decided to build a new medical building in the hospital. In 1933, the old St. Vincent Pavilion of the hospital was demolished to build a new one, which is today's Building 2.

In 1935, a grand ceremony, also presided over by Consul General Meyrier, was held to celebrate the completion of this fully equipped new St. Vincent Pavilion with 300 beds for poor Chinese male patients. Around 200 members of the French community and representatives of Chinese, British and American groups assembled in one of the larger rooms of the new building to attend the ceremony.

According to a report in *The China Press* on January 5, 1935, the main building has a frontage of over 200 feet and rises up four stories. The general offices of medicine and surgery occupy the three stories above the ground floor, which is allotted to ophthalmology and pediatrics. The "elegant though sober architecture" was to the credit of the firm Leonard, Veysseyre and Kruze.

"Spacious balconies surround all sides of the new building and will give patients a maximum amount of air and sunshine. The inner accommodation has been planned in collaboration with the best specialists in Shanghai: doctors of Ste. Marie's Hospital and professors of the faculty of medicine of the Aurora University. The arrangements for the clinic of ophthalmology are due to Dr. Motals, director of the clinic of ophthalmology, Cochin-China," *The China Press* report said.

Since 1912, Ste. Marie's Hospital has been a major teaching hospital for the adjacent Aurora University.

According to a full-page advertisement of the French architectural firm, in a 1934 local French newspaper, Leonard, Veysseyre & Kruze designed several other buildings for the hospital, including the Pasteur Pavilion and the Isolation Pavilion.

Leonard, Veysseyre & Kruze is an unfamiliar name to many but the firm's architectural works, such as the white, classic Okura Garden Hotel and the grand, chocolate-hued Bearn Apartments on Huaihai Road, are familiar to many eyes in Shanghai.

The firm was co-founded by two talented French architects, Alexandre Leonard and Paul Veysseyre in Shanghai in the 1920s. Its project in 1925, the new Cercle Sportif Francais project (today's Okura Garden Hotel) brought huge success to the firm. The third partner, Arthur Kruze, joined them in 1934.

As one of Shanghai's first Art Deco practitioners, this prolific firm had changed the look of the former French Concession during the "golden age" of Shanghai in the 1920s—1930s.

According to a new edition of *The Evolution of Shanghai Architecture In Modern Times* by Tongji University professor Zheng Shiling, it was estimated that more than 60 buildings still exist in Shanghai, including the twin buildings in the Ruijin Hospital.

"Leonard, Veysseyre & Kruze was the most important French architectural firm in modern Shanghai, which made a great contribution to the architectural design of modern architecture and tall apartment buildings in Shanghai. The firm has designed many public buildings and institutions in the French Concession. Their works demonstrate a variety of architectural genres and styles, including residences, apartments, offices, churches, cloisters, schools, hospitals, police stations, clubs and museums. Their work, which showcases a flavor of French culture, had largely influenced the forming of urban spac-

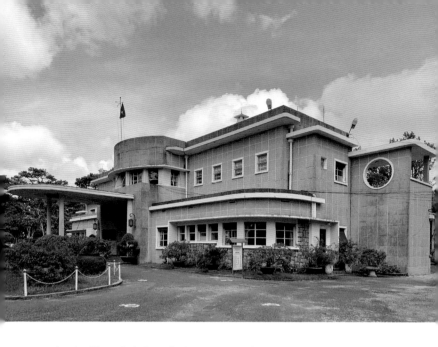

es in the Shanghai French Concession," professor Zheng writes in his book.

Another Tongji University Professor Liu Gang noted that Alexandra Leonard was an interesting man and a genuine internationalist. "He was gifted and free-spirited. I believe Leonard was the spirit of the firm," Liu commented.

However in 1934, just before the elegant, sober medical building was completed, Leonard's wife Elizabeth died of disease in the hospital at the age of only 35, according to *the North China Herald*. The architect later remarried but mysteriously disappeared from Shanghai in 1946. Veysseyre went to work in Vietnam in 1937, where he designed a large number of Art Deco buildings that mirrored the firm's Shanghai practice before returning to France. Kruze went to Hanoi and people never heard of him any more.

After the new St. Vincent Pavilion was completed in 1935, Ste. Marie's Hospital accommodated 700 beds, which made it "in the foremost plane among the largest hospitals in Shanghai" and constituted "one of the most important medical organizations in the Far East".

In 1940, St. Louise Pavilion, the second of the twin buildings, was built adjacent to the St. Vin-

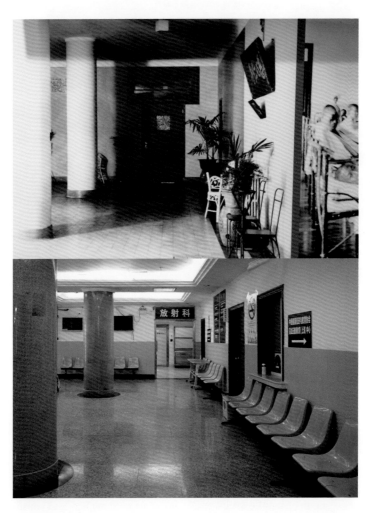

cent Pavilion for poor Chinese female patients.

"The twin buildings were built five years apart, but they were smartly designed as an entity," said Xu Shanhua, showing an un-noticeable crack between Building 2 and Building 3, which looked like one large building at a glance.

In 1951, the hospital was taken over by the Shanghai government, renamed several times and got its present name, Ruijin Hospital, Shanghai Jiao Tong University School of Medicine, in 2005.

The hospital archives reveal the twin buildings embraced a "peak time" in 1952 when they were combined and assigned to the internal department of the hospital.

Kuang Ankun, founder of this department, had nurtured five majors and numerous professionals of internal medicine in the buildings. A galaxy of China's renowned medical masters, including Chen Zhu and Chen Saijuan among the five academicians, have all worked and developed their career from here.

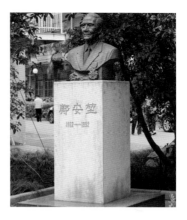

Today the garden-style compound of Ruijin Hospital is still sprinkled with several other historical buildings in classic style, including Building No. 8, the former maternity ward built in 1922 and Building No. 9, one of the only four structures built in 1907 upon the founding of the hospital. The latter now serves as a museum of hospital history.

And the Ruijin Hospital has developed to be a large hospital complete with medical treatment, education and research facili-

ties. Covering an area of 110,000 square meters, the hospital now has 4,402 employees, 1,893 beds and has won numerous awards for superb medical skills and services.

Today, the hospital's spirit "Guangbo Ci'ai, Zhuiqiu Zhuoyue" or "pursuit of excellence with extensive charity and love" is traced to its old Chinese name and medical spirit —"Guang Ci" (extensive charity and love).

The twin buildings, though mottled and worn-out, are still functioning as the department of internal medicine and witnessing a new chapter of care and love in this Shanghai hospital.

Yesterday: Ste. Marie's Hospital **Today:** Ruijin Hospital **Address:** 197 Ruijin Road **Architectural style:** Modern style **Architect:** Leonard, Veysseyre & Kruze
Tips: The entrance of the historical buildings might be restricted but the facades can be admired.

法国现代建筑中的先进设计实验室

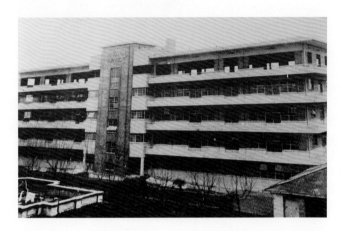

　　也许在全世界其他任何城市，都看不到在上海可以看到的建筑的差异性。在上海，这些差异性在法租界的建筑物中更加突出。在这方面，上海大都会是一个独特的城市，可以很好地充当现代建筑研究的"实验室"。

　　在该市的法国建筑师中，最重要的是赛安（A. Leonard）、韦西埃（P. Veysseyre）和克鲁兹（A. Kruze），他们对现代建筑需求的想法和现实诠释在法租界占有领导地位。

　　由这三位建筑师事务所设计的部分建筑物名录让人印象深刻。该名单包括：霞飞路格莱勋公寓（Gresham Apartments，今淮海中路光明公寓）、广慈医院（Pavilion des Marins）、法国总会（Cercle Francaise）、方西马公寓（F.I.C. Apartment Houses，今建安公寓）、广慈医院隔离病房（Isolation Pavilion）、福履理路道斐南公寓（Dauphine Apartments，Route Frelupt，今建国路建国公寓）、高恩路方西马A-B-C公寓（高安路公寓）、霞飞路盖司康公寓（Gascogne Apartments）、圣母圣心修道院（今长乐路上海社会科学院）、迈尔西南路法国球场总会（Cercle Sportif Francaise,今茂名南路花园饭店）、霞飞路培文公寓（Bearn Apartment, 今淮海中路上海市妇女用品商店）、圣伯多禄堂（St. Pierre's Church, Avenue Dubail，今重庆南路）、麦兰捕房（Poste Mallet of the French Police,今市公安局黄浦分局）、中汇银行大楼（Chung Wai Bank, 今中汇大楼）、雷米小学（Ecole Remi, Route Remi, 今永康路上海市第二中学）、祈齐路方西马住宅公寓（今岳阳路公寓）、高恩路福履理路方西马公寓D−E、方西马爱棠公寓（爱棠路，今余庆路）、萨坡赛小学（Primary Chinese School, Rue Chapsal，今淡水路416号）等。

前面的清单还很不完整，也没有显示三位建筑师的工作技巧。不用说，这些建筑代表了最先进的现代建筑类型。最低限度浪费空间、最多的光线、室内与外观的和谐，都与传统形式有所不同，但并不是公然的 "摩登"。最重要的是舒适性，进一步考虑使现代西方建筑适应上海和中国的环境。

写下现代法租界的发展史时，就不会少了对赛安、韦西埃和克鲁兹的天才的高度赞扬。

摘自 1935 年 7 月 14 日《大陆报》

Laboratory of Advanced Design Found In Modern French Buildings

Perhaps in no other city of the whole world will one find the contrasts in architecture to be seen in Shanghai, and in Shanghai these contrasts are accentuated in the buildings located in the French Concession. In this respect, metropolitan Shanghai is a city unique and can well serve as a sort of "laboratory" for the study of modern architecture.

Foremost among the French architects of the city are Messrs. A. Leonard, P. Veysseyre, and A. Kruze, whose ideas and realistic interpretation of the needs of modern architecture are to be found dominating the Concession.

A partial list of the buildings designed by the firm of three architects is indeed imposing. Such a list would have to include: Gresham Apartments Avenue Joffre; Hospital St. Marie, Pavilion des Marins; Foncim Apartments, Route Magniny; Cercle Francais, Route Vallon; Foncim Apartments, Routes Cohen and Frelupt; Hospital St. Marie, isolation pavilion; Dauphine Apartments, Route Frelupt; Foncim A-B-C Apartment, Route Cohen; Gascogne Apartments, Avenue Joffre; Sacred Heart Convent, Avenue Joffre; Cerele Sportif Francais, Route Cardinal Mercier; Bearn Apartment, Avenue Joffre; St. Pierre's Church, Avenue Dubail, Poste Mallet of the French Police; Chung Wai Bank Building, Avenue Edward VII; Ecole Remi, Route Remi; Foncim Residence Apartment, Route Ghisi; Foncim Apartments D-E, Route Cohen-Frelupt; Foncim Edan Apartments, Route Edan; primary Chinese School, Rue Chapsal; and Foncim Residences, Route Ghisi.

The foregoing list is far from complete nor do they indicate the technique of the work of the three architects. Needless to say, these buildings represent the most advanced types of modern architecture; a minimum of waste space, a maximum of light, harmonious interiors and exteriors which are departures from conventional forms and yet which are not blatantly "moderne" and above all, comfort. A further consideration ably carried out is the adaptation of modern Western architecture to conditions in Shanghai and in China.

When a history of the growth of the modern French Concession is written, it will not fall to include high tribute to the genius of Messrs. Leonard, Veysseyre, and Kruze.

Excerpt from *The China Press* on July 14, 1935

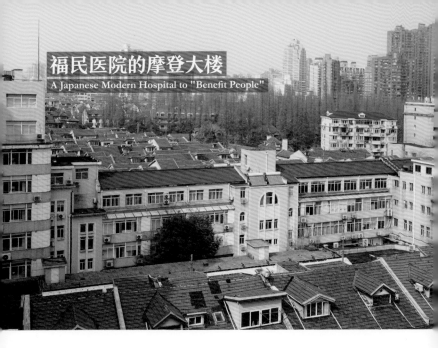

福民医院的摩登大楼
A Japanese Modern Hospital to "Benefit People"

上海市第四人民医院是上海北部最大的公立医院之一，很少有人知道它源自1921年成立的日本"福民医院"。医院位于四川北路的老院区里有一座摩登风格的米色大楼，曾经是福民医院引以为傲的新大楼。

上海医学史专家、原第四人民医院图书馆馆长陆明介绍，在老上海具有一定规模的西方医院中，福民医院在设施和医疗技术方面处于领先地位。医院吸引了包括作家鲁迅和演员阮玲玉在内的很多知名人士就医。

第四人民医院的档案里保存着昔日的广告。这则广告骄傲地称福民医院是上海同类医院中唯一的一家日本医院，新的七层大楼配备了美国、德国和日本的最新设备，使其成为远东地区出色的医疗中心之一。

这座"新的七层大楼"在上海市第四人民医院的老院区曾被用作2号楼使用，楼里常常奔波着医生、护士和病人，其中很多病人是虹口区的居民。

米色大楼历经沧桑，被加建了楼层，改变了部分外观。不

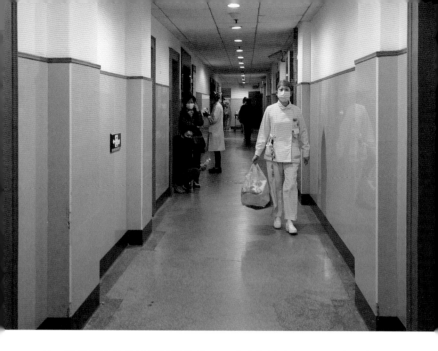

过，造型简洁的外墙仍保留着弧形入口和连续的长窗，展现20世纪30年代的建筑特征，那是上海这座城市的"摩登年代"。

1934年，米色大楼在一个"色彩缤纷的仪式"（colorful ceremony）中作为福民医院的新翼隆重开幕。

根据英文《大陆报》（The China Press）报道，大楼高达七层，造价为40万元，其中包括了购置最新的医疗设备。 楼为门诊部，二楼是儿童治疗室，护士都经过专门培训。产科病房和

一个专门治疗眼、耳、鼻、喉疾病的部门位于三楼。手术室配备了最先进的科学仪器。此外，医院还对病患提供日照治疗，并在新楼安装了三台X光机。

"新大楼的房间配备了充足的窗户，引入充足的阳光。福民医院一直为所有国籍的人士提供治疗，这次新的扩建将增强医院为上海市民抗击疾病的能力。"《大陆报》报道。

福民医院在广告中印制了新大楼的照片，并特别指出虽然医院的创始人兼院长顿宫宽医

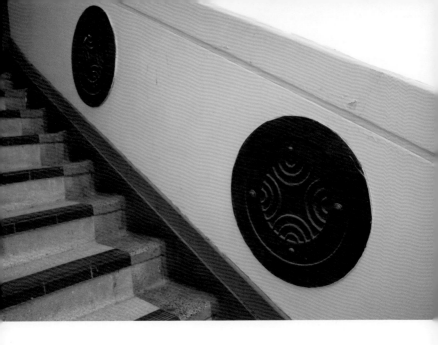

生（Dr. Yutaka Tongu)是日本人，但他的医院"绝对是国际性的"。当时，这位日籍院长还担任上海日本医学会主席。

南堀英二所著的顿官宽传记《奇迹的医师》一书记载，位于上海四川北路142号（现四川北路1878号）的福民医院新楼是一座钢筋水泥建筑，地下一层，地上七层，其设计与设备在当时是很先进的。大楼有170多张床位与门诊诊室，无论是隔断、空调、采光、隔音所有配置都很考虑周详。

除了院长顿官宽先生主持的外科与整形科，还有内科、小儿科、泌尿科、妇产科、眼科、耳鼻喉科、中医科、齿科、放射科等各科。医师有日本人、意大利人、德国人等，护士以华人为主，后勤工作人员多为印度人。福民医院共有员工超过200人，加上最新的医疗设备，让人很难想象这样一座国际化的综合医院是一位"东洋人"开设的。

陆明提到，上海著名画家王震（字一亭）与顿官宽交谊颇深，他向这位日本院长建议既然

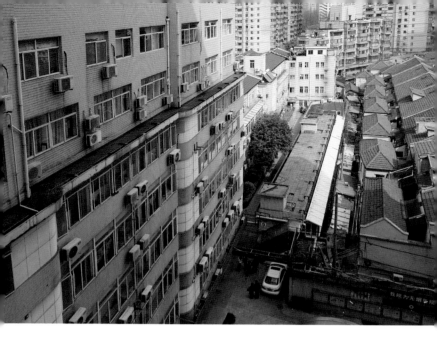

在中国开设医院，就该入乡随俗，取一个具有中国特色的院名。他为医院取名"福民"，意在造福于民，此建议遂为顿宫宽采纳。

这个美好的名字和先进的医疗服务为医院赢得许多中国病患的信任。著名作家鲁迅的家在虹口，又曾在日本留学，与福民医院有着许多渊源。鲁迅先生的儿子周海婴于1929年9月27日出生于福民医院，后来他多次带儿子去医院检查，同时也介绍亲戚朋友去福民医

院就诊。茅盾的妻子去福民医院就诊时鲁迅还帮忙翻译。鲁迅在1933年10月23日的日记中写道，他与内山完造等友人一起在福建路著名的杭帮菜馆"知味观"宴请顿宫宽与其他日籍医师，感谢福民医院医疗团队以精湛医术治愈了朋友张协和儿子的重病。他们一起品尝知味观的名菜"叫花鸡"和西湖莼菜羹，席间相谈甚欢。

根据上海社会科学院专家陈祖恩所著的《上海日本文化地图》，顿宫宽（1884—1974）

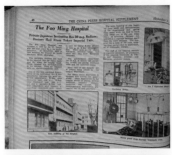

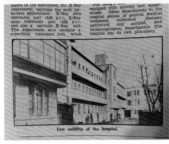

East building of the hospital.

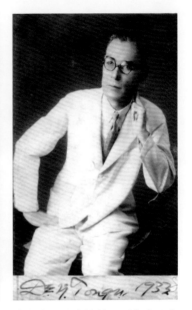

毕业于东京帝国大学医学部，曾在"汉冶萍煤铁厂矿公司"任医院院长。他于1921年创办的福民医院不仅成为上海著名的综合医院，其规模在当时日本国内也不多见。

"作为医生，顿官宽的理念是：患者都是医院的客人，没有人种和阶级差别。他打破了一般日本医院只为日本人服务的惯例，将华人作为主要的治疗对象，其次才是欧美人和日本人。"陈祖恩在书中写道。

1945年二战结束后，福民医院由中国政府接管，更名为"上海市立第四医院"，1949年再次更名为"上海市立第四人民医院"，1966年改名为"上海市第四人民医院"，2021年成为同济大学附属上海市第四人民医院。

如今，第四人民医院已发展为一家大型综合医院，拥有完整的科室、先进的设备，并结合了医疗、教学和科研。在悠久的发展历程中，医院引进了许多中国顶尖的医学专家。2020年，第四人民医院迁至三门路新址，新院区已拥有近1000张床位，约

2200名员工。

医院恪守"创新图强、造福于民"的核心理念，这与医院档案中保存的老广告里的一句话非常契合："顿宫宽希望他的医院不仅在上海抗击疾病的斗争中发挥重要作用，而且在巩固世界上这个国际大都市中所有居民之间的友谊纽带方面将起到很大作用"。

虽然上海第四医院已搬离这幢米色的现代分风格建筑，但源自这座大楼的医学精神会传承下去。

昨天：福民医院　**今天：**上海第四人民医院　**地址：**四川北路 1878 号　**建造年代：**1934 年
建筑风格：现代风格　**参观指南：**请欣赏米色大楼的弧形入口和历史楼梯。

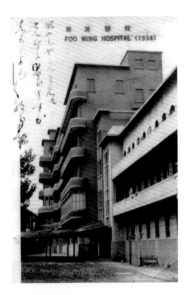

FOO MING HOSPITAL (1934)

"The Foo Ming Hospital is the only Japanese hospital of its kind in Shanghai and its new seven-storied building, equipped with the latest devices from America, Germany and Japan, makes it one of the outstanding medical centers in the Far East".

The "new seven-storied building" has been standing in the center of Shanghai No. 4 People's Hospital. It's been used as Building No. 2 for medical treatment, filled with busy doctors, nurses and patients, most of whom were residents of Hongkou District.

Renovations have added floors on top of the beige-hued building and changed some of its appearance. However, the simple-cut facade is still graced by a curved entrance and long, continuous windows, displaying architectural features of the 1930s, a modern era of Shanghai.

In 1934, this building was opened as the new hospital wing with a "colorful ceremony".

Shanghai No. 4 People's Hospital is one of the largest public hospitals in northern Shanghai. It's rarely known that it was founded as a modern Japanese hospital named "Foo Ming" in 1921.

"Among the dozens of Western hospitals of certain scales in old Shanghai, Foo Ming Hospital was a leading one in terms of facilities and medical skills. The hospital attracted many celebrities and social elites to seek medical care, such as Chinese writer Lu Xun and actress Ruan Lingyu," said Lu Min, a medical historian and director of No. 4 Hospital's library.

The hospital's archives preserve an old advertisement that claimed

According to a report in *The China Press*, the new wing was a seven-floor structure built at a cost of US$400,000, including the latest scientific equipment. The ground floor was reserved for the treatment of outgoing patients, while the second floor treated children, with specially trained nurses in charge. The maternity ward and a special department for the treatment of eye, ear, nose and throat diseases was located on the third floor. The operating room was equipped with up-to-date scientific apparatus. In addition, sunshine treatment for invalids was provided and three X-ray machines were installed in the new wing.

"The rooms of the new building were provided with ample windows and a plentiful supply of sunlight is let in. The Foo Ming Hospital has been giving treatment to all nationalities and its new expansion is bound to increase its efforts towards the combatting of all disease of which residents of this city might be inflicted," *The China Press* reports.

The hospital proudly printed a picture of the new building in the advert and noted that although Dr. Yutaka Tongu, the hospital's founder/president was Japanese, his institution was "decidedly international".

According to Dr. Tongu's biography entitled *A Magical Doctor*, Foo Ming Hospital's new building at 142 Northern Sichuan Road (today's 1878 Sichuan Road N.) was a steel-and-concrete structure housing more than 170 beds. The building was well designed with full consideration of partitioning, air-conditioning, lighting and sound insulation.

In addition to surgery and orthopedics departments of Dr. Tongu, there were various departments such as internal medicine, pediatrics, urology, obstetrics and gynecology, ophthalmology, otolaryngology, traditional Chinese medicine, dentistry and radiology.

The hospital was run by an international team of more than 200 employees. The doctors were Chinese, Japanese and Europeans. Most of the nurses were Chinese and the hospital porters were Indian.

Lu Ming notes that the hospital's name was given by famous Shanghai artist Wang Yiting.

"A friend of Dr. Tongu, Wang Yiting, suggested to him that a hospital in China should have a name imbued with Chinese characteristics. 'Foo Ming' means 'benefit people' in Chinese. His advice was well accepted by the Japanese doctor," Lu said, adding that Dr. Tongu was also president of Shanghai Japanese Medical Association.

Both this nice name and the advanced medical service won many Chinese patients and friends for Dr. Tongu. Foo Ming Hospital was often-visited by famous writ-

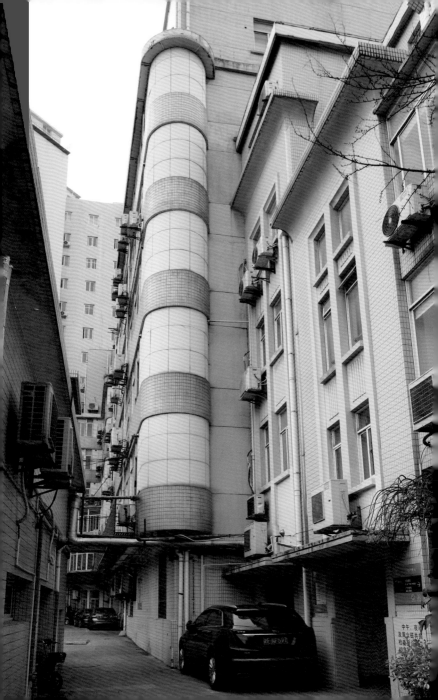

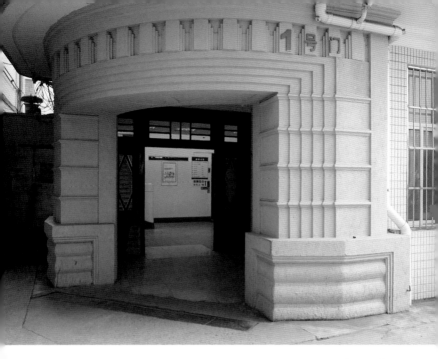

er Lu Xun, whose home was only several blocks away from the hospital. His son Zhou Haiying was born in the hospital on September 27, 1929.

Lu Xun wrote in his diary on October 23, 1933 that he invited Dr. Tongu and his fellow Japanese doctors to a banquet in a famous Hangzhou-style restaurant. The dinner was in gratitude to their efforts and superb skills for curing his friend Zhang Xiehe's second son who was seriously ill in the summer of that year.

According to the book *Shanghai Japanese Cultural Map*, Dr. Tongu was born in 1884 and graduat-

ed from the University of Tokyo's medical department. Foo Ming Hospital, founded by him in 1921, was not only a famous comprehensive hospital in Shanghai, its scale was also rare in Japan at that time.

"Dr. Tongu believed patients were all guests of the hospital, no matter what nationalities or classes they belonged to. He broke a tradition that Japanese hospitals generally served only Japanese and regarded Chinese as the hospital's major patients," Chen Zu'en, a researcher from Shanghai Academy of Social Sciences, wrote in the book.

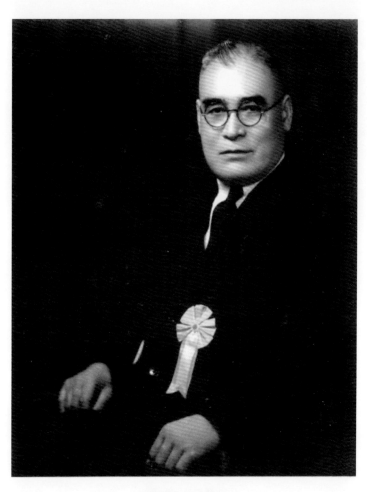

頓宮寬博士

Dr Yutaka Tongu　　　(1884~1974)

After World War II ended in 1945, Foo Ming Hospital was taken over by the Chinese government, renamed "Shanghai No.4 Municipal Hospital" in 1945, renamed again as "Shanghai No.4 Municipal People's Hospital" in 1949 and changed to Shanghai No.4 People's Hospital in 1966. In 2021, it became a hospital affiliated to the Tongji University School of Medicine.

Today, it's a comprehensive hospital with complete departments, advanced equipment, incorporating medical treatment, teaching and research. During the hospital's rich history of development, it has employed many of China's top medical experts. Later this year the hospital will move to Sanmen Road 1. and the new hospital compound has 1,000 beds with 2,200 employees.

The core value of the hospital is to "strive for better through innovations and benefit people", which mirrored a sentence from the 1930s advertisement preserved in the hospital's archives.

"Dr. Tongu hopes that his hospital will not only play an important role in Shanghai's battle against disease, but that it will do much toward cementing the bonds of friendship between all people resident in this most cosmopolitan city of the world," the advertisement said.

Shanghai No.4 People's Hospital has moved away from its original beige-hued modern building, but the medical spirit that originated there will be carried on at the hospital's new base.

Yesterday: Foo Ming Hospital   **Today:** Shanghai No. 4 People's Hospital affiliated to the Tongji University School of Medicine   **Address:** 1878 Sichuan Road N.
Built in: 1934   **Architectural style:** Modern style
Tips: Please note the curved entrance and the original staircase of the 1930s building.

医院的双重悲剧

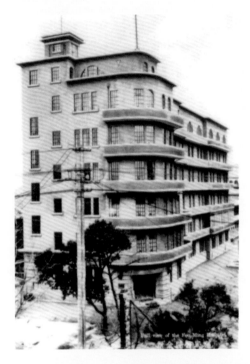

　　7月5日凌晨，四川北路福民医院发生了一起可怕的悲剧，一名菲律宾人开枪谋杀了一名躺在病床上的日本舞女，随后自杀。

　　7月4日，这名在维纳斯咖啡馆(Venus Cafe)担任舞女的女孩正在咖啡馆里。当时她的菲律宾情人出现了，两人发生了争吵，结束了几个月的恋爱关系。伤心欲绝的女孩失踪了，9点被发现已经服毒奄奄一息。

　　泰勒警长（Detective-Sergeant Taylor）从虹口警局赶来处理案件，女孩被送往公济医院（the General Hospital）。经过急救后，她被转移到四川北路日本福民医院101室。在这里，医生和警察都努力挽救了她的生命，大约两点钟时，负责治疗的村井医生（Dr. Murai）宣布她会康复。检查发现她吞下了54片钙莫汀（calmotine）。

凌晨3时许，经常光顾四川北路歌舞表演的另一名号称"强尼"（Johnny）的菲律宾人来到医院，要求探望病人。"强尼"是这位姑娘的前任男友。听说她企图自杀，他来到福民医院，恳求护士长让他在身边照顾她。护士没有怀疑他的企图，给了他照顾病人的机会。

不久后，护士要巡视病房，男人就留在了女孩身边。片刻之后，103号房间的病人们听到几声枪响，但因为被吓坏了，没有寻找原因。当护士在凌晨3点30分回来时，她发现女孩已经死了，一颗子弹击中她的头部，另一颗子弹穿过心脏。躺在她身边的是男人的尸体，也是中弹身亡，一颗子弹打进了他的脑袋，两颗子弹打进了他的心脏。他手里拿着一把小口径手枪。

7月8日，在美国领事法庭担任验尸官的克利斯戴（A. Krisel）专员做出了自杀判决：阿隆佐（Juan Y. Alonzo）被发现死在日本舞女的尸体旁边的福民医院。

根据判决，这位年轻的菲律宾人死于三处自残的枪伤。男孩留下了一张便条，解释了他希望和他以前的爱人一起"西行"。便条以愉快的"再见，强尼"（Cheerio, Johnny）结束。

摘自 1932 年 7 月 13 日《北华捷报》

2 dead in hospital shooting tragedy

A terrible tragedy was enacted early on July 5 at the Foo Ming Hospital, North Szechuen Road, resulting in the murder of a Japanese dancing girl and the suicide of a Fillipino after he had shot her as she lay helpless in her bed.

The girl, who worked as a dancing partner in the Venus Café, off Jukong Road, was in the café on July 4 when her Filipino lover appeared and the two had a quarrel, ending the relationship which had existed for several months. Broken-hearted the girl disappeared and at 9 o'clock was discovered in extremis from the effects of poison.

Detective-Sergeant Taylor arrived from Hongkew Police Station to handle the case and the girl was removed to the General Hospital. First aid was administered and she was then transferred to room 101 Foo Ming Hospital for Japanese, in North Szechuen Road. Here both doctors and police worked hard to save her life. And at about two o'clock, Dr. Murai, who was in charge of the case, announced that she would recover. It was discovered that she had swallowed 54 tablets of calmotine.

At 3am, another Filipino, who was known as "Johnny" among the cabarets of North Szechuen Road, to which he was a constant visitor arrived at the hospital and requested to see the patient. "Johnny" had been the predecessor of his compatriot in the affections of the girl. Hearing that she had attempted to commit suicide, he presented himself at Foo Ming Hospital and begged the nurse in charge to allow him to sit with her and look after her. The nurse having no suspicion of his intentions allowed him the privilege.

Shortly afterwards, the nurse had to proceed on her rounds of the wards and the man was left with the girl. A few moments later the patients in room No. 103 heard several shots fired, but being frightened made no effort to discover the cause.

When the nurse returned at 3:30am, she found the girl dead with one bullet wound in her head and another through the heart. Lying beside her was the body of the man, also shot, one bullet having entered his head and two into his heart. In his hand was a small caliber pistol.

A verdict of suicide was returned by Commissioner A. Krisel, sitting as coroner, in the United States Consular Court on July 8 in the case of Juan Y. Alonzo, found dead in the Foo Ming Hospital beside the body of the Japanese dancing girl.

According to the verdict, the young Filipino died from three self-inflicted bullet wounds. The boy left a note explaining his hope of going "Out West" with his former sweetheart and ending with a blithe "Cheerio, Johnny".

Excerpt from *the North-China Herald* on July 13, 1932

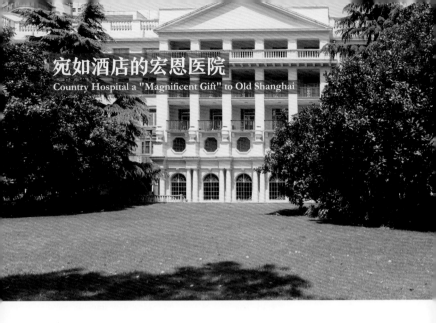

宛如酒店的宏恩医院

Country Hospital a "Magnificent Gift" to Old Shanghai

很多建筑源自梦想。一个多世纪前的上海，美国侨民雷纳（Charles Ernest Rayner）的梦想是为这座城市建造一座最好的医院。1926年，他梦想成真，捐资兴建的宏恩医院（The Country Hospital）隆重开业。这家美丽的医院宛如度假酒店，被媒体形容为"一件值得称赞的礼物"。

宏恩医院的建筑保存至今，位于延安西路华东医院的院落内，由东欧建筑师邬达克设计。

意大利建筑历史专家卢卡·彭切里尼（Luca Poncellini）在《邬达克》（Laszlo Hudec）一书中写道，1923年下半年，因已年迈，又无子嗣和家人继承财产，美国富商雷纳决定把财产留给这座让他获得巨额财富的城市。他决意为居住在上海的侨民建造一所现代化的医院，然后捐赠给当时管理公共租界的上海工部局（Shanghai Municipal Council），但有一个条件：他的身份必须保密。因此雷纳跟邬达克签订了一份奇怪的合同，约定建筑师不得透露客户的姓名。如若泄露，邬达克将立刻被解雇，失去这个项目。

宏恩医院是一座钢筋混凝土结构的大楼，高达五层，局部六层，占地面积约2300平方米。在20世纪20年代的上海，医院的选址"大西路"（Great Western Road，今延安西路）十分理想，既避开闹市的尘嚣，距离城市中心也不远，到外滩不过15分钟车程。

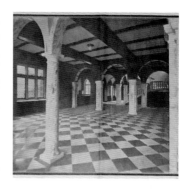

宏恩医院的外观设计为意大利文艺复兴风格。邬达克在一次采访中透露设计时采用了意大利的氛围和风格，主要是考虑到医院的捐赠者曾在意大利生活多年，对意大利风格既欣赏又相当了解。

这家医院美奂美轮，呈现一种简单素朴的优雅。主立面有三组凉廊，顶部装饰有三角形山花，可以为病房引入更多日照。

最让人印象深刻的是医院的门厅。走进宏恩医院，就仿佛走进了一家富有设计感的度假酒店，明亮开放，宁静而有格调，与传统医院冰冷幽暗的气氛迥然不同。邬达克大量使用进口的黑、白、灰色大理石来设计立柱、楼梯和地坪。门厅的天花以原木装饰，给空间增加一种温暖轻松的度假氛围，也与大理石材质形成有趣的对比。

宏恩医院竣工时，上海媒体纷纷报道。英文《上海星期天时报》（Shanghai Sunday Times）的记者写道，"田园式的、闲适的，意大利文艺复兴初期风格，令人仿佛置身于托斯卡纳的别墅庭院和房间里"。1928年，美国知名期刊《建筑论坛》（Architectural Forum）也出版了关于宏恩医院项目的特刊，这是该期刊首次如此关注非美国本土建筑。

宏恩医院不仅环境优美，所用的设施设备也是当时最先进的。病房全部朝南布置，北面安排手术室和设备用房等。病房带有独立卫生间，配备了进口卫生三件套。大楼还安装了瑞士苏尔寿的冷气系统，保证在炎热的夏天也能进行手术。

1926年6月13日，英文《大陆报》（*The China Press*）报道称宏恩医院致力于为病人提供家庭般的氛围。病房用浅色木质家具、玫瑰色窗帘、深色印花棉布软椅布置，窗外可以眺望大花园，景色宜人。

医院儿科病房的墙壁上装饰着童谣图画，还有购自美国的白色小床。柔和的光线透过绿色百叶窗和精美的窗帘照射进来。旁边的一个大凹室里，是一间阳光明媚的游戏室，里面有适合儿童尺寸的奶油色珐琅桌椅，孩子们可以在一尘不染的橡胶地板上画画或玩游戏。

设备精良、超现代的产科病房是宏恩医院的骄傲之一，新生儿在婴儿室里得到照顾，那里"像现代发明所能想象的那样干净、清新、舒适"。

医院的楼上还有卫生手术室和药房等，所有的玻璃瓶和其他器具都是从日本运来的。

作为建筑师邬达克的早期作品之一，宏恩医院一直被认定为意大利文艺复兴风格的古典主义建筑。《上海邬达克建筑地图》作者、同济大学华霞虹教授研究发现，这家医院其实是"一个古典外衣遮蔽下的功能主义实践"。

"我在2000年撰写的硕士论文中也将宏恩医院归入'古典风格的延续'一章。通过更多历史文献的研究发现，这种判断属于'以貌取人'，是一种典型的误读。"华教授说。

她发现，为实现捐资者强烈而美好的理想，无论是平面布局、立面风格还是材料设备的选择，宏恩医院始终遵循"形式追随功能"的现代主义原则，甚至连古典风格的外立面和接待大厅也非保守美学或追逐时尚的结果，而是为应对上海夏季高温、创造友好的医疗氛围和寻求上海国际社区的普遍认同所作的理性选择。南立面那三组顶部饰有山墙的巨大凉廊并非纯粹造型，而是用来遮挡夏季毒辣阳光，到了冬天，太阳高度角减小时，又不会妨碍日照。

"作为一种功能性极强，需要大量设备投入、人流量很大的公共建筑类型，医院跟工厂一样需要经济实用。因此，其建筑往往布局紧凑、形式简洁，也往往是较早采用现代风格的类型。比如稍晚建成的仁济医院（德和洋行）、虹桥结核病疗养院（奚福泉）等。即使仍沿用复古风格，也不会在公共空间、材料、装饰上浪费资金，比如邬达克后面设计建成的宝隆医院和西门外妇孺医院。"华教授在"古典外衣遮蔽的功能主义实践：重读邬达克设计的宏恩医院"一文中写道。

宏恩医院是邬达克离开美商克利洋行独立执业后的第一个重要作品。由于他遵守了那份奇怪的合同，对医院捐建者的身份守口如瓶，雷纳得以享受在医院开业典礼时站在前排，却无人知晓他就是神秘捐建者的快乐。

雷纳的人生与另一位同样没有子嗣继承财产的旅沪英国富商雷士德十分相似。他们都在上海凭借头脑与才干"点石成金"，又选择将获得的财富回报给这座城市，并且主要用于公共卫生事业。建筑师出身的雷士德是地产大王，他去世前留下遗嘱，用遗产捐建了仁济医院大楼和雷士德医学研究院。雷纳曾为德商礼和洋行工作，后来拥有自己的公司（Housser & Co.），他为上海外侨社区建造了这家当时条件最好的医院。

宏恩医院开业后赢得了良好声誉，美好的环境和优越的医疗吸引了很多中外病患。1946年3月的《文汇报》报道，宋美龄曾到宏恩医院探望端纳（William Henry Donald, 1875—1946）。澳大利亚人端纳担任蒋介石顾问多年，在著名的"西安事变"过程中，曾受宋美龄之托，亲赴西安斡旋。同年11月，端纳在宏恩医院去世。宋美龄还曾陪同美国将军马歇尔（George Marshall）的夫人到宏恩医院看病。

如今，昔日的宏恩医院成为华东医院一号楼，主要作为老年科病房使用。华东医院现有1300多张床位，医疗特色是治疗老年疾病。

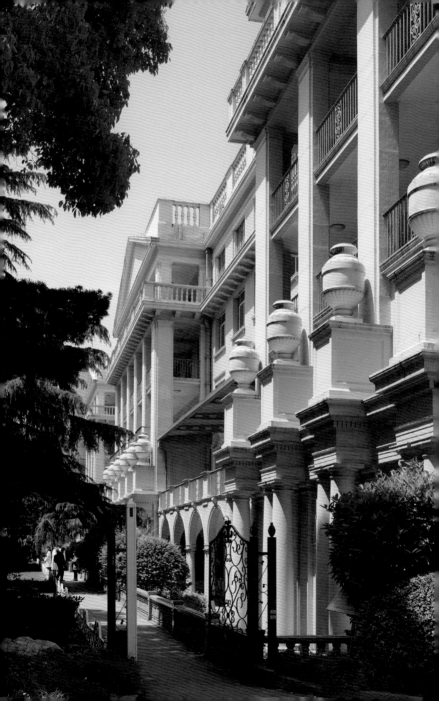

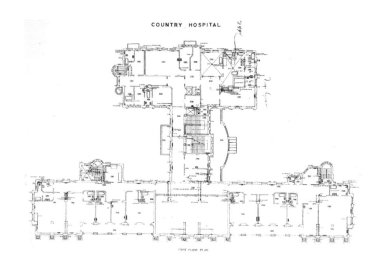

初夏是适宜探访昔日宏恩医院建筑的季节。穿过繁忙的院区，在院落深处有一个大花园，点缀着古松、玉兰，有时还有几位安静坐在轮椅上晒太阳的百岁老人。

1926年6月9日《大陆报》报道，宏恩医院的花园和美景也是捐赠者用"爱的劳动"创造出来的礼物。自从两年半前确定医院选址以来，树木、花卉和灌木都是他本人亲自规划并照料的。

如今，花园已郁郁葱葱，阳光将它染成金色，成为欣赏这家传奇医院的完美背景。

昨天：宏恩医院　**今天：**华东医院1号楼　**地址：**延安西路221号　**建造年代：**1926年
建筑师：邬达克　**参观指南：**1号楼不对外开放，但可以欣赏美丽的花园与建筑主立面。

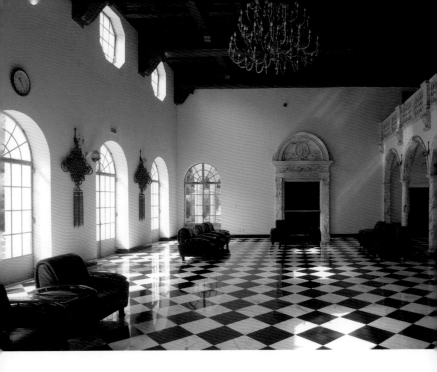

Buildings are sometimes built from dreams. For American merchant Charles Ernest Rayner, who lived in old Shanghai, the dream was to build the best hospital for the city. With a donation of funds and his efforts to supervise the construction, the dream became a reality with the Country Hospital, which still perches in the compound of Huadong Hospital on Yan'an Road.

A 'magnificent' gift

The hospital was called a "magnificent gift" by local media when it opened its doors in 1926. Un-

like other barrack-like structures, as many hospitals were, it was an unusually beautiful building designed by Slovakian-Hungarian architect Laszlo Hudec.

"The benefactor who asked Hudec to design an upper-class hospital for Shanghai expatriates insisted on the highest standards and the best facilities. And there was no budget limit — a perfect project for an architect. He also asked Hudec to keep his identity a secret, or the contract would be canceled," said Professor Hua Xiahong from Shanghai Tongji University, author of the book *Shang-*

Covering 2,300 square meters, the five-story steel-concrete building had an ideal location, far away from the noise and bustle of the city but close enough to the heart of Shanghai to be within 15 minutes' drive of the Bund.

As one of Hudec's early works, the building was an Italian Renaissance-style design. According to a study by Italian architectural historian Luca Poncellini, Hudec chose an Italian Renaissance style due to the preference of the hospital's benefactor who had spent much of his life in Italy.

The hospital is beautiful in every way. The southern facade features a tripartite vertical composition with balanced east and west wings.

The ground floor consists of double-columned arched windows and an arcade, while the second to fourth floors are treated with a unified approach. The fifth floor and the parapet are designed as three imposing pediments and make a powerful impression on visitors.

The most striking part of this hospital is the reception lobby, which in no way looks like a hospital's ground floor. It's more like a stylish hotel lobby, quiet and elegant. Hudec made extensive use of imported black, white and gray marbles on classical columns, the large staircase and flooring. The patterned wooden ceiling makes an interesting textural contrast with the smooth marble as sunlight pours into the lobby from a row of French windows.

"Hudec created a bright and open lobby for the hospital, which totally changed the usual cold, dim decor of a hospital," said Hua, noting the Country Hospital was widely reported by Chinese and international media at the time for its scale and advanced facilities.

The old *Shanghai Sunday Times* newspaper wrote: "The rural, restful early Italian Renaissance effect reminds visitors of the courtyard and rooms of a villa in Tuscany."

It was also the only hospital outside U.S. territory to be discussed in the hospital section of the American journal Architectural Forum in December 1928.

"Bathroom and air-conditioning in every room were also rare and luxurious at the time. The benefactor wanted patients to feel at home in the hospital. Air-conditioning was so important because the temperature of operating rooms in Shanghai could reach 42 degrees Celsius in summer," she said.

According to a report in *The*

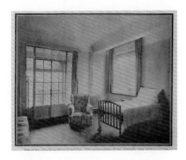

China Press on June 13, 1926, an atmosphere of a home was carefully created for this dream hospital.

The wards were decorated with light enameled woodwork, rose curtains, big deep flower-cretonne overstuffed chairs, bed lights and a restful outlook over the gardens.

The children's creche featured nursery rhyme pictures painted all around the walls and little white beds brought from America. Dainty cross-barred curtains at the window let in a soft light from green blinds outside. In a large alcove off the nursery was a sunny playroom with jolly little child-size tables and chairs in cream enamel where one could draw pictures or play jacks on the rubberized, immaculate floor.

Upstairs in the sanitary operating rooms, dispensary and prescription rooms, all the glassware bottles and other utensils were brought in from Japan.

The splendidly equipped and ultra-modern maternity ward was one of the prides of the hospital and the infant nursery, where newborn babies were cared for, was "as clean and fresh and comfortable as modern invention can conceive".

A modern architectural practice

For a long time, the Country Hospital was classified as a classic-style architecture. But Professor Hua finds that it's a modern, functional architectural practice disguised in "a classic coat".

"I have also classified the hospital as a classic building in my master's paper written in 2000. But after studying more historical archives, I found it was a misunderstanding. To realize the benefactor's intensive ideal, the design of the Country Hospital always followed the principles of modernism which was 'form follows function,' whether in terms of the layout, the façade style, or the selection of materials and equipment," Professor Hua said.

She discovered the classic-style façade and reception hall were not merely designed to pursuit fashion or conservative aesthetic beauty. It was "a rational selection" to deal with Shanghai's summer heat and create a friendly medical ambience. The three sets of gigantic porches topped by gables were used to prevent summer sunlight.

"Like factories, hospital buildings are required to be economical, practical and designed in a concise, simple-cut layout style, which as later adopted by Renji Hospital, built in 1932, Hongqiao Sanatorium in 1933, Paulun Hospital and Margaret Williamson Hospital both designed by Hudec in the 1920s. But the dream of the benefactor was to build an upper-class, comfortable country sanatorium. So Hudec thoughtfully designed furniture, floor decorations and selected materials and colors to create a cozy, tranquil atmosphere of home," Hua said.

It was the first project Hudec was in full charge of and the first important work after he left American architect R. A. Curry's firm to start his own business.

Since Hudec had obeyed the agreement, the benefactor was so satisfied that he enjoyed standing in the front row of the opening ceremony with no one knowing that he built the hospital.

Rayner's life mirrored that of another heir-less wealthy old Shanghai resident — British merchant Henry Lester. Both of them had made money out of Shanghai and wanted to put it back into the

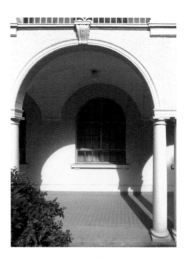

metropolis for the benefit of the community. And they both emphasized charity projects for medical purposes.

A successful architect and landlord, Lester was the main contributor to the Lester Chinese Hospital (today's Renji Hospital), and Lester Institute of Medical Research. Rayner, who had worked for German firm Carlowitz Co. and owned a company named Housser & Co., thought of building a hospital for the international community.

The Country Hospital had enjoyed a favorable reputation after it opened, whose quality services attracted both foreign and Chinese patients. According to reports in Chinese newspapers Wenhui Dai-

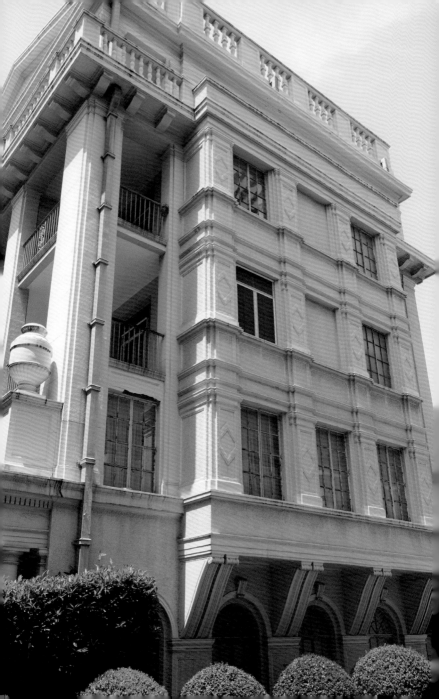

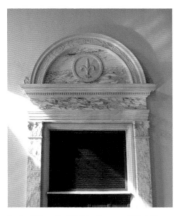
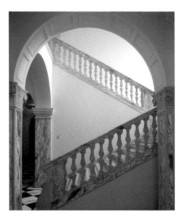

ly in March 1946, Soong Mei-ling, wife of Kuomintang leader Chiang Kai-shek, came to the hospital to visit her husband's famous Australian consultant William Henry Donald, who passed away in the hospital in November of that year. Song also accompanied American General George Marshall's wife to the hospital for medical treatment.

Today the former Country Hospital serves as the No. 1 Building in Huadong Hospital, where many of the city's VIPs received medical treatment. The hospital grew to house more than 1,300 beds and is specialized in treating diseases for the elderly.

Early summer is a nice time to visit Huadong Hospital. Walking past the busy nurses, you will find a huge garden in the depth of the hospital. It is dotted with century-old pines, magnolia trees and centenarian patients sitting peacefully in wheelchairs.

According to *The China Press* on June 9, 1926, the gardens and beauty surrounding it were also the gifts of the benefactor who created them with "a labor of love". It was him who planned and nursed the trees, flowers and shrubs ever since the hospital site was decided upon two and a half years before.

Now the lush lawn is a perfect setting to appreciate a hospital of love and care, sprayed in gold by the summer's sunlight.

Yesterday: The Country Hospital   **Today:** No. 1 Building of Huadong Hospital
Address: 221 Yan'an Rd W.   **Built in:** 1926   **Architect:** L. E. Hudec
Tips: The entrance to the building, might be restricted. However, it is possible to appreciate the building from the garden.

仁慈捐赠者的承诺

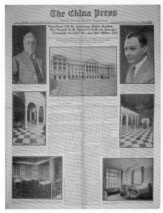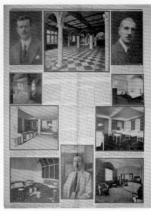

应《大陆报》的要求，捐助者向上海公众传达以下信息：

捐助者和他的妻子在中国度过了最好的工作时光，为这个国际化社区建造了宏恩医院并为配置好设备，希望以此在某种程度上为加强这种友善与友好合作的精神而做一点贡献。多年来，正是这种精神将许多在这里生活和工作的不同国家和种族的人们团结在一起，为了共同的利益并肩工作。

宏恩医院的舒适性得到了扩展，没有国籍、种族或宗教的歧视，所有人都可能受到健康不良的折磨。而捐助者所要求的回报无非是对所有人都怀有这种开朗的善意精神，而对任何人都不会恶意相加，如此就会逐步坚定地团结所有将要居住在这座城市的人们。

医院为没有钱的病人提供了两个病房，这两个病房以上海有史以来最富有公共精神的慈善的医生命名。对捐助者来说，没有什么比看到这里成为其他类似捐助的榜样更令人欣慰了，比如捐助一张病床或整个病房。

摘自 1926 年 6 月 9 日《大陆报》

Benevolent benefactor's city pledge

At the request of *The China Press* the donor gives the following message to the public of Shanghai:

The donor and his wife, having spent the best part of their working lives in China, have erected and equipped the Country Hospital for the use and benefit of this cosmopolitan community, hoping thereby to contribute in some small measure to the reinforcement of that spirit of goodwill and cordial cooperation which has for many years united for the common good the many nationalities and races living and working here side-by-side.

The comforts of the Country Hospital are extended, without distinction of nationalities, race or religion, to all may be afflicted with ill health, and the donors ask for no greater reward than that this same spirit of cheerful goodwill for all and malice towards none may gradually and firmly unite all those whose lot it is to dwell in this city.

Provision has been made for those without means in two wards commemorating the names of two of the most public-spirited and charitable doctors Shanghai has ever known, and nothing would be more gratifying to the donors than to see the example thus set followed by other similar endowments of single beds or of entire wards.

Excerpt from *The China Press* on June 9, 1926

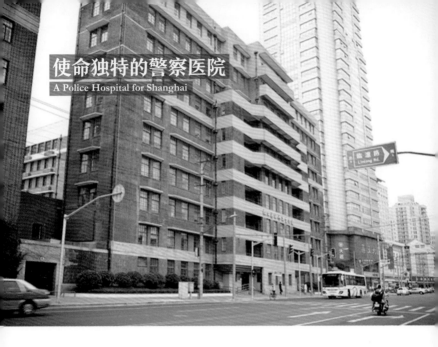

使命独特的警察医院
A Police Hospital for Shanghai

上海虹口区疾控中心是一座巧克力色的大楼，位于著名的提篮桥监狱旁。这座大楼始建于1932年，原来是一家为华人巡捕和印度巡捕提供医疗服务的医院。

"这座大楼原来是医院，立面呈现出原始的外观，加建过两层，现在变成公共卫生大楼。如今这里有许多实验科室，内部结构已改变了。"上海医学史专家、原上海市第四人民医院图书馆长陆明说。

《上海地方志》记载，1909年11月，工部局在海能路开设华捕医院，专门为华人巡捕提供医疗服务，此后又开设印捕医院。1932年起设立一家较正规的巡捕医院，主要收治华印籍巡捕和犯人中的病患者，其门诊部对外公开营业。该院还承担工部局候补职员的体格检查。1939年4月的统计显示有50张印捕病床和122张华捕病床。

1845年旧英租界成立时还没有警察管理社会治安，只有负责火灾警报的华人更夫。1854年上海工部局（Shanghai Municipal

Council）成立，负责公共租界的市政管理，很快就把租界的警察局(巡捕房)设立起来，以维持社会秩序和公共治安。

根据张斌所著的《上海英租界巡捕房制度及其运作研究（1854—1863）》，上海英租界巡捕房是仿照19世纪20年代末出现的英格兰现当代警察组织建立的。

"上海英租界开辟之后的将近九年时间内，一直施行华洋分局政策，租界内人少事简。上海小刀会起义爆发后，上海地方政府自顾不暇，百姓则大量涌入英租界中，使租界局面为之一变。租界内的外侨为了自己的商业利益，不愿撤离上海。在战争环境下，他们同时又希望能保证租界的安全和秩序，于是决定成立租界自治政府。巡捕房也随之应运而生。"张斌写道。

从今天的眼光来看，老上海的巡捕队伍相当国际化，分工合作得也不错。巡捕房由以欧洲人为主的西捕领导管理，擅长包打听的华捕负责采集消息，大胡子的印度锡克族巡捕指挥交通，日

籍巡捕则管理日本工厂较多的虹口和普陀一带。

根据徐家俊撰写的《上海警察医院小史》，1909年开设的两座巡捕医院主要为华籍巡捕和印籍巡捕进行疾病治疗、体检和防疫，由于两座医院均为租借他人的房产，需要归还，而且设备简陋，病床不足，医院的业务跟不上工作的需要。为此，工部局考虑在华德路(今长阳路)197号、毗邻提篮桥监狱处重建巡捕医院，经多年筹备于1929年破土动工，耗资40万银元，与今上海市监狱总医院8层高的新大楼一起建造。上海巡捕医院与提篮桥监狱医院的新楼均高达8层，仅一墙之隔。

"关于为中国和印度巡捕提供的医院住宿，委员会曾一度使用一些普通的建筑物作为医院，但后来在 1929 年，现在的这座现代医院就建在了华德路。监狱医院也有类似的历史，监狱最初只是提供一个病房，而护理工作由其他犯人完成。直到 1933年，监狱医院才在华德路的监狱内建立起来。" 1937 年 6 月 13

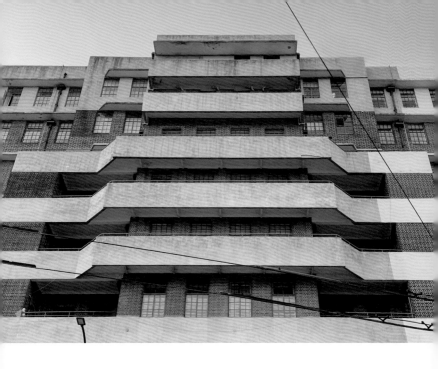

日《大陆报》(*The China Press*)报道介绍。

巡捕医院由上海成泰营造厂承建，1932年竣工，同年10月启用。它是一幢钢筋混凝土结构的楼房，楼高8层，建筑面积5000多平方米。启用时，把原先的华捕医院和印捕医院一起并入，由上海工部局卫生处管理。

关于这座新医院建筑的记录很少，但其建设期间的一些英文报道显示，大楼设计精良，配备了现代化、先进的设施。

1932年5月19日的《大陆报》称，电梯的安装工作正在进行中，所有楼层的固定家具都准备好了。

"所有房间都涂上了墙壁底漆，预制水磨石和褐色石灰岩护墙板正在固定到位。电灯安装已经完成。排水和排污工程进展顺利。"《大陆报》报道写道。

1932年9月29日，巡捕医院六楼的地板和手术室的橡胶地板已经铺设完毕。

"医院五楼的犯人病房和六

楼的办公室已经完成，手术室的空调设备已经交付准备使用。"报道写道。

根据《上海警察医院小史》，上海巡捕医院的首任院长为英国人，医院的主要任务是负责华籍、印籍巡捕的疾病诊治和体检防疫工作。同时，巡捕医院还对公共租界各巡捕房和提篮桥监狱的部分犯人进行治疗。建院初期，医院设特等病床2张、二等病床10张、普通病床160张。工作人员60余人，其中医务技术人员30余人。巡捕医院的年平均门诊达到25000人次，住院病员2500人次左右，手术170人次左右。

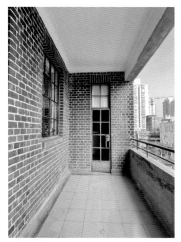

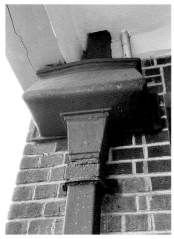

研究上海公共租界卫生史的朱德明指出，当时上海的警员工作努力，1930年破获谋杀、绑票、抢劫、纵火、盗窃等大小刑事案件共15664起。在侦破案件时警员们受伤率较高，巡捕医院成为了他们的坚强后盾。巡捕医院和华德路监狱医院都配备了解剖实验室、X光室、药品室、化验室、候诊室、诊室、手术室、病房、戒烟所、瘰病施诊所、皮肤病诊所、花柳病诊所等，设备较为先进，医务人员技术较高，成绩斐然。

"上海公共租界警务处和卫生处通过各种医疗措施，使警员

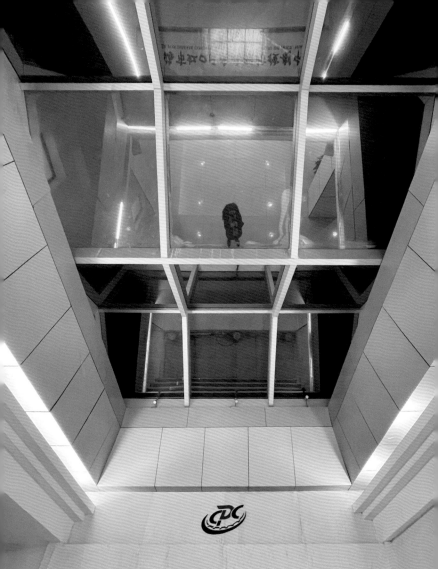

和囚犯的死亡人数大幅度下降，40多种疾病得到有效的医治，这些实绩在当时贫穷落后的旧中国十分罕见，这对近代上海医院卫生事业的发展大有裨益，应该在中国警政、医学发展史上为其写上一笔。"他在《三十年代上海公共租界警政机构的医疗状况》一文中评价。

1941年12月太平洋战争爆发后，日军占领上海租界，次年巡捕医院由日本医师接管，1945又由上海市警察局管辖，改称上海市警察局警察医院。

1951年，上海警察医院更名为上海市公安局公安医院，主要服务上海地区的公安干警。1994年，医院历经几次合并变化，又更名为上海市中西医结合医院。

2005年，昔日警察医院大楼移交给上海市虹口区卫生局及虹口区疾病预防控制中心等单位使用。这里的工作主要是促进公共卫生健康，楼内各项工作与昔日一样繁忙。

昨天：巡捕医院（警察医院）　**今天：**虹口区疾病预防控制中心　**地址：**长阳路 197 号
建筑风格：现代风格　**参观指南：**在长阳路可以欣赏建筑立面。

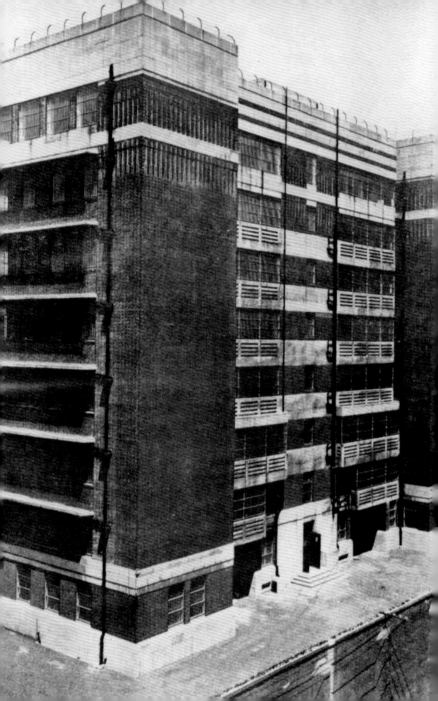

The chocolate-hued building for the Center for Disease Control & Prevention in Hongkou District perches next to the former Tilanqiao Prison. It was built in 1932 as a hospital for Chinese and Indian policemen in old Shanghai.

"It's a public health building today with labs and offices. The facade shows an original look. It has been added two more floors and the internal structure has been changed as well," says Lu Ming, an expert on Shanghai Medical History from Shanghai No. 4 People's Hospital.

According to Shanghai Annals, the Shanghai Municipal Council opened a hospital on Haineng Road for Chinese policemen in 1909 and later opened another for the Indian policemen. In 1932, a formal police hospital was founded to offer medical service for the Chinese and Indian policemen as well as some sick prisoners.

The outpatient department of the police hospital was open to the public. It also conducted physical examination for candidate employees of the Shanghai Municipal Council. In 1939, the hospital had 50 beds for Indian policemen and 122 beds for Chinese policemen.

The police system of old Shanghai was established in 1854 to maintain social orders and pub-

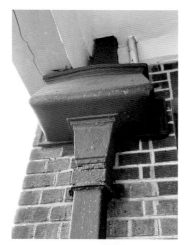

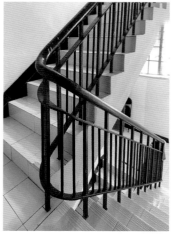

lic security. According to Zhang Bin's book *A Study of the police system and its management in the former Shanghai British Settlement (1854—1863)*, Shanghai's police organization has directly referred to the England modern police system originated in the 1820s.

"During the first decade of the former British settlement, foreigners and Chinese lived separately. There were only a few foreign residents and civil affairs. After the Small Sword Society Uprising in 1853, some 20,000 Chinese refugees flooded into the settlement. The expatriates, who profit from leasing houses to the Chinese, found emerging problems when refugees drank a lot, fought and caused traffic jams. So there was an urgent need to restore social orders," Zhang Bin wrote in his book.

That led to the immediate founding of Shanghai Municipal Council and its police station in 1854. The police team was rather international from today's point of view. European sergeants and constables were in charge of the management. Chinese constables were good at gathering information and managing Chinese-related cases. Sikh constables were responsible for guiding local traffics while Japanese constables covered Hongkou and Putuo areas where many Japanese factories were located.

According to Xu Jiajun's article "The Little History of Shanghai Police Hospital", the two old police hospitals were formed to provide medical treatment, physical examination and epidemic prevention for Chinese and Indian policemen. Both hospitals operated on leased properties lacked medical facilities and accommodations for patients.

In 1929 it was decided to build a new police hospital beside the Shanghai Municipal Goal (now Tilanqiao Prison) at 197 Ward Road (today's Changyang Road). At a cost of 400,000 taels, the new police hospital was constructed along with the new jail hospital. Both the new hospitals were eight-story buildings separated by a wall.

"With regard to hospital accommodation for the Chinese and Indian police, the council for a while used some ordinary buildings for hospitals, but later in 1929 the present modern hospital was erected on Ward Road. The Jail Hospital has a similar history, the jail at first being merely provided with a 'Sick Bay' and the nursing being done by other convicts. It was not until 1933 that a Jail Hospital was erected inside the jail countries on Ward Road," *The China Press* reports on June 13, 1937.

The new police hospital is a steel-and-concrete structure with a floor area of more than 5,000 square meters. After its comple-

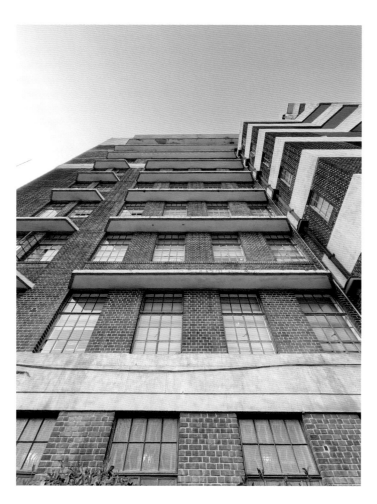

tion in 1932, both the two old police hospitals were merged in.

There was little record of this
new hospital architecture, but
newspaper reporting during the
construction period revealed that
the building was well-designed

with modern, advanced facilities.

The China Press on May 19, 1932
said the erection of lifts was in
progress and fixed furniture being
prepared for all floors.

"The priming coat to walls has
been applied to all rooms, and the

precast terrazzo and Caen stone jadoos are being fixed in position. The electric lighting installation has been completed. The drainage and sewerage works are well advanced," *The China Press* reported.

On September 29, 1932, *The China Press* noted that the patent floors on the sixth floor and the rubber flooring to the operation theaters at the Police Hospital had been laid.

"The work in the Prisoners' Ward on the fifth floor of the hospital and all staff rooms on the sixth floor has been completed, the air conditioning plant to operation theaters has been handed over for occupation." the newspaper said.

According to "A Short History of Shanghai Police Hospital," this new police hospital on average received 25,000 outpatient visits, 2,500 hospitalized patients and operated 170 surgeries every year. The hospital also treated some prisoners from the municipal goal or other police stations.

Another researcher Zhu Deming noted that the police hospital served as a strong backing for hard-working policemen who were mostly likely to get injured during work. "Both the police hospital and the jail hospital were equipped with autopsy room, X-ray room, drug room, laboratory, waiting room, clinic, operating Room, wards, smoking cessation, tuberculosis clinic, dermatology clinic, STD clinic etc. The hospitals made remarkable achievements for the advanced equipment and highly skilled medical staff.

"The police and health departments of Shanghai Municipal Council adopted various medical measures and the number of deaths of police officers and prisoners had been greatly reduced. More than 40 kinds of diseases had been effectively treated. These achievements were very rare in old China, which was poverty-stricken and backward at that time. It was of great benefit to the development of the health cause of modern Shanghai hospitals. It well worths a record in the history of Chinese police and medical development," Zhu comments in an article named "Medical Conditions of Police Agencies in Shanghai International Settlement in the 1930s".

After the outbreak of the Pacific War, the police hospital was taken over by the Japanese and received by the Chinese government in 1945. Despite the changes, it had been serving as a police hospital for decades.

In 1951, the Police Hospital

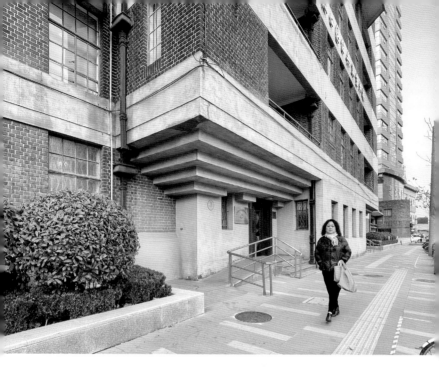

changed its name to the Public Security Hospital which served local public security officers and expanded its size. After some merging and changes, it was renamed Shanghai TCM-Integrated Hospital in 1994. However in 2005, the building was handed over to Shanghai Hongkou District Health Bureau and Hongkou District Center for Disease Control and Prevention for use. During the Covid-19 pandemic since 2020, medical officers working in the former police hospital building were busy supervising the prevention work of institutions and enterprises in the region.

Yesterday: Police Hospital   **Today:** The Center for Disease Control & Prevention in Hongkou District   **Address: 197** Changyang Road   **Architectural style:** Modern style
Tips: The building's facade can be appreciated on Changyang Road.

印度囚犯死于肺结核：在巡捕医院不治

昨天下午，验尸官海恩斯（C. H. Haines）在英国警察法庭宣告判决，大意是印度人马汉·辛格 (Mahan Singh) 于 7 月 11 日在巡捕医院死于肺结核，他当时正在服刑 10 个月期间。

在审讯中提供证据的唯一证人是监狱医生休伯特·史密斯（Dr. Hubert Smith）。史密斯医生说，这名囚犯自 1932 年 8 月 10 日入狱以来一直由他照顾，医生经常看到辛格。5 月 24 日，辛格被转移到巡捕医院，此前他曾在监狱的病囚房待过一段时间。

辛格被发现患有肺结核。他的咳嗽从二月份开始，一直在观察治疗，但没有好转，夜里开始发烧。在他去世前两个月发现了细菌感染，X 光片显示病情加重。

根据史密斯医生的说法，当时辛格没有治愈的可能，他作为一个没有希望的病例被转移到巡捕医院，7 月 11 日在那里死于肺结核。当他在巡捕医院治疗时，一名工作人员每天照顾他，一名中国医生每周为他治疗 3 次，史密斯医生每周为他诊疗一次，如有必要也会增加治疗频率。

最后，史密斯医生表示，这种疾病在这个年龄、这种类型的印度人中非常普遍。验尸官随后通过了判决。

摘自 1933 年 7 月 15 日《大陆报》

Indian Prisoner Dies of Tuberculosis Here: Succumbs in Police Hospital

A verdict to the effect that an Indian, Mahan Singh, died at the Police Hospital on July 11 from tuberculosis while serving a sentence of 10 months' imprisonment, was returned by Coroner C. H. Haines in the British Police Court yesterday afternoon.

The only witness to give evidence at the inquest was Dr. Hubert Smith, physician of the Municipal Jail. Dr. Smith stated that the prisoner had been under his care since he was first admitted to the prison on August 10, 1932. The doctor saw the prisoner frequently. Mahan Singh was transferred to the police hospital on May 24, although he had been in a hospital cell at the jail for some time previous.

The prisoner was found suffering from tuberculosis of the lungs. His cough started in February. He was kept under observation and treatment, but did not improve and begun to run an evening temperature. Two months before he died germs were found and an x-ray showed the disease advanced.

There was no hope of saving the prisoner at the time, according to Dr. Smith, and Mahan Singh was transferred to the police hospital as a hopeless case. He died of tuberculosis at the Police Hospital on July 11. A dresser attended him once a day, a Chinese doctor three times a week and Dr. Smith once a week and more frequently if necessary, while he was in a hospital cell.

In conclusion Dr. Smith stated that this sickness was very common among Indians of this age and type. The coroner then passed the verdict.

Excerpt from *The China Press* on July 15, 1933

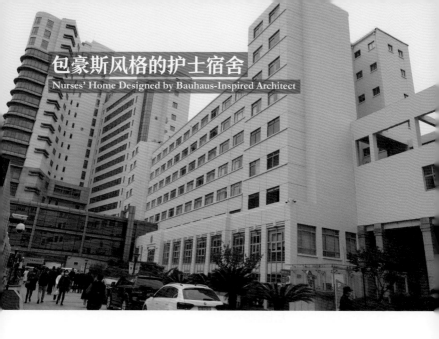

包豪斯风格的护士宿舍

Nurses' Home Designed by Bauhaus-Inspired Architect

上海华东医院的一号楼曾是著名的宏恩医院（The Country Hospital），但院区里还有一座不为人所知的老建筑——延安路高架边的5号楼。1933年，这座摩登现代的大楼作为新的"维多利亚护士之家"（Victoria Nurses Home）开幕，设计师是受到包豪斯风格影响的德国建筑师汉堡嘉（Rudolf Hamburger）。

1933年10月25日，英文《北华捷报》（The North-China Herald）刊登大楼落成的照片，

说明文字写着："新的维多利亚护士之家(Victoria Nurses Home)"。这座引人注目的建筑高达八层，带有长而贯通的阳台，是管理旧公共租界的上海工部局（Shanghai Municipal Council）为宏恩医院而建造的，位于医院附近的一块基地。

"维多利亚护士之家"是一座专门为护士而建的宿舍，这座摩登大楼历经变迁。《上海市第六人民医院纪事（1904—2013）》一书记载，1937年抗战爆发后，原上海工部局所属医院

都迁至苏州河以南地带。位于老靶子路（Range Road，今武进路）的西人隔离医院租借宏恩医院病房，收治肺病病人，其护士就入住工部局建造的这座护士宿舍，二楼住华人护士，三楼住西人护士。1942年，为了彻底改善西人隔离医院的就医环境以及接纳犹太难民传染病人入院，工部局决定将隔离医院从大西路63号迁至大西路23号维多利护士之家（今延安西路251号华东医院北楼）。这里曾发展为上海第六人民医院，如今由华东医院作为特需病房使用。

1933年"维多利亚护士之家"开幕前夕，英文《大陆报》（The China Press）在10月20日刊登报道，详细介绍了这家机构的历史背景。

1897年为庆祝维多利亚女王即位60周年，一个由本地英国侨民组成的委员会募集资金，在工部局位于老靶子路附近的一块土地上修建了维多利亚护理院（Victoria Nursing Institute），后改名为维多利亚疗养院（Victoria Nursing Home），

1901年对外开业。捐款者主要是英国人，也包括其他外国侨民。

时光流转到1927年，随着环境条件更好的宏恩医院开业，疗养院收治的病人越来越少。1928年，维多利利亚疗养院因为经济原因关门停业。1933年，新的维多利亚护士之家在宏恩医院附近竣工。

英文老报纸透露，这座护士宿舍有着深红色的面砖，由上海工部局工务处的一位建筑师设计。这位建筑师就是汉堡嘉，1930年从德国来到上海担任工部局的建筑师。

汉堡嘉出生于德国下西里西亚的小镇"Landeshut"，1924年移居德累斯顿学习，并在那里结识了见习建筑师鲍立克（Richard Paulick）。汉堡嘉和鲍立克成为密友，日后他们又在上海相聚。

1925年，汉堡嘉和鲍立克转到柏林工业大学学习，导师是德国现代设计大师汉斯·珀尔齐格（Hans Poelzig）。汉堡嘉在毕业后留在柏林工作，1928年又成为柏林艺术学院珀尔齐

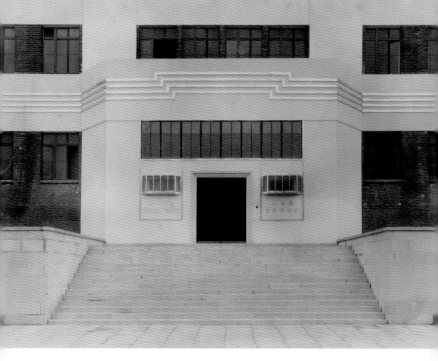

格工作室的硕士研究生。1930年，他应征了一则刊登在柏林当地报纸上的招聘广告，获得前往上海工部局担任建筑师的工作合同。1930年7月，他与妻子乌苏拉·库钦斯基（Ursula Kuczynski）前往上海定居。

"维多利亚护士之家"是汉堡嘉设计的第一个大项目，被媒体誉为"可能是上海的第一座现代建筑"。这座护士宿舍楼里的公寓经过高标准装修，装有暖气片和带纱窗的窗户，1933年10月23日开业后受到医务人员和媒体的广泛赞誉。

根据德国学者华纳（Torsten Warner）所著的《德国建筑艺术在中国》一书，宿舍楼高八层，长约60米，可供100名护士住宿，为钢筋混凝土楼层框架承重结构。因为担心房间会因此而不隔音，所以在内部装修时采用炉渣石和隔音材料作地面铺层。建这座宿舍楼使用了680根约20米长的木桩做支柱。护士宿舍楼显然是采用了德国包

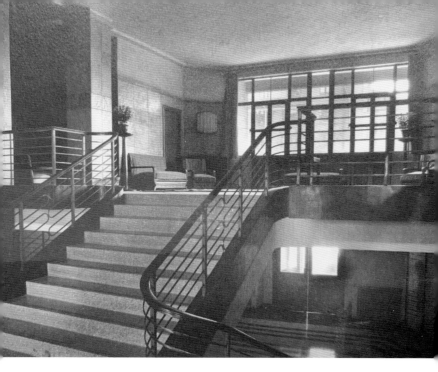

豪斯流派的建筑形式，立面朴实无华，用明快的水平线条稍加点缀，横贯南立面的阳台连廊表现了这种横向划分的艺术手法。

研究上海医疗历史建筑的同济大学博士研究生黄钰婷发现，这座现代主义风格的大楼与汉堡嘉在上海的其他几座建筑的风格保持一致。大楼高八层，整体呈倒凹字形，各层设置朝南向贯通的阳台长廊，白色的栏杆在立面上形成简洁的横向线条强调出建筑横向的体量与节奏感。

汉堡嘉设计生涯最重要的委托项目都是1930至1936年在上海期间完成的。维多利亚护士之家、新加坡路（今余姚路）女子学校和华德路监狱展示了建筑师的想象力、他对现代知识和材料的利用，以及对细节的关注。

1933年《大陆报》的报道透露，维多利亚护士之家使用的设备都是当时最先进的。底层安装着最现代化的烹饪用具和食品制冷设备，设有主厨房和食品准备室。锅炉房和中国员工宿舍也位

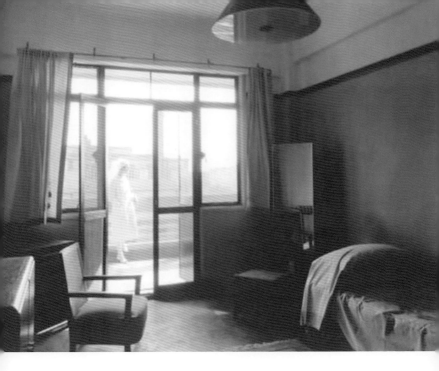

于底楼。

　　一楼有一个宽敞的休息室，可通往修女、全职护士和见习护士的餐厅、图书馆和茶室，这些地方都可以欣赏花园美景。休息室旁边是访客的等候室和衣帽间，还有驻院修女的办公室。

　　二到六层都是相同的布局，为护士提供单独的卧室宿舍。这些宿舍共享阳台，可俯瞰花园。每一层的西端设有供资深修女使用的两室公寓，而东端则是给护士长和修女的小公寓。每间公寓均有客厅、卧室、浴室、储藏室和私人阳台。

　　七八层是见习护士的宿舍，也提供独立的卧室。八楼有一个凉台和屋顶花园。每层楼的两端都有铺设瓷砖的浴室，阿姨和男孩的工作间靠近每层的中部位置。

　　1933年的报道特别提到，"新的护士之家向上海所有的外国护士开放，并且与原来的维多利亚护理院一样，具有国际性"。

设计现代护士之家的建筑师汉堡嘉在上海迎来了新的命运。他的妻子乌苏拉·库钦斯基被招募到苏联情报部门工作，并成为著名的间谍。据说汉堡嘉一直支持妻子的间谍工作，直到1939年两人离婚。

1933年时，这对夫妇邀请老朋友鲍立克来中国发展。汉堡嘉于1936年离开上海，但鲍立克一直留在这座城市工作，直到1949年。他在上海经历丰富，担任建筑师、室内设计师、舞台设计师和圣约翰大学教授，1945年成为参与起草"大上海都市计划"（Greater Shanghai Plan）的核心成员。

今天，昔日护士之家的入口和北立面基本保持历史旧貌，南立面外墙标志性的长阳台已被拆除。

大楼如今用作高端医疗的特需部使用，一间间护士宿舍被改造为条件舒适的私人病房。在白衣修女护士住过的房间里，穿着淡蓝色制服的护士们也在忙碌着。

昨天： 维多利亚护士之家　**今天：** 华东医院五号楼　**地址：** 延安西路 221 号
建筑风格： 现代风格　**建筑师：** 汉堡嘉（Rudolph Hamburger）
参观指南： 在延安西路可以欣赏建筑立面。

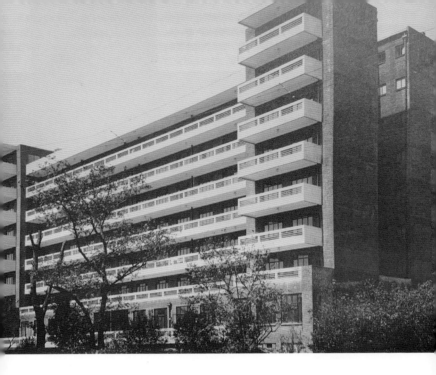

Huadong Hospital's Building No. 1 is well known throughout Shanghai for being the former Country Hospital, designed by Laszlo Hudec in 1926. But it also has another historical building rarely known and easy to miss — Building No. 5 adjacent to the Yan'an elevated highway.

When the doors of this modern building opened in 1933, it was the new Victoria Nurses Home designed by German Bauhaus-inspired architect Rudolf Hamburger.

On October 25, 1933, *the North-China Herald* published a picture of the building with long, continuous balconies. It was an imposing eight-story structure built for the Country Hospital by Shanghai Municipal Council. The caption reads, "The New Victoria Nurses Home. A general view of the striking building erected on a site adjacent to the Country Hospital".

"This medical building has endured many changes," said Lu Ming, an expert of Shanghai medical history, from Shanghai No. 4 People's Hospital.

"The Victoria Nurses Home" was built as a new hostel for nurs-

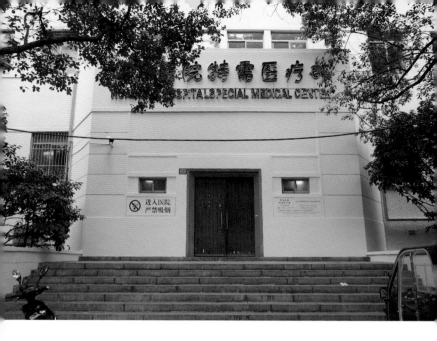

es. In 1937, the Isolation Hospital on Range Road (today's Wujin Road) rented wards off Country Hospital to receive tuberculosis patients while its nurses resided at the Victoria Nurses Home.

"In 1942, the Isolation Hospital moved into the nurses' home and developed into Shanghai No. 6 People's Hospital. In 1956, Shanghai Public Medical Treatment Hospital transferred here, was renamed Yan'an Hospital but relocated to Kunming of Yunnan Province in the 1970s," Lu says.

Shortly before its official opening, *The China Press* published a report on October 20, 1933 to introduce the historical background of the Victoria Nurses Home.

In 1897, a committee of local British residents raised funds to provide a memorial of Queen Victoria's Diamond Jubilee. Subscribers were mainly British, but included other foreign nationals. These funds were used to erect a building on land owned by the Shanghai Municipal Council (SMC) near Range Road. Upon completion the building was delivered to the SMC and named the Victoria Nursing Institute (later Victoria Nursing Home), which opened in 1901.

However in 1927, with the opening of the Country Hospital, the Victoria Nursing Home received less patients. In 1928, it was closed under economic measures. In 1933, the new Victoria Nurses Home was built on land adjacent to the Country Hospital. The report recorded that the nurses' hostel, faced with dark red tiling, was designed by one of the architects at the SMC Public Works Department.

The architect was Rudolph Hamburger, who came to Shanghai from Germany in 1930, to work for the SMC.

Born in Landeshut, a small town of Lower Silesia Germany, Hamburger moved to Dresden in 1924 where he studied and met trainee architect Richard Paulick. They became close friends and their careers would become later entwined in Shanghai.

In 1925 Hamburger and Paulick moved to study in the Technical University of Berlin, where Hans Poelzig taught them. After graduating, Hamburger stayed in Berlin to work. In 1928 he became a Master's student at the Arts Academy studios with Poelzig. In 1930, Hamburger responded to a job advertisement placed in a local Berlin newspaper and won the contract to work as an architect with the SMC. In July 1930, he emigrated with his wife, Ursula Kuczynski, to Shanghai.

The Victoria Nurses Home was his first major project, which has been described as "probably the first modern building in Shanghai". The block occupied a dominating site directly beside the Great Western Road, today's Yan'an Road W. Imaginative design features compensated for the essentially rectangular shape of the building. The apartments were finished to high standard, with radiators and insect nets for the windows. The "Victoria Nurse Home", which opened on 23 October 1933, was widely praised both by medical workers and local media.

According to Torsten Warner's book *German Architecture in China*, the eight-floor structure consisted of reinforced concrete floor frames and stands on 680 wooden piles. Slag stone and noise-insulating floor coverings were used to prevent noise.

"The building is a manifest expression of the German Bauhaus school's clearly-formulated architectural idiom. It is simple, stark and extremely horizontal," Warner writes in the book.

Huang Yuting, a Ph. D researcher on Shanghai medical architecture from Tongji University, finds Hamburger's Shanghai buildings were all in modern style.

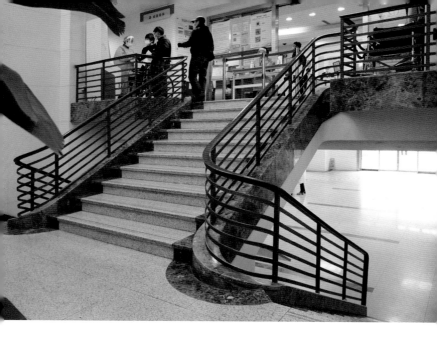

"In the Victoria Nurses Home, every floor was designed with a long, continuous balcony that faces the south. White railings form simply-cut horizontal lines on the facade, emphasizing the horizontal volume and rhythm of this building," she said.

Many of Hamburger's most important commissions were undertaken in Shanghai where he lived and worked between 1930 and 1936. The Victoria Nurses Home, as well as his Secondary Girls' School in the Singapore Road (now Yuyao Road), and the vast cruciform Ward Road Jail complex displayed the architect's exploitation of modern knowledge and materials, imagination and attention to detail.

A China Press report in 1933 noted the new Victoria Nurses Home was equipped with "Everything Up-To-Date".

The interior was done in plain and ornamental plaster. The most modern cooking appliances and food refrigeration devices were installed on the ground floor, which housed the main kitchen and food-preparation rooms. The boiler room and Chinese staff quarters were also located on this floor.

The first floor featured a large lounging hall, giving access to the sisters, staff nurses and proba-

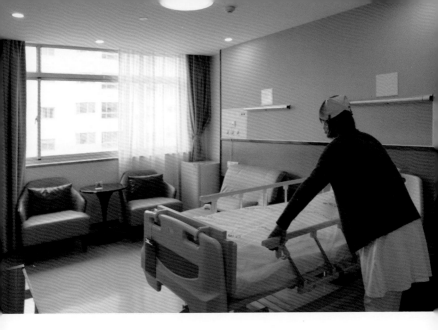

tioners' dining rooms, library and tea room, all of which had garden views. Adjacent to the lounge were the visitors' waiting and cloak rooms and the resident sister's office.

The second to sixth floors were identical and provided accommodation for the nursing staff in individual bedrooms with a common veranda overlooking the gardens. The west end of each floor had a two-room apartment for senior sisters, while a small flat occupied the east end of every floor for matrons and the home sister. Each flat consisted of a living room, bedroom, bathroom, box room and private veranda.

Both ends of each floor on the north side had tiled bathrooms, with amah and boys' work rooms located near the center of each floor.

The seventh and eighth floors served as quarters for probationer nurses and provided individual bedrooms. The eighth floor also had a sleeping porch and roof garden.

"The new nurses home is open to all foreign nurses in the city and is entirely international in character as it was when the original home was built," the 1933 report said.

In Shanghai, architect Hamburger's wife was recruited to work for the Soviet intelligence and became a famous spy. It is said he supported her espionage related activities till their divorce in 1939. In 1933, the couple invited Richard Paulick to China.

Hamburger left Shanghai in 1936 but Paulick stayed in the city until 1949, where he worked actively as an architect, interior designer, stage designer and a professor at St. John's University. In 1945 he was commissioned by the Kuomintang government as a core member for drafting postwar Greater Shanghai Plan in the 1940s.

Today, the entrance and the northern facade of the Victoria Nurses Home were largely unchanged. The southern facade had been renovated and the long balconies removed.

The building served mainly as a VIP clinic. The former nurses' rooms were turned into private wards designed in a comfortable decor. Chinese nurses in green uniforms were busy working in these rooms, which were once resided by nurse sisters in white robes.

Yesterday: Victoria Nurses Home   **Today:** Building No. 5 of Huadong Hospital
Address: 221 Yan'an Road W.   **Architectural style:** Modern style
Architect: Rudolph Hamburger
Tips: The building's entrance and northern facade can be admired from Yan'an Road W.

化装舞会

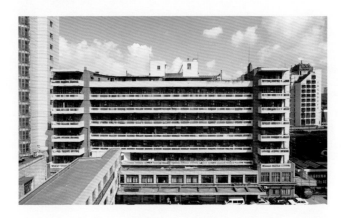

随着新年的到来，化装舞会似乎越来越受欢迎。上周，"维多利亚护士之家"的修女和护士们举办的舞会是一件令人愉快的事情，这有力地证明了医学界并不缺乏创意。负责护士之家的修女约翰斯通小姐（Miss M. Johnstone）小姐接待了来宾，不过很多人她很难认出来。这里一把胡子，那里的眉毛多一点，以及其他地方的彩色斑点，将改变那些最熟悉的面孔。出席活动的有沙逊爵士（Sir Victor Sassoon）、麦克纳腾准将（E. B. Macnaghten）、麦克纳腾小姐（Miss Audrey Macnaghten）、兰姆夫妇（Mr. and Mrs. W. P. Lambe）、博文医生（Dr. E. Bowen）、邓恩医生和夫人（Dr. and Mrs. T. B. Dunn）、邓斯康比医生（Dr. W.K. Dunscombe）、马什医生（Dr. D. L. March），至少三位医生和许多其他人。

摘自 1935 年 2 月 13 日《北华捷报》

Another Fancy Dress Party

Fancy dress parties seem to be increasing in popularity as the New Year grows older. The dance given by the sisters and nurses at the Victoria Nurses Home last week was a delightful affair, and positive proof that the medical profession are not lacking in originality of ideas. Miss M. Johnstone, sister in charge of the home, received the guests, some of whom she had a good deal of difficulty in recognizing. A moustache here, a little more eyebrow there, and a hectic spot of color somewhere else, will transform the most familiar face. Amongst those present were Sir Victor Sassoon, Brigadier General E. B. Macnaghten and Miss Audrey Macnaghten, Mr and Mrs W. P. Lambe, Dr. E. Bowen, Dr. and Mrs T. B. Dunn, Dr. W. K. Dunscombe, Dr. D. L. Marsh, no less than three doctors and many others.

Excerpt from *the North—China Herald* on February 13, 1935

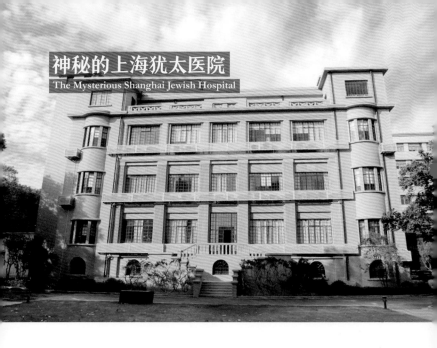

神秘的上海犹太医院
The Mysterious Shanghai Jewish Hospital

上海眼耳鼻喉科医院汾阳路院区深处有一座灰色大楼，面向着恬静的花园。在20世纪40年代，这里曾是上海犹太医院（Shanghai Jewish Hospital），由俄国建筑师李维·戈登士达（Livin Goldenstadt）设计。这家医院存续的历史不长，却很丰富，它的前身是神秘的圣裔社医院（The B'nai B'rith Polyclinic and Hospital）。

上海地方志记载，19世纪中叶至20世纪30、40年代，有三次犹太人移居上海的浪潮，分别是19世纪中叶至20世纪初叶的中东塞法迪犹太人、20世纪初至20世纪30年代末的俄罗斯犹太人、20世纪30、40年代来自德、奥等中欧国家的犹太难民。三批犹太人逐渐形成了上海犹太人社区。

"犹太民族十分注意卫生保健工作，视之为民族赓续的重要保证之一。旧上海的犹太人也不例外"，《上海犹太文化地图》作者、上海社会科学院王健教授说。

1929年，上海塞法迪犹太人建立犹太圣裔社，序号为1102号（Shanghai Lodge No.1102 B'nai B'rith），开展慈善救济。1934年2月，圣裔社开设诊所，发展成为圣裔社医院，院址设在浦石路（Rue Bourgeat，今长乐路）514号。施坦因曼医生（Dr. I. M. Steinman)担任院长。

二战爆发后，上海俄罗斯犹太人社区接管了医院。1942年，圣裔社医院得到犹太富商嘉道里家族的资助，迁到毕勋路（Route Pichon，今汾阳路），扩建为上海犹太医院（Shanghai Jewish Hospital）。

曾担任上海犹太医院院长的伊斯雷尔·基彭(Israel Kipen)在自传*A Life to Live*中透露，位于毕勋路的上海犹太医院大楼原属于天主教会。波兰外交使团一度占用过大楼，后来又因战争而撤离。后来，上海犹太社区租下大楼创办犹太医院，当时有60张床位、一个手术室和其他配套设施。

如今，医院保留着1931 年李维绘制的建筑图纸副本。同济大学郑时龄院士评价李维（一译列文·戈登士达，1878—？）是"在上海作品最多的一位俄国建筑师"。

"李维原名弗拉迪米尔·戈登士达，1915年改名'列文'，曾获中山陵名誉奖第五名。1878年出生于海参崴（今符拉迪沃斯托克），毕业于圣彼得堡建筑工程学院，曾设计海参崴的中央饭店（1907）。1922年以后移居上海，在上海工作了13年。1930年以前曾经在永安地产公司工作，他的代表作有克莱门公寓（Clements Apartments, 1929）、亚尔培公寓（King Albert Apartments, 1930，今陕南邨）、圣心教堂（1931）和阿斯屈来特公寓（Astrid Apartments, 1933，今南昌大楼）"。郑时龄院士在《上海近代建筑风格》（新版）中写道。

他提到，李维的大部分作品有着装饰艺术派建筑风格，局部以线条和图案作为装饰。

毕勋路的灰色大楼最初是为天主教三德堂（Missions Etrangeres de Paris）而建造

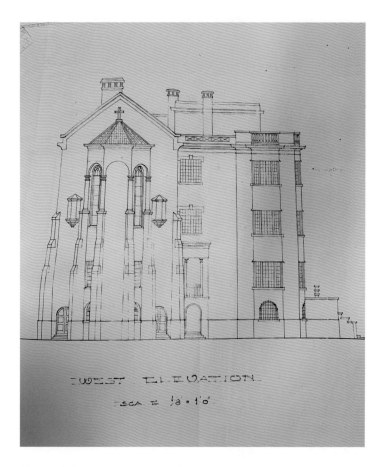

的。三德堂是 1659 年在巴黎成立的天主教会。作为最早在海外传教的天主教组织之一，在上海购置了多处房产。

灰色大楼是一幢功能完善的现代化建筑，共有三层。原始图纸显示，一楼设有接待室、办公室、台球室、客厅、餐厅和储藏室，二楼是图书馆、小教堂和卧室。男仆房、车库、厨房、储藏室、锅炉房、煤炭箱和仓库位于地下室。楼前有一个大花园，花园里有水塔。大楼改建为医院后，大花园也保留下来。

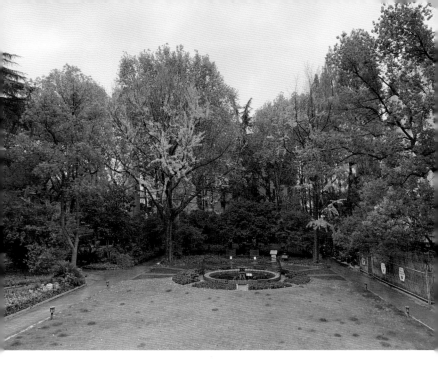

王健教授提到，犹太医院配备了X光机、电疗机和高压灭菌器等辅助设施。主楼四周环绕着美丽而开阔的花园，环境十分幽雅。上海犹太医院由名誉董事组成的董事会领导，董事长为来自里加的艾萨克·克利洛维奇·卡根（Isak Kirilovich Kagan），副董事长西蒙·利伯曼（Simion Liberman）原是专业会计师，祖籍波兰的俄罗斯犹太人斯坦曼博士（Dr. Steinman）担任院长。医护人员大多是俄罗斯犹太人和

德国犹太人。护士长维拉·亚历山大罗芙娜和会计师库巴·克罗宁伯格均是俄罗斯犹太人，外科医生马库斯、外科和妇产科医生布伦戴尔兄妹和住院医生克林格则来自德国。

1941 年，年轻的难民基彭从波兰来到上海，1942 年获任管理这家犹太医院。这份新工作提供给他一个自己的房间，还有膳食供应和一些现金报酬。当时，在医院工作并居住在医院宿舍的人可免受日军对犹太难民的

管束规定，留在自己的工作地。

"当大多数人搬进虹口狭窄而拥挤的环境时，我搬到了毕勋路的花园，在自己的房间安顿下来，满怀热情地投入到新的任务中。"基彭在自传中写到。

根据他的回忆，在犹太医院工作的医生群体堪称上海欧洲侨民的缩影。

"许多杰出的德国犹太外科医生在那里做手术。马库斯医生（Dr. Marcuse）的名字很容易浮现在脑海中。他是矮个子，总是很幽默，而且吹口哨都是经典音乐的曲调。他也是一位音乐家和交响乐队指挥，给人的印象是音乐才是他的最爱，而做手术只是谋生手段。另一位优秀的外科医生是希尔本（Dr. Heilborn）。他个子很高、沉默寡言、性格内向。他从来不大声说话，却能让手下不折不扣地执行他的每个指令。"他在自传中回忆。

"一方面，上海公济医院（Shanghai General Hospital，今上海市第一人民医院））远离犹太人居住的法租界。欧洲人和中国人生活水平的差异是另一个因素。此外，相当多的犹太家庭负担不起医疗或住院费用。因此，需要一家可以为贫困人口服务的医院。归根结底，也许是社区自助的概念推动了人们建立医院和其他服务机构。"他写道。

王健教授研究发现，除了经营这家犹太医院，上海犹太人还捐款在公济医院和宏恩医院（Shanghai Country Hospital，今华东医院)设置犹太病床，并建立了中山医院皮肤病防治所。犹太富商艾里·嘉道里（Elly Kardoorie，又名坎大利)资助颜福庆建立了上海第一家专门胸科医院——澄衷医院（今上海市肺科医院）。为纪念嘉道里的资助，颜福庆将医院内一幢红砖绿色琉璃瓦的大楼，取名为坎大利爵士茶厅（Sir Elly Kadoorie Tea Pavilion）。

"二战期间，上海犹太人还在虹口每个收容所设立了门诊间，建立了三家医院。其中一所难民医院和一所产科医院设在华德路（今长阳路）的第一难民营。隔离病院设在兆丰路收容

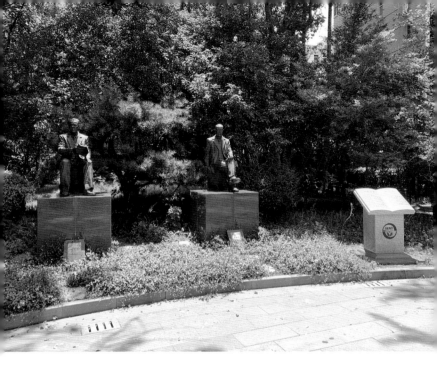

所。这些难民诊所和医院虽然设备简陋，但医生工作十分认真热情。在住房拥挤、人员混杂的难民收容所中几乎没有发生过传染病和流行病。"他补充道。

1952年，耳鼻喉科教授胡懋廉与眼科教授郭秉宽在上海犹太医院旧址创办上海医学院眼耳鼻喉科学院。这家医院如今是复旦大学附属眼耳鼻喉科医院，经过多年变迁与发展，已发展成为中国领先的集医疗、教学、科研为一体的专科医院，有汾阳、宝庆、浦江、浦东四个院区。医院有700多张床位，1400多名员工，其眼科和耳鼻喉科均为国家重点学科及临床重点专科。

如今，灰色大楼是10号楼，用于行政办公。大楼前是郁郁葱葱的花园，矗立着高大的水塔，还有两位创始人教授的雕像。

这座灰色大楼和外滩沙逊大厦、南京路哈同大楼、几座犹太教堂一样，成为上海犹太历史文化遗迹之一。

1994年4月23日《文汇报》

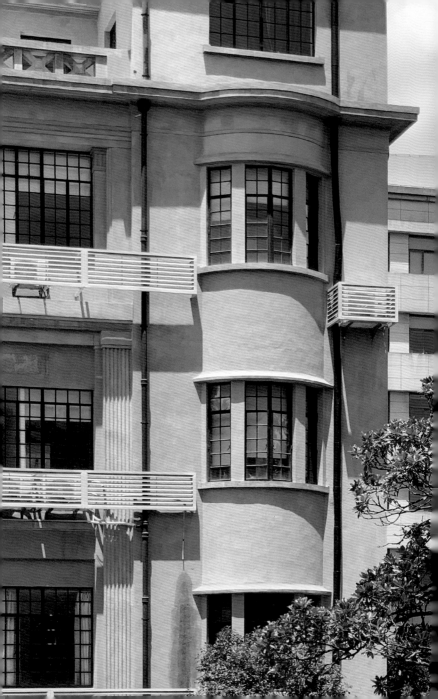

报道，第二次世界大战期间犹太难民在虹口区聚居，上海人民当时与犹太难民有着患难与共的经历。为重温历史、增进友谊，上海市邀请世界各地重要犹太人民间组织和知名人士来沪参加重聚活动。前来赴会的犹太友人们参观了原犹太商会、犹太教堂、犹太俱乐部，还有这座历史独特的犹太医院。

昨天： 上海犹太医院　**今天：** 复旦大学附属眼耳鼻喉科医院　**地址：** 汾阳路 83 号
建筑风格： 现代风格　**建筑师：** 李维（Livin Goldenstaedt）

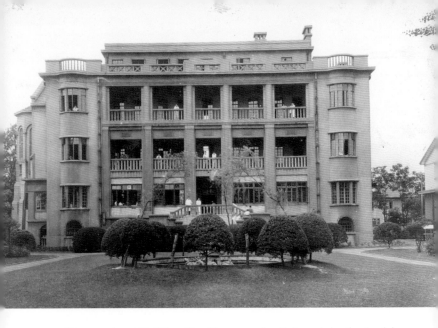

The gray-hued Building No. 10 of the Eye & ENT Hospital of Fudan University on Fenyang Road was the Shanghai Jewish hospital in the 1940s. It was a work of Livin Goldenstaedt, the most prolific Russian architect in old Shanghai.

"Jewish people paid great attention to public health. The hospital was moved from today's Changle Road to Fenyang Road in 1942," says Professor Wang Jian from Shanghai Academy of Social Sciences who authored the book *Shanghai Jewish Cultural Map.*

According to Shanghai local annals, in 1929, the city's Sephardie Jews founded the Shanghai lodge of B'nai B'rith, a religious organization to conduct charity and relief work in the Jewish community with D. E. J. Abraham as the leader. They opened the B'nai B'rith Polyclinic and Hospital on Rue Bourgeat (today's Changle Road) in February 1934 with funds donated by the prominent Jewish businessman Elly Kadoorie. Dr I. M. Steinman served as the director.

After the outbreak of World War II, the Russian Jewish community in the city took over the clinic in 1942, moved it to the current site on Route Pichon (now Fenyang Road) and expanded it to become the Shanghai Jewish Hospital.

According to Shanghai Jewish Hospital's former manager Israel Kipen's autobiography *A Life to Live*, the new hospital building on Route Pichon belonged to the Catholic Church and was occupied by the Polish diplomatic mission which vacated it as a result of the war. The Jewish community took out a lease and established a hospital with 60 beds, an operating theater and other support facilities.

Today, the hospital still preserves copies of original drawings of the gray building which was designed in 1931 by Goldenstaedt.

In the new edition of *The Evolution of Shanghai Architecture in Modern Times* published months ago, Tongji University professor Zheng Shiling praised Goldenstaedt as "the most prolific Russian architect in old Shanghai" who won an honorary prize of the design competition for Sun Yat-sen's Mausoleum in Nanjing in 1925.

"Born in 1878 in Vladivostok, the architect graduated from the Architectural Engineering Institute of St. Petersberg, designed the Central Hotel in Vladivostok and moved to Shanghai in 1922, where he worked for 13 years. His signature works include the Clements Apartments in 1929, the King Albert Apartments in 1930, the Sacred Heart Church in 1931 and Astrid Apartments in 1933.

Most of Livin's works were Art Deco "with lines and patterns in the part", Professor Zheng writes in the book.

The Sacred Heart Church was built for the Sacred Heart Hospital in Yangpu District which was featured in this column last November.

The gray building on Route Pichon was originally built for "Missions Etrangeres de Paris", a Catholic church founded in Paris in 1659.

As the earliest Catholic organization to conduct overseas missionary work, "Missions Etrangeres de Paris" acquired many properties in old Shanghai.

It was a modern, functional building of three major floors.

According to the original drawings for the Catholic church, the ground floor featured reception room, office, billiards room, parlor, dining room and pantry while the first floor housed a library, chapel and bedrooms. The boys' room, garage, kitchen, store room, boiler room, coal box and godown were in the basement. The building had an attic and a water tower in a large garden.

When the building was converted into the hospital, the large garden was retained. Professor Wang Jian says the Jewish hospital

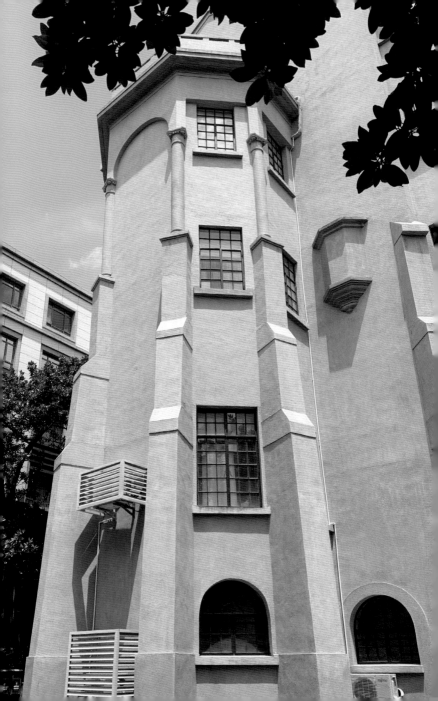

was well equipped with X-ray machines, electrotherapy machines and autoclaves. The main building was surrounded by beautiful gardens, and the environment was very elegant.

"The hospital is led by a board of directors composed of honorary directors. The chairman is Isak Kirilovich Kagan originally from Riga. Vice Chairman Simion Liberman was formerly a professional accountant. Dr. Steinman, a Russian Jew with Polish ancestry, served as the director. Most of the medical staff in the hospital were Russian or German Jews," Professor Wang says.

With this new job in 1942, Israel Kipen, a young refugee arriving in Shanghai in 1941 from Poland, was provided with a room, full board and some payment in cash. At that time, people working in hospitals with quarters on the premises were exempted from the general regulations for Jewish refugees by the Japanese and permitted to remain at their place of work.

"When most people moved into the restricted and overcrowded conditions of Hong-Kew (Hongkou), I moved to the gardens of Route Pichon, settled into my room and threw myself into the new task with enthusiasm," Kipen

writes in the autobiography.

According to his narration, the doctors who worked at the hospital represented a microcosm of European settlement in Shanghai.

"A number of outstanding German Jewish surgeons operated there. The name of Dr. Marcuse comes readily to mind. He was a short man, always in good humor and forever whistling a tune from the classics. Being a musician of note and an orchestral conductor, he gave the impression that music was his first love while surgery served as a means of making a living. Another excellent surgeon was Dr. Heilborn, tall, thin, taciturn and withdrawn. He never spoke above a whisper but he had the staff hanging on to his every word and responding to every twitch of a muscle," he recalls.

Kipen outlined the reasons for establishing a Jewish hospital.

"For one, the general Shanghai Hospital was far from the French Concession where the Jews lived. The difference in standards of living between Europeans and Chinese was another factor. In addition, a considerable number of Jewish families could not afford medical or hospital care; consequently, a hospital was needed which could waive feeds for the indigent. At bottom, perhaps, was

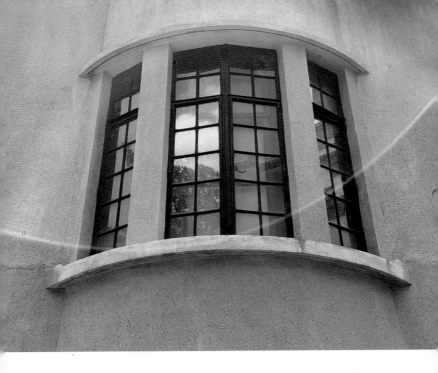

the whole concept of communal self-help that gave impetus to those who brought the hospital and other service institutions into being," he writes.

In addition to operating this hospital, Shanghai Jewish merchants also donated to install beds for Jewish patients in Shanghai General Hospital and Shanghai Country Hospital.

"The Jewish people in Shanghai also established a research institute to research on the prevention of skin disease for Zhongshan Hospital and sponsored medical educator Yan Fuqing to found Shanghai's first chest hospital — Ching Chong Hospital. During World War II, Jewish people in Shanghai set up clinics in every ghetto and opened three refugee hospitals. Though these clinics and hospitals for refugees were poorly equipped, the doctors worked enthusiastically. There were few pandemics in the crammed ghettos," Professor Wang adds.

In 1952, the hospital became the Shanghai Eye and ENT Hospital, Shanghai Medical College and today it's attached to the Fudan University. After changes over the years, it has developed to be one of China's leading hospitals that integrates medical care, education, and research, providing patient care for the health of eye, ear, nose, throat, head, and neck, with more than 1,400 employees. In addition to the Fenyang Road site, the hospital has two branches on Baoqing Road in Xuhui District and on Jiangyue Road in Minhang District.

The gray building is now used for administration. The building is still fronted with the spacious lush garden, graced by a tall, historic water tower and statues of Eye and ENT professors Hu Maolian and Guo Bingkuan, early founders of the hospital.

It's also one of the city's major Jewish sites along with Sassoon House on the Bund, the Hardoon Building on Nanjing Road and several surviving synagogues. According to a Wenhui Daily news report published on April 23, 1994, Shanghai invited former Jewish refugees to revisit the city. During the event, the Jewish people visited many synagogues, clubs, and chambers as well as the hospital.

Yesterday: Shanghai Jewish Hospital   **Today:** Eye & ENT Hospital of Fudan University
Address: 83 Fenyang Road   **Architectural style:** Modern style
Architect: Livin Goldenstaedt

一个帮助所有人的使命

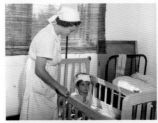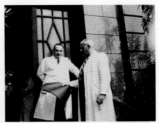
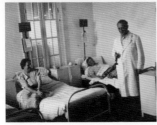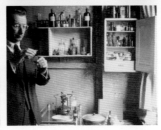

圣裔社医院由上海会堂（Shanghai Lodge）于 1933 年创立，八年来一直为上海穷人提供医疗援助，并在需要时给予有用的建议，没有任何歧视。医院的入口位于蒲石路，非常朴素，但院内的医疗活动既安静，又严肃紧张，医生和护士们努力为病人和体弱者减轻痛苦，恢复健康。医院的牙科室、做小手术的手术室、药剂科和电疗科等，虽然规模较小，但与任何一流医院的设施都是一样的。对于那些宗教不允许他们吃普通食物的人来说，医院的一种特色和福音是提供由犹太厨师制作的犹太饮食（Kosher diet）。

担任院长的斯坦曼医生（Dr. I.M. Steinman）在过去的七年中将自己的时间和学识投入到这家医院。他持续的热情与合作为医院的稳步发展和顺利运行做出了不少贡献。医院有一批称职的专家，包括负责五官科的科若斯医生（Dr. A. Korosi）、皮肤科医生佩沙霍夫（Dr. A. M. Peisahoff）、神经和精神科曼德尔医生（Dr. Mandel）、妇产科昆夫医生（Dr. T. Kunfi）、肺科卡佩尔医生（Dr. L. Karpel）和内科麦道斯基医生（Dr. M. Madorsky）。

1940 年，医院接待门诊病人 15635 人次，比上一年增加了 637 人次，其中 35% 是非犹太患者。牙科诊所的访问量比上一年增加了 140 人次，1940 年的总数为 3460 人次。住院人数也大幅增加，收治患者268人次，共计4778天，比上年增加767天。病床几乎从来没有空过。不仅在过去的一年里，而且在诊所开业以来的每一年，接受治疗的患者人数都有明显的增加。

布朗牧师（The Rev. M. Brown）对于他在创办维护这家机构中的贡献非常谦虚。他花费了无穷无尽的时间精力来募集捐款和捐赠，这是一项不太令人愉快的任务，因为每年都有更多的病人来要求免费治疗。如今，生活费用上涨，尤其是食品和药品费用，大大增加了每个月必须支付的账单。

"管理委员会的目的是鼓励开展增加床位的运动，这将减轻他们的巨大负担。"布朗牧师昨天对《北华捷报》记者说。"我们的一些患者支付了他们负担得起的费用，但超过 60% 的患者得到了免费治疗。"这家机构不会拒绝任何需要医疗服务的男人、女人或儿童，无论是欧洲人还是亚洲人。它值得大家好好支持。任何捐赠，无论多么小，都将被充满感激地接受。委员会希望一旦得到足够的资金就能搬入更大的场地，以便他们扩大已经在做的这些好工作。

摘自 1941 年 5 月 28 日《北华捷报》

A mission to help all, no matter who

The B'nai B'rith Polyclinic and Hospital, founded by the Shanghai Lodge in 1933, has been rendering medical assistance and, where needed helpful advice, to Shanghai's local poor without any discrimination whatsover, for eight years. The hospital itself possesses a very unostentatious entrance on Rue Bourgeat but inside there is silent, intense activity as doctors and nurses seek to alleviate pain and restore good health to the sick and the weak. The dental room, the surgical room where minor operations are performed, and the pharmaceutical and electro-therapy departments are equal to those of any first-class hospital, although on a smaller scale. One specialty and a boon to those, whose religion will not permit them to partake of any ordinary food, is the Kosher diet which is prepared by a Jewish cook.

Dr. I. M. Steinman, who is the medical superintendent, has devoted his time and knowledge to the hospital for the last seven years and has continued enthusiasm and cooperation has contributed in no small way, to the steady progress and smooth running of this institution. There is a staff of qualified specialists including Dr. A. Korosi, eye, nose and throat; Dr. A. M. Peisahoff, skin; Dr. A, Mandel, nervous and mental; Dr. T. Kunfi, midwifery and gynecology; Dr. L. Karpel, lung diseases; and Dr. M. Madorsky, internal diseases.

During the year 1940, 15,635 visits were made by out-patients to the Polyclinic, an increase of 637 visits over the previous year, 35 per cent of these visits were by non-Jewish patients. Visits to the dental clinic showed an increase over the previous year of 140, the total for 1940 being 3,460. In the hospital there was also a substantial increase, 268 patients were taken care of, making a total of 4,778 days, which is 767 days more than the year before. The hospital beds were practically never empty. Not only in the past year, but in each year since the polyclinic has been opened, there has been decided increase in the number of patients treated.

Excerpt from *the North–China Herald* on May 28, 1941

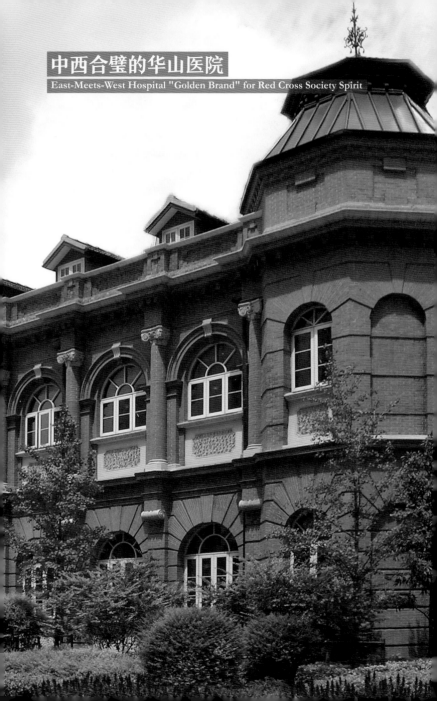

中西合璧的华山医院

East-Meets-West Hospital "Golden Brand" for Red Cross Society Spirit

上海华山医院的建筑风貌很独特，中西合璧。医院的标志建筑——西式"红会老楼"坐落于中式园林"周家花园"旁，红砖券窗与红木凉亭相映成趣。

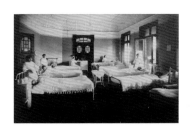

中西合璧的建筑风貌映射了百年医院独特的历史。华山医院前身——中国红十字会总医院是上海第一家中国人创办的西医院，由沈敦和先生创办于1907年，曾与美国哈佛大学医学院合作办学。

"沈敦和先生早年留学剑桥，专攻法政，回国后历任要职。1904年，日俄战争爆发，为救援东北战地难民，以他为首的上海慈善家，筹集钱款，发起成立了上海万国红十字会，这也是中国红十字会的前身。1907年在上海，沈敦和呈给京城的奏折在沉寂三年后批了下来，'中国红十字会总医院暨医学堂'成立，这成为华山医院历史的开始。"华山医院原院长徐建光在《沈敦和与华山医院的100年》一文中写道。

沈敦和（1866—1920）是晚清著名的社会活动家、慈善家。他从英国留学回国后受到刘坤一、李鸿章、曾国荃、左宗棠、张之洞等清朝大员器重，历任张家口和山西省洋务局督办、山西大学堂督办、金陵同文馆教习、江南水师学堂提调、吴淞自强军营机处总办、上海记名海关道、四明公所董事、上海总商会董事等职，履历丰富。沈敦和虽然官阶不高，但在上海是一位很有社会影响力的人。1904年，他发起成立中、英、美、德、法五国合办的上海万国红十字会，被推举为中方办事总董，成为中国红十字会的缔造者。

华山医院院史档案显示，1909年沈敦和等人购置徐家汇路7号土地14亩作为院址，动工建造医院和医学堂，翌年竣工落成。1911年10月14日，"中国红十字会总医院暨医学堂"正式开业。1913年，医院

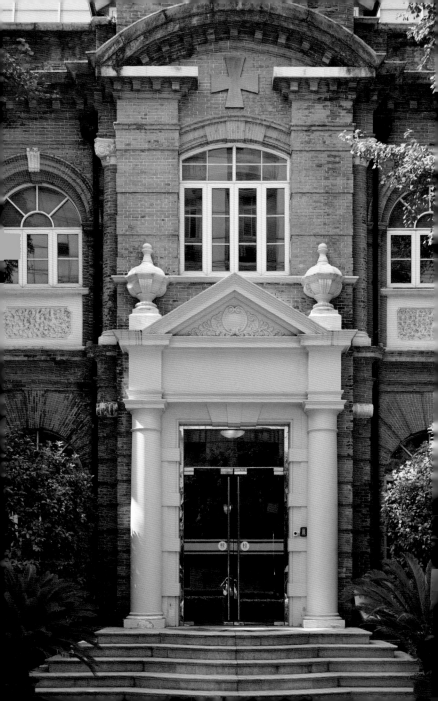

与中国哈佛医学院（Harvard Medical School of China）合作办学，签约五年，由美国人胡恒德（Henry Houghton）担任院长。1921年，红会总院与美方合约期满后，收归国人自办，由名医牛惠霖担任院长。1928年，医院成为国立中央大学医学院（上海医学院前身）实习医院，由医学院院长颜福庆兼任院长。

"医院建院时，规模小、设备差，但在旧上海，当时多数医院由教会所办，这样一所由国人筹款自办的医院，确实具有一定时代意义。"上海医学史专家、上海第四人民医院原图书馆长陆明评价。

红会老楼

如今，华山医院的标志性建筑就是百年前中国哈佛医学院的校舍，被称为"红会老楼"或"哈佛楼"。这座建筑今日犹存，楼前的铭牌写着红十字会精神："人道、博爱、奉献精神。"

"红会老楼"是一座二层高的外廊式砖木结构建筑。红砖铺设的外立面生动地装饰了古典建筑元素：带拱心石的白色券窗、爱奥尼克窗间柱和屋顶小巧的老虎窗。

这座楼缘起于哈佛大学医学院的上海项目（the Harvard Medical School at Shanghai）。根据1915年11月1日美国教会在华出版的英文杂志《教务杂志》（The Chinese Recorder）报道，该项目当年共有5个班级的13名教师，约25名学生。该机构"向东方的年轻人提供医学和外科方面的指导，为希望成为公共卫生官员的医学毕业生提供预防医学和公共卫生方面的培训，并发展研究部门，在那里可以研究中国和东方的疾病"。

文章提到，上海被选中出于多种原因：上海这座城市对于医疗工作的兴趣；以上海为中心的能讲英语的学生人数众多；上海与其他东方港口的紧密联系；以及上海高效的公共卫生部门。

"根据与中国红十字会的协议条款，学校使用位于徐家汇7号设备优良的大型校舍、医院和宿舍。主楼内有设施齐全的用于

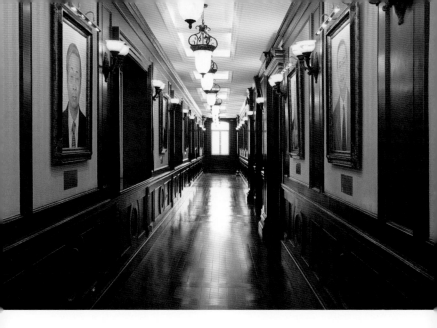

物理、化学、生理、生物化学和细菌学等学科的实验室、一个大型研究实验室和一个设备很好的X光室。教室、阅览室和图书馆在同一栋楼里。主楼的二楼由私人病房组成，还有一个很好的手术室，那里是外科诊所。"1915年的报道透露。

百年老楼历经修缮后加建了一层，室内现在仍为西方古典风格装饰，一楼的墙上挂着历任院长和终身教授的画像。一楼和二楼现在用于华山医院院史陈列室和会议室，顶楼是终身教授的办公室。

"我们大概计算过，华山医院100年间救治过近4000万病人，这个惊人的数字正是用100年的'人道'写成的。如果从技术角度，华山医院已经是一家值得许多人自豪的医院，但这并不影响我们继续追究一下这家医院的'人文内核'。仅从占地面积来看，现在的华山医院肯定不能算大医院，甚至我们一直与100年前的原址同一圆心，固守着那栋'红会老楼'的精神。"徐建光院长写道。

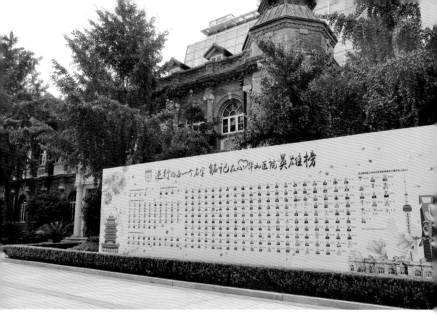

周家花园

华山医院位于上海的黄金地段——华山路与乌鲁木齐路之间。在这寸土寸金的地段，医院虽然不算大，但却有一座占地面积达26680平方米的中式花园。这里曾是上海著名的私家花园，园内亭台楼阁、小桥流水，是闹市里的一方净土，对医院的病人开放。

"华山医院西边的花园至今人们仍习惯称之为周家花园，因为在1945年以前是周纯卿的，叫'莼庐'，占地40亩，园中花木四时缤纷，有小桥流水和亭台楼榭之胜，荷花池中种着菱藕，当年纯卿一家每年夏天来此避暑。"研究老上海家族史的作家宋路霞在《上海望族》中写到这个花园。

周家花园后来卖给另一位上海商人虞洽卿。经颜福庆多方奔走，周家花园后来由华山医院使用。

复旦大学历史系高晞教授在原复旦大学医学院的校史陈列馆中，发现一张20世纪50年代上医老教授们在华山医院周家花园聚会的合影照片。她提到，照片上荟集了当时中国医学界的各界

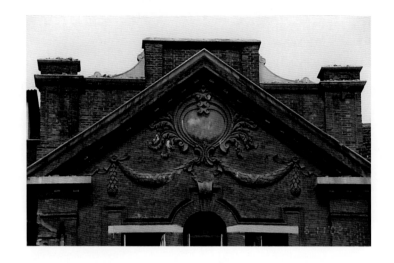

精英：上海医学院的创始人颜福庆、儿科专家陈翠贞、眼科专家郭秉宽、耳鼻喉科专家胡懋廉、病理学家谷镜汧，以及上海第一医学院院长兼党委书记陈同生等。

"20世纪50年代初期，许多从旧时代过来的老教授对党的知识分子政策并不了解，甚至产生误解，往往以消极情绪对待学校的工作，有些有困难的老教授与党的领导干部有隔膜。于是，陈同生院长委托颜福庆副院长，通过举办各类学术活动和聚餐活动，将老教授们集聚在一起，在轻松愉快的学术派对中，让教授们了解党的知识分子政策，拉近学校领导干部与知识分子之间的联系。50年代初期的许多个周末，这类聚餐派对常在华山医院的周家花园和颜福庆在肇嘉浜路的私家花园内举行。"高晞教授在题为《颜福庆与中国现代医学》一文中写道。

研究中国近代医学史的上海中山医院杨震教授认为，华山医院是中国红十字的一块"金字招牌"。

"1923年，日本关东大地震，时任院长牛惠霖就带领中国红十字救护队前往日本救援，这是中国第一次海外救援。华山医院有非常漂亮的哈佛楼老洋房，还有历史悠久的虞家花园。他们家的特色就是：'头大皮厚手长'（神经科、皮肤科、手外科）。"他说。

如今，华山医院已经发展为一家大型综合医院，现有浦东、虹桥等多个院区，床位从初建时的50个增加到2000多，是国内最著名、最具国际化特色的医教研中心之一。

2020年疫情期间，华山医院将院里273位参加抗疫的医护人员姓名列在一个巨大的光荣榜上，就展示在红会老楼百年沧桑的砖墙前。

昨天：中国红十字会总院老楼　**今天：**复旦大学附属华山医院红会老楼

地址：乌鲁木齐中路 12 号　**建造年代：**1910 年　**建筑风格：**古典风格

参观指南：红会老楼不对外开放，可以欣赏红砖立面。周家花园对医院病人开放，适宜漫步。

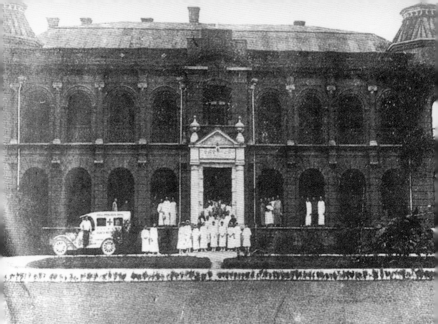

Huashan Hospital boasts a unique East-meets-West architectural scene. Its signature "Harvard Building", a red-brick Western-style structure, perches next to the "Zhou Family Garden" of Chinese pavilions and white lotus.

The architectural scene mirrors the history of the century-old hospital. The predecessor of Huashan Hospital was the Chinese Red Cross General Hospital, the first Chinese-run Western hospital in Shanghai.

"It was Shen Dunhe who among others founded Shanghai International Red Cross Society in 1904 and his application for founding a red cross hospital was granted by the Qing government in 1907. That kicked off the history of Huashan Hospital," former Huashan Hospital president Xu Jianguang wrote in an article in the now-defunct Oriental Morning Post on December 21, 2006.

An influential official and successful merchant of the late Qing (1644—1911) Dynasty, Shen had studied law and politics at Cambridge University in the United Kingdom and took many important prominent positions after returning to China.

According to Huashan Hospital archives, Shen purchased a

9,338-square-meter plot of land at No. 7 Siccawei Road (now Huashan Road) for building the hospital in 1909. The construction was completed in 1910.

In 1913, the hospital signed a five-year contract with Harvard University for founding the Harvard Medical School at Shanghai. In 1921, the hospital was fully operated by Chinese nationals with Dr. Niu Huilin (Way-ling New) as its president.

In 1928, the hospital became a teaching hospital affiliated to the College of Medicine of the National Central University, which later became Shanghai Medical College. It was under the charge of Dr. Yan Fuqing (F. C. Yen).

At the beginning, the hospital merely had 50 beds. As a Red Cross hospital, it charged only a clinic fee and poor patients were treated free of charge.

"To begin with, the hospital was small in size and lacking medical equipment. But as most Western hospitals in old Shanghai were founded by churches, such a hospital built with Chinese funds was significant," said Lu Ming, a medical historian from Shanghai No. 4 People's Hospital.

The Red Cross Old Building

"The Red Cross Old Building"

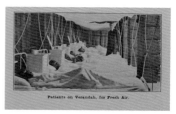

Patients on Verandah, for Fresh Air.

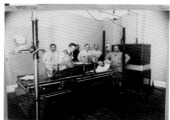

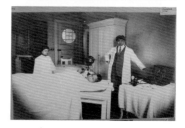

is featured on the hospital logo today and regarded as a symbol of the famous medical institution. A nameplate in front of the building is engraved with the spirit of the Red Cross Society — "humanity, fraternity and dedication".

The building, a brick-and-wood structure, which has been used as a medical ward, was constructed upon the founding of the hospital. The red-brick facade is vividly graced by classic architectural details, from white-framed arched windows with key stones, Ionic columns between windows and small dormer windows over the top. The entrance is flanked with two Doric columns and topped by a grand gable. The facade is half shaded by green trees.

The structure is also related to the "Harvard Medical School at Shanghai" project.

According to an article, named "Medical Education in Shanghai" in the Chinese Recorder on November 1, 1915, there were 13 instructors with five classes and about 25 students for this project in the academic year.

The purposes of this institution was "to give instruction in medicine and surgery to young men of the Orient, to give training in preventive medicine and public health to graduates of medicine desiring to become public health officers and to develop departments of research, where the disease of China and the Orient may be studied". And Shanghai was recommended as a location for the institution for the interest in medical work in the city, the number of English-speaking students about Shanghai as a center, the ready touch of the city with other Oriental ports and the efficient organization of the Shanghai Department of Public Health.

"Under the terms of an agreement with the Red Cross Society of China, the school occupies the large and well-equipped school buildings, hospital and dormitories of the society situated at No. 7 Siccawei Road. In the main building there are fully equipped laboratories for class work in physics, chemistry, physiology, bio-chemistry and bacteriology, etc., a large research laboratory and a well-equipped X-ray room. Classrooms, a reading room and a library were in the same building. The second floor of the main building is made up of private wards and contains an excellent operating suite, where surgical clinics are held," the 1915 report revealed.

During a renovation years ago, the two-story building added another floor. The interior is now decorated in a classic Western style. The walls of the ground floor are graced by portraits of the hospital's presidents and lifetime tenured professors.

The two ground floors are used as a hospital history museum and conference rooms. The top floor serves as offices for lifetime professors.

"We estimated that Huashan Hospital has treated 40 million patients within a century. This amazing figure is written with 'humanity' for 100 years. Today it is not a large hospital in terms of the size, but it's been a hospital with pride in terms of medical skills. We have maintained the same 'circle center' 100 years ago, to adhere to the spirit of the 'Red Cross old building'," former president Xu said.

The Zhou Family Garden

Huashan Hospital sits on a prominent location between Huashan Road and Wulumuqi Road. The not-so-big hospital compound has a 26,680-square-meter Chinese garden, which is elegantly designed and open to patients.

"The garden in the west of Huashan Hospital is widely called Zhou Family Garden because it belonged to Chinese merchant Zhou Chunqin before 1945. The garden named 'Chun Lu' features flowers and wood of the four seasons, a small bridge, flowing water and pavilions. The lotus pond was planted with water chestnuts and lotus roots. The Zhou family spent summer days here," Song Luxia, a historian/writer, writes in her book *The Prominent Shanghai Families.*

The garden was later sold to the family of another Shanghai tycoon Yu Yaqing. It was Dr. Yan Fuqing who tried to get this garden for the hospital to use.

Fudan University professor Gao Xi discovered a group photo of Shanghai Medical College professors gathering in the Zhou Family Garden. The party was joined by a galaxy of Chinese medical elites, including Yan Fuqing, founder of Shanghai Medical College, pediatrician Chen Cuizhen, ophthalmologist Guo Bingkuan, otolaryngologist Hu Maolian, pathologist Gu Jingli and Chen Tongsheng, dean of Shanghai First Medical College.

"In the early 1950s, many professors from old Shanghai did not understand the new government's policies for intellectuals. Therefore, Chen Tongsheng entrusted Yan Fuqing, who was deputy dean of Shanghai First Medical College, to host gatherings for better communications. Through academic activities and dinners, Yan tried to make them understand the policies in a more relaxing atmosphere. On many weekends in the early 1950s, such dinner parties were often held in the Zhou Family Garden of Huashan Hospital or in Yan's private garden on Zhaojiabang Road," professor Gao wrote in an article titled "Yan Fuqing and Chinese modern medicine".

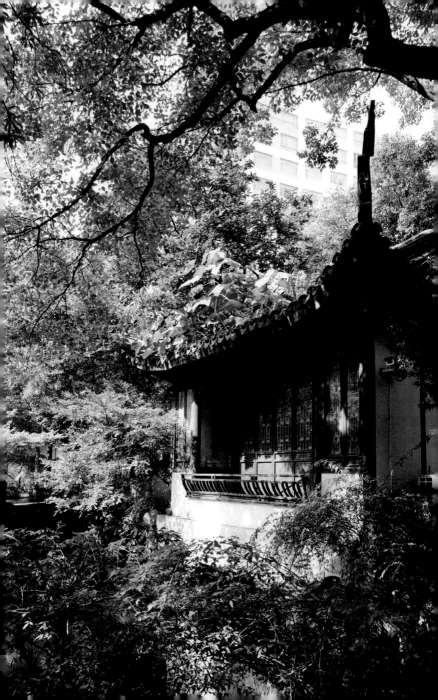

"Huashan Hospital has been a golden brand for the China Red Cross Society. The special skills of the hospital can be described as 'big head, thick skin and long hand', which means they have a superb nerve unit, dermatology unit and unit of hand surgery," said Yang Zheng, a medical historian from Shanghai Zhongshan Hospital.

Today Huashan Hospital has developed into a large comprehensive hospital with 2,092 beds. As a designated medical institution of 10 foreign consulates in Shanghai, it has received more than 600,000 foreign patients from more than 100 countries.

"During the Japan earthquake in 1923, the then president Dr. New led a China Red Cross medical team to aid Japan. It was China's first overseas medical aid," he added.

During the past century, the hospital has also sent many medical teams to assist where disaster has struck, including the Tangshan earthquake in Hebei Province in 1976 and Wenchuan earthquake in Sichuan Province in 2008.

Huashan Hospital's most recent mission was to treat COVIC-19 patients. On January 24, 2020, the red-brick building witnessed the departure of the hospital's first medical team to Wuhan.

Yesterday: Chinese Red Cross General Hospital
Today: Huashan Hospital, Fudan University   **Address:** 12 Wulumuqi Road M.
Built in: 1910   **Architectural style:** classic style
Tips: The "Red Cross Old Building" is not open to the public but the facade can be admired. The garden is open and it's really nice for a walk.

沈敦和去世：一位战士、政治家、改革家

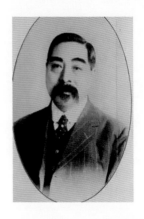

"我们很遗憾地宣布，上海最重要的中国商人、慈善家和人道主义工作者之———沈敦和先生去世。不幸发生在周一下午5点，他在白克路（Burkill Road, 今凤阳路）34号的家中去世。更令人痛苦的是，沈先生在心愿即将实现——中国传染病医院开业之际离开人世。

沈先生今年64岁，是宁波人。他已经患病多年，但到近三周才病情严重。

他在红十字会的光辉事业掩盖了他所有其他的成就，以至于今天很难对他的人生有合适的描述。他曾在剑桥大学学习，在清政府担任官职，在泰安府任职相当长的时间。他还与军队保持联系，晋升为少将军衔。他想法开明，走在时代的前沿。如果没有弄错，他成功地为吴淞军营获得重型枪械。

1911年发生革命那年，他在红十字会的工作与成功赢得了来自华人和外国侨民的钦佩之情。当时的中国军队，无论是保皇派还是革命派，医务人员和医药用品的配备都很少。但沈先生带来的红十字会的善举极大地弥补了缺医少药的状况。在不断壮大的中外医护队伍的帮助下，他在减轻战争带来的痛苦方面取得了很大成就。

沈先生也积极参与商业活动。他曾经与轮船招商局有联系，是华安联合保险公司的创始人，并且在过去的15年间担任中国总商会会员。此外，他还担任过许多其他组织或慈善机构的负责人。唯有能够帮助开展一些慈善工作，他才感到满足。

柯师太福医生（Dr. Stanford Cox）在日内瓦作为中国红十字会顾问代表参加红十字大会。他与沈先生有多年深厚交情，曾见证新的红十字会成立，并了解到红十字会未来工作的计划，其中包括和平、疫情、洪水、饥荒、地震等方面未来的救济工作，其中大多数代表们

印象中从未尝试过。当柯师太福医生站起来告诉他们沈先生多年来在这些方面所做的杰出工作时，与会代表们都感到震惊。

摘自 1920 年 7 月 10 日《北华捷报》

Death of Mr. Shen Tun-ho, Soldier, Statesman and Reformer

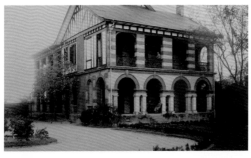

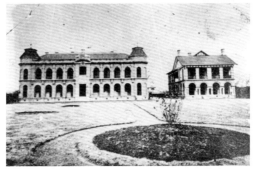

We regret to announce the death of one of Shanghai's foremost Chinese merchants, philanthropists, and humanitarian workers, Mr. Shen Tun-ho.

The sad event occurred at his home, No. 34 Burkill Road, at 5 o'clock on Monday afternoon. What makes it the more painful is the fact that just as Mr. Shen was about to see a great desire of his life accomplished-the opening of the Chinese Infectious Diseases Hospital-he passed away.

Mr. Shen, who was 64 years of age, was a native of Ningpo. He had been ailing for several years past, but it was not until the past three weeks that he had been seriously ill.

His career as an officer of the Red Cross has so over-shadowed all his other achievements that it is difficult today to obtain an adequate account of his life. He was educated at Cambridge and under the Manchu regime held official rank, being stationed at Taianfu for some considerable time. He was also connected with the army, rising to the rank of General, and was surely in the forefront of enlightened opinion in his day, for if we are not mistaken it was he who demanded and succeeded in obtaining the heavy guns for Woosung Forts.

In the year 1911, when the revolution took place, he aroused the admiration not only of his fellow countrymen but of foreign residents by his activity and success in Red Cross work. The Chinese army-whether royalist or revolutionary was ill-equipped with medical staff or stores, but Mr. Shen brought as a great substitute the benevolence of the Red Cross. Aided by an ever-growing band of foreign and Chinese workers, he accomplished great deeds in the relief of suffering. To him, China owns a very great debt. Again in 1913 when rebellion was afoot was he to the fore and once more his ministrations brought comfort to the wounded who otherwise were too likely to be left untended. His was an example which we trust will have many followers, and in course of time stand as an example to his nation.

He also carried the spirit of the Red Cross into peace, and there was his work on behalf of famine relief during the Chihli floods at Hupeh and countless other places to be borne in mind.

Mr. Shen also took an active part in business. At one time, he was connected with the China Merchants Steam Navigation Co. While he was the founder of the China United Assurance Company and was for the past 15 years member of the Chines General Chamber of Commerce. Besides this he was director of numerous other organizations or philanthropic institutions. He was never satisfied until he was able to help in some charitable work.

When in Geneva attending the Red Cross Convention as advisory delegate for the Red Cross of China, Dr. Stafford M. Cox, who has for many years past been closely associated with Mr. Shen, saw the formation of the new League of Red Cross Societies and heard their plans for future work. These included plans for work in peace, pandemic diseases, floods, famines, earthquakes, etc. Which work most of the delegates were under the impression had never been tried before. They were astounded, however, when Dr. Cox stood up and told them of the great work that MR. Shen had been carrying on for many years in these very lines.

Excerpt from *the North—China Herald* on July 10, 1920

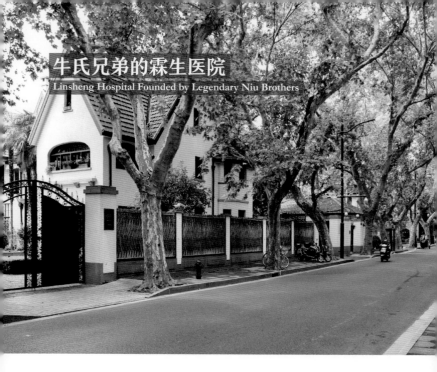

牛氏兄弟的霖生医院

Linsheng Hospital Founded by Legendary Niu Brothers

　　上海的岳阳路美丽幽静，梧桐树后掩映着一座座花园别墅，位于190号的米白色别墅曾是著名的"牛氏兄弟"创办的霖生医院。

　　牛惠霖（1889—1937）、牛惠生（1892—1937）兄弟是近代中国医界一对闪耀的双子星座。1920年，他们在祈齐路（Route Ghisi，今岳阳路）开办私营诊所，从各自的名字取最后一字为诊所命名"霖生医院"。

　　医院的旧址是一座三层高的英式风格花园住宅，斜屋顶覆盖着红瓦，与米白色墙面形成对比。建筑的外立面点缀着券窗、露台和阳台，弧形门厅装饰有多立克柱式和宝瓶型栏杆。别墅面向一个安静的花园，有喷泉和棕榈。

　　1937年11月20日，牛惠霖在这座小楼里去世，年仅48岁。6个月前，他45岁的弟弟牛惠生也因病早逝。

　　在上海近代医学史中，牛氏兄弟的名字频频出现。他们创办

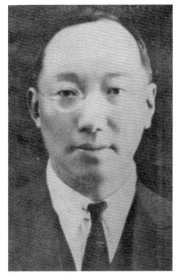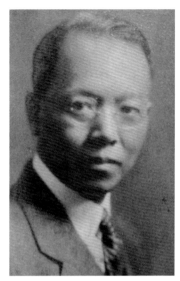

或参与管理多家医疗机构，用精湛医术拯救了无数生命。在短短四十多载的人生中，牛氏兄弟完成了这么多工作，取得了不起的成就，令人惊叹。

牛氏兄弟的优秀源自他们的父亲牛尚周。1872年，中国近代著名教育家、外交家容闳（Yung Wing，1828—1912）招考的第一批30个官费留美幼童从上海乘船出发赴美留学，来自嘉定的牛尚周（1862—1917）是其中之一。牛尚周美国学成回到上海后，成为中国电报业的拓荒者之一，后来到江南制造总局担任帮办。

在美国留学期间，牛尚周与波士顿一家丝茶店老板的养子宋耀如（Charlie Soong）结为好友。他们回国后分别娶了徐光启后裔、中国牧师倪韫山的长女倪桂清和小女儿倪桂珍。宋耀如和倪桂珍是"宋氏三姐妹"的父母。

根据中华医学会原办公室主任张圣芬的研究，牛氏兄弟的求学经历极其相似。

"两人都是在18岁以优异

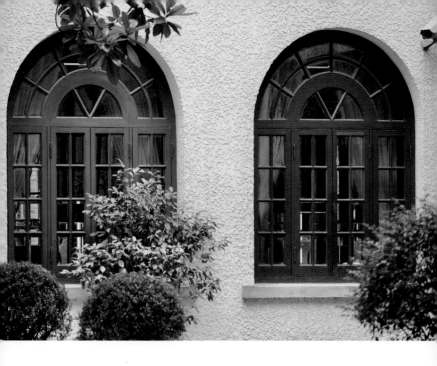

的成绩从上海圣约翰大学毕业。哥哥毕业后远赴英国剑桥大学医学院深造，弟弟则选择了美国的哈佛大学医学院。国度不同，学费同样昂贵。两人又先后走上勤工俭学之路。哥哥到银行充当职员，弟弟烧锅炉、扫楼道、摆餐具、刷试管，用辛勤的劳动换得的报酬支撑各自学业的完成。"张圣芬在《民国医界翘楚牛氏兄弟》一文中写道。

　　1914年，牛惠霖获剑桥大学医学博士学位，在伦敦执医。

一战爆发后，他担任伦敦叶普斯惠区医院（Ipswich Military Hospital）重伤病主任医师，1916年到1918年转任伦敦密它瑟斯重伤兵医院（Middlesex Hospital），协助著名苏顿医生（Sir John Bland Sutton）担任外科医生。

　　1914年这一年，牛惠霖的弟弟牛惠生也从哈佛大学医学院博士毕业了。他在大学期间就有医疗实践经历，毕业后担任美国马萨诸塞州新贝福德市（New

Bedford）圣卢克医院（St. Luke's Hospital）的住院医师。

牛氏兄弟学成后都回到祖国工作。1915年，弟弟牛惠生先回国在上海哈佛医学院（Harvard Medical School of China in Shanghai）任教，负责病理科。上海哈佛医学院是哈佛大学和中国红十字会总院（华山医院前身）合作的项目。

回国任教后，牛惠生发现当时中国还没有西医骨科专家和骨科专科。为了挽救更多的骨疾病患，他于1916年再次赴美学习，1918年回国后成为北京协和医院首位骨科医生。

1918年，哥哥牛惠霖回国后担任雷士德华人医院（the Lester Chinese Hospital，仁济医院前身）副院长兼外科主任，1920与弟弟联合创办了霖生医院。

研究上海家族史的作家宋路霞提到，霖生医院是中国早期的西医医院之一，抗战前名气很大。

"他们的医院开张不久，适逢英国驻香港的总督病重垂危，电请英国政府派良医前去救治。英国政府的卫生部回电说，用不着从伦敦派医生，请上海霖生医院的牛惠霖医生去就行了，牛惠霖是英国剑桥大学的医学博士，刚回上海不久。他在伦敦期间，经历了第一次世界大战的全过程，在大战中担任了重伤外科手术主任医师，英国医学界了解他的实力……牛惠霖医生远赴香港出诊，为港督治病，果然手到病除，香港、上海为之轰动。消息传出，这也在客观上为霖生医院做了个大广告。"宋路霞在《从霖生医院到上海医院的故事》中一文中写道。

此后，慕名而来的病人越来越多。牛惠霖为方便病患就医，除了祈齐路的霖生医院本部，又在南京路和成都路都设立了诊所。

1927年，霖生医院的成都路诊所就来了一位腿伤病人——不幸负伤的陈赓大将。他的左腿连中三弹，胫骨、腓骨都被打断，行军途中未得到妥善治疗，辗转来到上海就医时伤势恶化，腿部严重肿胀。牛惠霖医生看到是枪伤以为病人是强盗，陈赓遂表明身份，说明了自己的负伤过程，希望不要截肢。牛氏兄弟安排陈赓将军在霖生医院住了下来，经过悉心治疗，为他保住了这条腿。

牛惠霖还曾担任中国红十字会总院院长兼红十字会时疫医院、西藏路时疫医院院长。1937年11月21日英文《大陆报》（*The China Press*）为他刊登的讣告透露，牛惠霖经常参与志愿急救任务。

"1923年日本大地震期间，他出于同情带领一支中国医护人员组成的医疗队前往日本救助。1926年江浙战争时，他又领导了红十字工作。由于与著名的宋氏家族的关系，牛氏兄弟在西安事变后接待了蒋介石与宋美龄。"《大陆报》报道写道。

牛惠霖的职业生涯蒸蒸日上之时，牛惠生也在医学界扮演着举足轻重的角色。

1923年，美商《密勒氏评论报》（*The China Weekly Review*）在其名人栏目"Who's Who in China"就报道过牛惠生。1928年，牛惠生在海格路（今华山路）创办了中国第一家西医骨科专科医院。后来，他还为骨结核病患儿在上海创办了儿童骨科医院，让许多伤残儿童通过整形矫治重获健康。此外，他还在多家重要医疗卫生机构担任要职及医事顾问，如中华医学会会长（the Chinese Medical Association）。

1937年牛惠生去世时，英文《北华捷报》（*the North-China Herald*）评价"中国失去了一位伟人"。

"年仅46岁的牛惠生医生于凌晨在他位于徐家汇路852号的家中去世。中国不仅失去了一位医学界有影响力的人物，而且失去了一位富有远见卓识和勇气的人。他全力以赴地推动着这个国家医疗机构的工作，白天想着它，晚上想着它。

即使在他生命中的最后一周，他虽然病重，但醒来时仍然不断提到该协会(注：指中华医学会)的工作。牛医生是杰出的组织者和协调者，他是一个勇于进取、勇于面对困难的人，但在

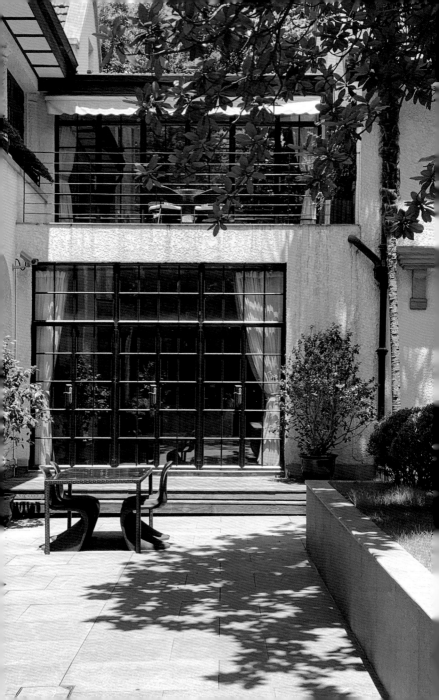

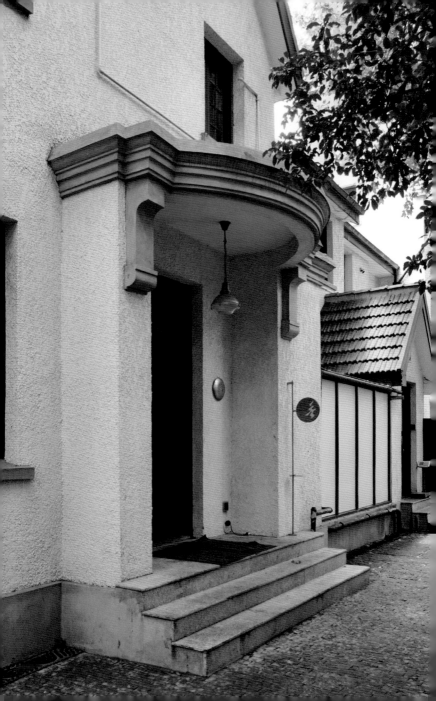

对待难相处的人与困难处境时总是很有风度。" 1937年5月12日《北华捷报》报道。

1937年4月，中华医学会第十二次大会召开，上海医事中心落成典礼和中山医院开幕典礼也同时举行，身染重病的牛惠生坚持亲临盛会。大会闭幕三周后，他于5月4日离开人世。牛惠生在去世前留下遗嘱："所用棺木绝不可逾四百元。余生平用血汗所换得之金钱应用于有益社会人群之事业，不当抛掷于无用之地。"

2015年10月26日，上海仁济医院的袁蕙芸主任接待了牛恩美女士，她是牛惠霖的女儿，归国整理父亲和亲属的遗物。

"八十多岁的她精神矍铄，在专人陪同下兴致勃勃参观了仁济东、西两院院区，尤其是看到那栋建于1932年的仁济西院的独特病房建筑时，她激动不已。她在父亲牛惠霖曾经工作过的仁济西院病区看了又看，摸了又摸，与在场医护人员和病人们亲切交流，亲身感受百年仁济的深厚历史底蕴和新装修病区的现代化功能，感受着古老与经典在这家百年老院的融合。"袁蕙芸回忆道。

在参观过程中，牛恩美决定将父亲牛惠霖的一些珍贵文物捐赠给仁济医院，包括生前使用过的金丝边眼镜、烟灰缸和茶杯，还有患者赠送的"今世华佗"刺绣牌匾。她透露，牛家后人受父辈善举的影响，也大都走上从医道路，为中国医疗卫生事业的发展和人民的健康做出了贡献。

米白色的霖生医院规模不大，但创办它的牛氏兄弟曾经为中山医院、华山医院和仁济医院等上海大医院的发展奉献专业心力，打下坚实基础。他们的生命虽然短暂，但是成就的事业和留下的精神却很长久。

昨天：霖生医院 **今天：**餐厅 **地址：**岳阳路 190 号 **建造年代：**1920 年
参观指南：岳阳路可以欣赏建筑外立面，隔壁画廊的二楼可以眺望花园。

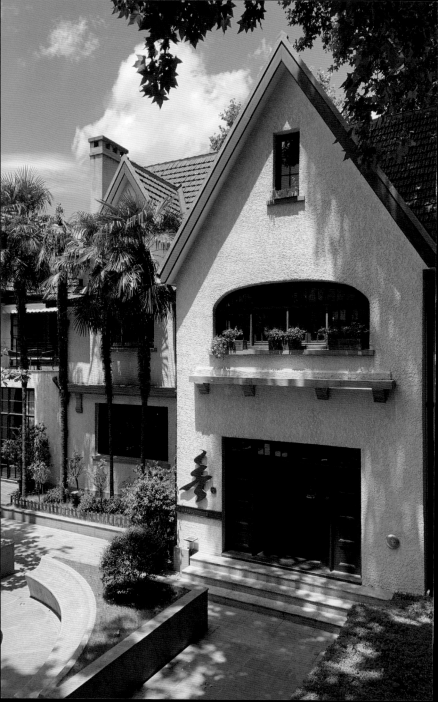

Yueyang Road is flanked by plane trees and a rainbow of garden villas. A century ago, the creamy-hued villa at No. 190 was a private hospital founded by the famous "New Brothers", both of whom had been dedicated medical practitioners and contributed to Chinese health care. The hospital name "Linsheng" comes from their names — "Huilin" and "Huisheng".

"It was a small hospital, but there were many figures and stories behind the building. As one of China's earliest Western hospitals, it was founded in 1920 by Dr. Niu Huilin (Way-ling New) and Dr. Niu Huisheng (Way-Sung New), sons of Niu Shangzhou (Shang-Chow New) who had been sent to study in the US by the Qing's royal government," said writer and historian Song Luxia.

The Linsheng Hospital, also known as Ling Sung Hospital, is located in a British-style three-story villa. The steep roof capped by red tiles contrasts with the creamy-hued walls. The facade is graced by arched windows, a terrace, a lovely balcony and a curved porch of Doric columns and vase-shaped railings. The villa faces a garden with a fountain and palm trees.

On November 20, 1937, Niu Huilin, the elder brother, passed away in the hospital building at the age of 48, six months after his younger brother Niu Huisheng died, aged 45.

In many books about Shanghai medical history, their names crop up everywhere. They founded, managed, operated and participated in several medical institutions and saved so many lives. It's incredible how the brothers achieved so much during their short lives.

The excellence of the siblings undoubtedly lies with their father, Niu Shangzhou, who was one of the first Chinese students to study in America. On his return Niu was made secretary of the Jiangnan Dock and Engineering Works of Shanghai.

In the US Niu met another Chinese young man named Charlie Soong and they became good friends. After returning to China, they married two sisters from the Ni Family. Charlie Soong's three daughters later became the famous Soong sisters who married Dr. Sun Yat-set, Kuomintang leader Chiang Kai-shek and minister H.H.Kung.

According to a study by scholar Zhang Shengfen from Chinese Medical Society, the lives of Niu's two sons mirrored each other.

Both Huilin and Huisheng studied medicine overseas after graduating from Shanghai St. Johns School at the age of 18. Huilin studied in the medical college of Cambridge University in the United Kingdom while Huisheng chose the medical college of Harvard University in the US.

In 1914 Huilin had his early medical training at London Hospital after graduating from Cambridge University with a Ph.D degree in medicine. As the Great War broke out, he joined the staff of the Ipswich Military Hospital (1914—1916) where he acted as superintendent. From 1916 to 1918, he was the house surgeon at the Middlesex Hospital under the famous surgeon Sir John Bland Sutton.

Also in 1914, Huisheng graduated from the Medical School of Harvard University with a M.D. degree (Medical Doctorate). During and after his college years, Huisheng had considerable practical experience, being house physician and surgeon of St. Luke's Hospital, New Bedford from 1914 to 1915.

Both Niu brothers returned to China after gaining experience overseas. In 1915, Huisheng was the first to go back to China where he took charge of the Department of Anatomy at the Harvard Medical School of China in Shanghai, which was a cooperative project between Harvard University and Chinese Red Cross General Hospital, predecessor of today's Huashan Hospital.

However after witnessing the suffering of many Chinese patients with fractures, he went to the US again to study orthopedic medicine from 1916 to 1918 and returned to take charge of the department of orthopedic surgery, Peking Medical College.

Huilin returned to China in 1918 and later became head of the Lester Chinese Hospital surgical department, which developed into today's Renji Hospital. In 1920 he founded Linsheng Hospital on Route Ghisi (today's Yueyang Road) with his brother.

Shanghai historian and writer Song Luxia says soon after Linsheng Hospital was opened, the English governor of Hong Kong, who was severely ill, telegraphed the British government to send a good doctor.

"The ministry of health replied that there was no need to dispatch a doctor from London. Dr. Niu Linsheng of Shanghai Linsheng Hospital graduated with a PhD of medicine from the Cambridge University. The British

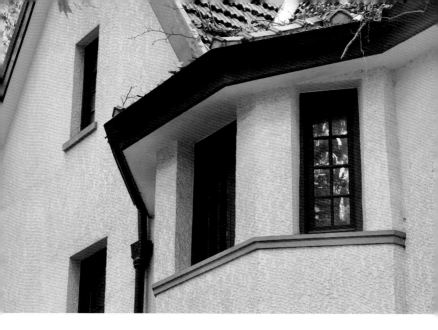

medical circle knew about Niu's skills through his performance as a surgeon during World War I. So Niu was invited to Hong Kong and cured the governor. That won him a reputation in Hong Kong and Shanghai and Linsheng Hospital became a renowned medical center," said Song, who has researched Shanghai prominent families for decades.

In 1927, Linsheng Hospital received a heavily injured patient whose left leg had been shot three times. His bones were broken and set wrong. According to Mu Xin's article named "Chen Geng In Shanghai", Niu Huilin suspected the patient was a robber and was reluctant to treat him. The patient then claimed to be General Chen Geng, who was shot during a battle in Nanchang of Jiangxi Province some two months before. Niu was touched by Chen's honesty and the brothers used their superb medical skills to save the general's left leg from amputation.

From 1924—1927, Niu Huilin was honorary superintendent of the Chinese Red Cross Hospital on Avenue Haig, which is today's Huashan Road. It was largely due to his efforts and labor that the Red Cross Hospital grew in importance. From 1921—1927 he was also superintendent of Cholera Hospital under the Chinese Red Cross Society. At the same time, he directed the Cholera

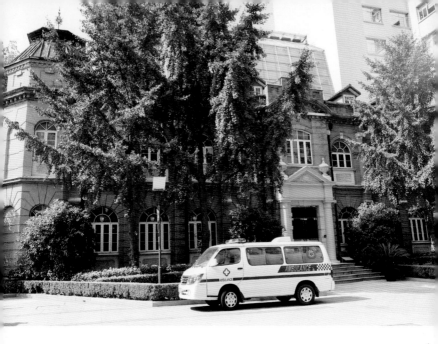

Hospital on Yu Ya Ching Road, which is Xizang Road now.

Apart from his hospital duties and practices, he would volunteer from time to time to do emergency work, according to his obituary published on *The China Press* on November 21, 1937.

"In 1923 he headed a red cross unit to Lincheng to render medical aid to foreign and Chinese captives in Shantung. During the great earthquake in Japan in 1923, he took a group of Chinese doctors and nurses to Japan on an errand of mercy. During the Kiangsu-Chekiang civil war in 1926, he again headed the red cross work. Related to the famous Soong fam-

ily, the brothers entertained Generalissimo and Madame Chiang Kai-chek when China's foremost couple came to Shanghai following the Sian coup," the report says.

When Huilin's medical career was flourishing in old Shanghai, his younger brother also played important roles in the medical circle.

According to his obituary in *the North-China Herald*, on May 12, 1937, Niu Huisheng had held office as secretary and counsellor in several national medical bodies. He became the first president of the new Chinese Medical Association.

In 1923, Huisheng was introduced into the "Who's Who in China" column by *The China Weekly Review* on November 24.

In 1928, he founded China's first medical orthopedic hospital on today's Huashan Road. He also founded a children's orthopedic hospital for little ones who suffered from bone tuberculosis.

When Niu Huisheng passed away in 1937, a local English newspaper commented that "China has lost a great human personality".

"The death of Dr. Way-sung New at his home at 852 Route de Siccawei, at the age of 46, early morning removes not only a man influential in medicine, but one who was a man of vision and courage in all human relationships. He devoted his energy to pushing forward the work of this national medical body, thinking of it by day and dreaming of it by night.

Even during the last week of his life, while lying desperately ill, he woke up continually to mention the work of the association. Dr. New was conspicuous as an organizer and coordinator, a man of courage and firm in facing difficulties, but always full of grace in his approach to difficult human personalities and situations," the newspaper said.

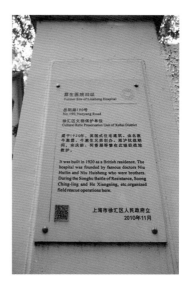

According to Zhang Shengfen's research, a severely ill Huisheng attended the Chinese Medical Association's 12th grand meeting, which was hosted along with the completion of Shanghai Medical Center and Shanghai Zhongshan Hospital. He passed away three weeks after this important meeting.

In 2015, officer Yuan Huiyun of Renji Hospital received a visitor named Niu Enmei, who was daughter of Dr. Niu Huilin.

"She was in her eighties and was very energetic. She visited Renji Hospital with great interest, especially when she saw the building built in 1932. She watched and looked and touched the ward of

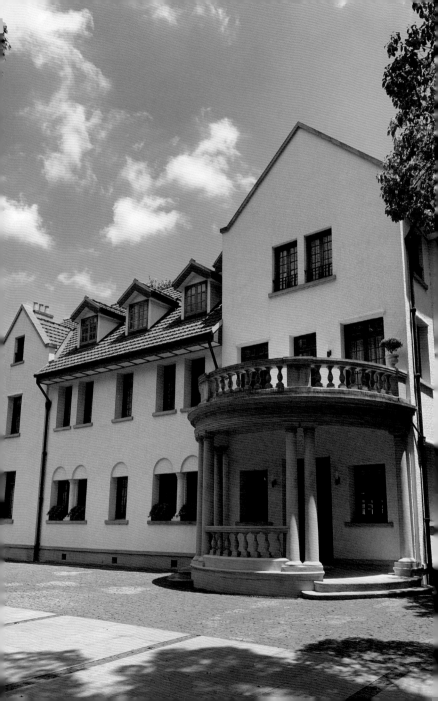

the building where her father Niu Huilin had worked. She spoke cordially with the medical staff and patients present, and took in Renji Hospital's profound historical heritage and the modern functions added to the newly renovated ward area," Yuan said.

During the visit, Niu Enmei decided to donate several precious cultural relics to the hospital, such as gold-rimmed glasses, ashtrays, tea cups and an embroidered plaque by Niu's patients to admire his superb medical skills.

She said most of the Niu descendants had embarked on a medical career and made contributions to the development of China's medical and health care services.

The creamy-hued Linsheng Hospital on Yueyang Road is small and quiet, but its founding brothers provided a solid foundation of the city's largest hospitals, previously introduced in this column, such as Renji Hospital, Huashan Hospital and Zhongshan Hospital. The medical brothers' lives were short, but their achievements and spirits are everlasting.

Yesterday: Linsheng Hospital   **Today:** a Chinese restaurant
Address: 190 Yueyang Road   **Built in:** 1920
Tips: The facade can be admired from Yueyang Road. The second floor of an adjacent gallery/cafe offers a good view of the villa garden.

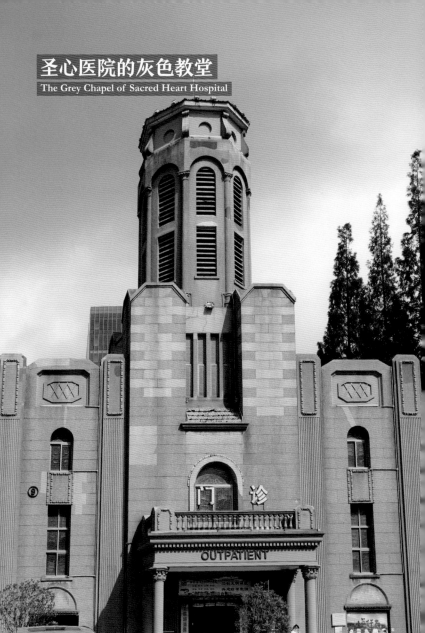

OUTPATIENT

上海是中国建造教堂最多的城市，上海市第一康复医院的院区内就有一座引人注目的灰色教堂，透露了医院不寻常的历史。

一个多世纪前，天主教慈善家、企业家陆伯鸿（1875—1937）租用几间民房作为临时诊所，为看病难的杨浦工人开办了圣心医院。1923年，因民房不敷使用，陆伯鸿等人在宁国路购地，兴建5幢新型病房，1932年又建造了这座圣堂和产科病房。

1934年3月7日，英文《北华捷报》（*The North-China Herald*）报道，新的产科病房是在陆伯鸿之子、圣心医院副院长陆隐耕（Lo Yin-kung）的指导下建造的。医院举行了隆重的新病房启用仪式，包括上海市长吴铁城在内的中外来宾都出席了盛典。

"新病房是一幢三层楼高的建筑，从柔和的墙壁到高效的手术室，各方面都很现代。病房可容纳80多张床位，其中30张为一等病房，其余为二等病房。病房确保有明媚的阳光，可以俯瞰一大片将以绿树花卉美化的空地。

产房和手术室位于顶层。"《北华捷报》报道。

负责修缮康复医院历史建筑的建筑师王凌霄调研发现，原圣心医院的圣堂和产房大楼为钢筋混凝土结构建筑，均由俄国建筑师李维·戈登士达（Livin Goldenstadt）设计。院区内还有其他几幢分别建于20世纪20年代和70年代的砖木结构建筑。目前教堂已被列为上海市优秀历史建筑，其余均为杨浦区文物保护单位。

同济大学郑时龄院士在《上海近代建筑风格》（新版）中写道，俄国建筑师李维（一译列文·戈登士达，W. Livin-Goldstaedt，1878—?）原名弗拉迪米尔·戈登士达，曾获中山陵设计竞赛名誉奖第五名。他主持的李维建筑工程师（W. Livin Architect）位于四川路29号，作品除了圣心医院圣堂（Sacred Heart Church），还有五官科医院汾阳路院区的三德堂及水塔、大胜胡同（Victory Terrace）、白赛仲路19号住宅以及几座公

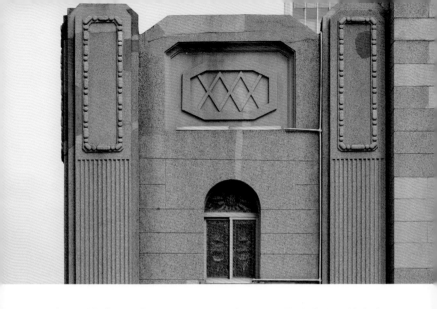

寓——克莱门公寓（Clements Apartments）、伊丽莎白公寓（Elizabeth Apartments，今复中公寓）、亚尔培公寓(King Albert Apartments，今陕南邨)、阿斯屈来特公寓（Astrid Apartments，今南昌大楼）。

王凌霄发现李维的设计独具匠心。阿斯屈来特公寓是一座横向空间为主的建筑，他在街道转角的立面设计了突出的竖向装饰物，其中轴线的立面构图与圣心医院教堂主立面有异曲同工之妙。这位俄国建筑师常常在古典复兴和装饰艺术派风格之间摇摆。他为古典复兴的克莱门公寓

中采用了装饰艺术派的室内设计，但在装饰艺术派风格的阿斯屈来特公寓上则使用强烈的古典风格的中轴装饰物。

圣心医院的灰色教堂采用巴西利亚布局，装饰艺术风格的塔楼以垂直线条装饰，立面设计有精美的彩绘玻璃玫瑰窗。大厅的两侧是两个柱廊，铺设有两种色彩明快的地砖。柱廊、地砖、天花和主楼梯的水磨石栏杆都是历史原物。

周进博士在《上海教堂建筑地图》一书中点评道，"圣心医院的教堂因与医院合建，沿用了医院建筑的样式，但大厅的教

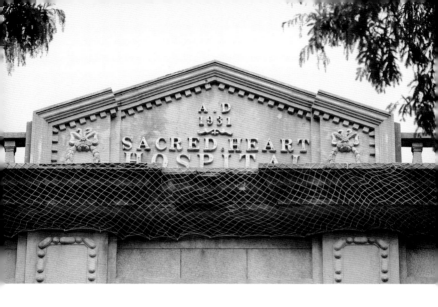

堂氛围依然非常强烈，中部设有象征哥特教堂的八边形钟塔，侧立面则模仿了罗马风教堂惯用的扶壁和半圆券，彩色玻璃非常漂亮。"

如今，与圣心教堂同期建成的产科大楼外墙上仍有医院的旧英文名：Sacred Heart Hospital (圣心医院)。在院区里，一座座建筑围绕着一个中央花园布置展开，体现了当年的科学规划。

圣心医院是陆伯鸿创办的众多慈善项目之一。上海宗教史专家，复旦大学李天纲教授认为，陆伯鸿是上海近代史上的重要人物。

"他出生于南市的一个天主教家庭，家族受徐光启的影响而皈依天主教。陆伯鸿擅长与法国人做生意，创办了多个公司、宗教机构和慈善项目。"李天纲说。

陆伯鸿曾任闸北水电公司、上海华商电气公司、大通仁记航业公司、和兴码头堆栈公司、新和兴铁厂、浦东电气公司、上海内地自来水公司的董事长或董事，1927年当选为上海法租界最早的5位华人董事之一。

意大利建筑历史学者卢卡·彭切里尼（Luca Poncellini）在《邬达克》一书中写道，他的

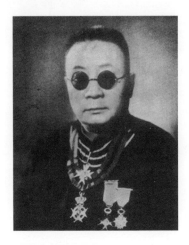

慈善活动扩展到了社会各个阶层。因为运营着一个庞大的慈善捐赠网络，陆伯鸿成了一个权势很大的人。与此同时，他还在上海的商业活动中发挥着关键作用，他在贸易和工业企业中拥有的头衔跟在教堂和教育机构的一样多。他被任命为上海天主教小学和中学的董事会主席，中国最大的水电供应商的主管以及航运和钢铁行业公司的主管。

"陆伯鸿天生有种本事，能在上海经济与政治生活的利益网络中如鱼得水，这些网络部分是公开的，部分则是秘密的，隐藏在操控这个城市的秘密群体背后。"彭切里尼评价道。

除了圣心医院，陆伯鸿还创办了圣心女子学校，并委托建筑师邬达克（L. E. Hudec）设计，就是今天距医院不远的眉州路长城宾馆。热心公益事业的陆伯鸿还创办了普慈疗养院、中国公立医院、南市时疫医院、北京中央医院等慈善医疗机构。

除了为穷苦的杨树浦工人疗愈病痛，圣心医院内还开办过中比镭锭研究所，在上海医学史上具有重要意义。1937年3月31日，《北华捷报》报道称这个由中比庚子赔款资助的项目是"中国第一个抗癌中心"。

不幸的是，同年12月30日，陆伯鸿在（Avenue Dubail，今重庆南路）遇刺，年仅63岁的他在送往广慈医院（今瑞金医院）的途中死亡。他被暗杀的原因至今仍是未解之谜。

幸运的是，陆伯鸿为上海留下的医疗事业遗产今日犹存。他创办的普慈疗养院曾是中国最早的现代精神病院之一，如今已成为上海市精神卫生中心闵行分院。中比镭锭研究所治疗院发展为复旦大学附属上海肿瘤医院。

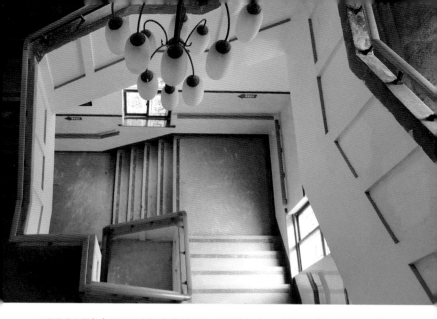

而圣心医院内不同时代建造的历史建筑大部分都被保存了下来，今天仍作为医疗功能使用。

1949年后，圣心医院历经变迁，一度为适应老龄化社会而改为杨浦区老年医院。由于2008年汶川地震后社会对康复护理的需求日益增长，2012年老年医院又转型为上海首家康复专业医院。

上海市第一康复医院原院长周明成介绍，这里是华山医院的临床基地，很多康复医学大家从这里走出。上海市第一康复医院目前有500多张床位，50多名康复医生，160名治疗师，拥有包括机器人、VR、心脏康复和儿童感觉统合评估在内的世界顶尖设备。作为杨浦滨江段一座重要的历史建筑，灰色教堂修复后被打造为一个集医学图书馆、展览、活动为一体的重要文化地标对公众开放。这家传奇的百年医院计划成为亚洲康复医疗中心，为历史建筑带来新的发展。

昨天：圣心医院　**今天：**上海市第一康复医院　**地址：**杭州路 349 号
建筑师：李维（Livin Goldenstadt）　**参观指南：**小教堂对病人开放。可以在杭州路欣赏建筑立面。

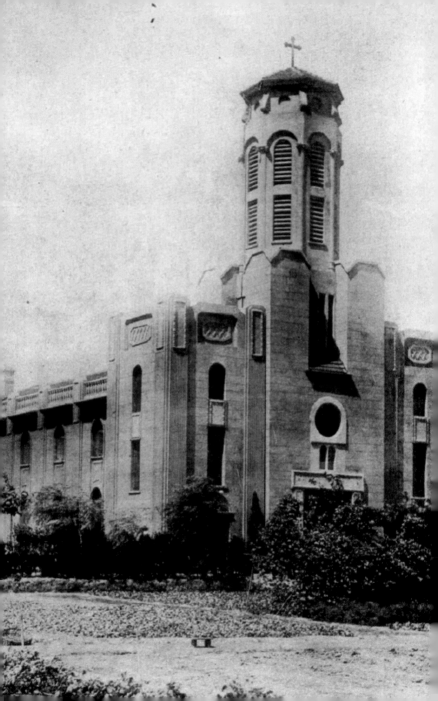

It's kind of ironic that a man who had a religious zeal to save lives should die tragically at the hands of an assassin. Yet this was quite common of the tumultuous times during the warring times.

Lu Bohong, also known as Joseph Lo Pa Hong, was a well-known Catholic entrepreneur and philanthropist, who founded several hospitals and businesses in Shanghai. Yet in 1937 he was murdered in the French Concession under mysterious circumstances.

Lu founded the Sacred Heart Hospital, predecessor of the First Rehabilitation Hospital of Shanghai. A stylish chapel and a modern maternity ward both built in 1932 showcase the history of a hospital built for poor Chinese workers.

Hospital archives reveal Lu founded the Sacred Heart Hospital in 1923 for Chinese people who worked in the nearby factories in Yangpu District.

The hospital used several Chinese houses as a temporary dispensary. As the houses struggled to take in more patients, Lu and some other philanthropists purchased a site on Ningguo Road and built five new-style ward buildings in 1923. In 1932, the chapel and a maternity ward were added to the hospital.

The North-China Herald reported on March 7, 1934, that the new maternity ward was constructed under the instruction of Lo Yin-kung, son of Lu Bohong and vice-president of the Sacred Heart Hospital. The hospital's authorities on 41 Ningkuo Road celebrated the formal opening of the new ward with a ceremony attended by a big gathering of foreigners and Chinese people, including Shanghai mayor Wu Tiecheng.

"Modern in every respect, from the soft-toned walls to the efficient operation rooms, the new ward is a three-story building capable of accommodating more than 80 beds, of which 30 are for first-class patients while the remaining for second-class. Pleasant sunshine is guaranteed as it overlooks a large piece of vacant ground, which will be beautified with trees and flowers. The maternity ward and operation rooms are on the top floor," the 1934 report said.

Shanghai H. N. A. Architects. Co. Ltd. reveals the chapel and maternity ward building are concrete-and-steel structures both designed by Russian architect Livin Goldenstadt. The hospital compound also features several other brick-and-wood buildings built in the 1920s and 1970s. Among them, the chapel has been listed as a Shanghai historical building while the others are all heritage sites under the preservation of Yangpu District.

"Born in 1878 in Vladivostok, the architect moved to China and worked in Shanghai for 13 years. The styles of his Shanghai works switched between classic revival and Art Deco styles. In addition to the Sacred Heart Hospital, he also designed the Astrid Apartments, a striking building of apartments in an Art Deco style situated on the corner of Maoming and Nanchang roads. The composition of an axis on the facade mirrors the chapel of the Sacred Heart Hospital," said Wang Lingxiao from H. N. A. Architects. Co., Ltd, whose firm researched the hospital's architectural history for a restoration project.

"It's interesting that this architect adapted an Art Deco style for the interior design of another of his work, the Clement's Apartments in classic revival style on Fuxing Road M. But he used a strong classic style axis decoration on the Art Deco Astrid Apartments."

The chapel in a basilica layout features an Art Deco tower decorated with vertical lines. The facade formerly had an exquisite stained glass rose window. The interior hall is still flanked by two colonnades. The original colorful tiles on the floor and the ornamental ceiling are well preserved. The maternity ward building also bears the original English name on the facade. The hospital buildings are placed around a central garden, which displays a scientific planning of the hospital. The Sacred Heart Hospital was one of Lu Bohong's major philanthropic projects.

"Lu Bohong was a famous figure in the modern history of Shanghai," said Fudan University professor Li Tiangang, an expert of Shanghai religious history.

"He was born into a family in the old Nanshi district of Shanghai and a neighbor of another renowned Chinese Catholic Family, Xu Guangqi, a Ming Dynasty (1368—1644) minister whom Xujiahui was named after. Lu's family was influenced by Xu to convert to Christianity. Adept at doing business with the French, Lu founded a galaxy of companies, religious institutions and philanthropic projects," he said.

A famous Chinese entrepreneur and leader in modern Shanghai, Lu founded the first Chinese-invested iron factory and was elect-

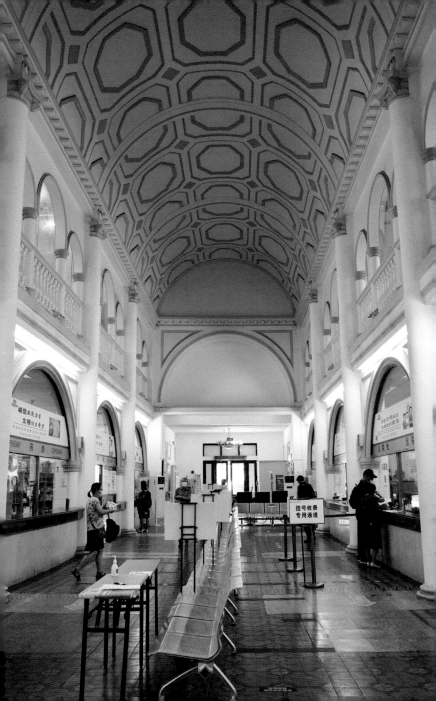

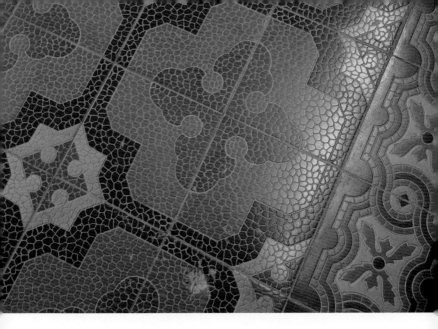

ed as one of the first five Chinese members of the former French Municipal Council.

He was appointed president of the board of Shanghai's Catholic primary and secondary schools, the director of the largest Chinese water and electricity providers and the director of companies in the shipping and steel industry.

Lu's humanitarian activities extended to all layers of society. He was the founder and director of several colleges and hospitals, and co-operated with other Catholic and international charity and educational organizations. In addition to the Sacred Heart Hospital, Lu also founded the Sacred Heart School for Women and commis-

sioned architect L. E. Hudec to design the building, which is the Changcheng Hotel on Meizhou Road today near the hospital.

"Managing an extensive network for charity donations, Lu Bohong became a man of great power. At the same time he played a key role in Shanghai's business life, holding numerous titles in trade and industrial businesses as well as in church and educational institutions. Lu Bohong had a natural talent for successfully liaising in a web of interests in Shanghai's economic and political life, part of which was public, the other part clandestine, hidden behind secret societies that operated in the city," Italian architectural historian

Luca Poncellini said in his book *Laszlo Hudec*.

In addition to saving the lives of Chinese workers, the Sacred Heart Hospital is significant in Shanghai medical history for hosting a physio-therapeutical department of the Sino-Belgium Radium Institute in its grounds. *The North-China Herald* called the project founded with the Boxer Indemnity Fund "the first anti-cancer center in China", on March 31 1937.

However, later that year on 30 December, Lu Bohong was assassinated on Avenue Dubail (today's Chongqing Road S.). The 63-year-old man died on his way to Saint Marie's Hospital, now Ruijin Hospital. The reason of his assassination remains a mystery. No one was arrested for the murder and the case remains unresolved.

It was tragic but Lu's medical legacy lives on in Shanghai. His Shanghai Mercy Hospital, a modern hospital for mentally ill patients, became the Minhang branch of Shanghai Mental Health Center. The physio-therapeutical department of the Sino-Belgium Radium Institute developed into Fudan University Shanghai Cancer Center. Historical buildings built in different eras for the Sacred Heart hospital are largely preserved and still used for medical function today.

After 1949, the Sacred Heart Hospital endured changes and developed into the city's first professional hospital of rehabilitation since 2012.

"Our hospital was founded to answer the growing need and attention for rehabilitation care following the 2008 Sichuan Earthquake. Now we have more than 500 beds, 54 rehabilitation doctors, 160 therapists and the world's most cutting-edge equipment, including robots, VR, heart rehabilitation and children's sensory integration assessment," said Zhou Mingcheng, director of the First Rehabilitation Hospital of Shanghai.

After the restoration, the hospital plans to open the chapel to the public as a cultural venue with a medical library and spaces for exhibitions and activities. The goal is to build a rehabilitation medical center of Asia and seek new development on historical buildings.

Yesterday: the Sacred Heart Hospital   **Today:** The First Rehabilitation Hospital of Shanghai   **Address:** 349 Hangzhou Road   **Architect:** Livin Goldenstadt
Tips: The chapel is open to patients. The facade can be admired on Hangzhou Road.

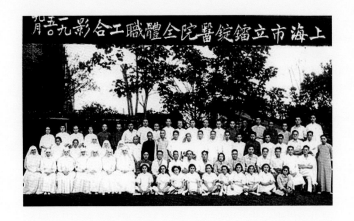

上海市立镭锭医院全体职工合影九五吾月

民元之夏，上海陆伯鸿先生等因鉴于杨树浦一隅，工厂林立，工人患病者，以窘于资，无处求医，爰就近赁屋数椽，请方济各会姆姆，施诊给药。每日踵门求治者，有五六百人之多。每逢主日，公教进行会亦遴派会员，前赴宣传要理。同时虹口天主堂，亦有神父前往讲道。由是弃邪归正者，为数不鲜。民十二，以所租屋宇不敷应用，由陆君与其他热心慈善家，集资在宁国路，购进良地六十余亩，建造新式病房，计男女各一座，内分头、二、三等。又幼稚院一座，修女住院一座，小堂附设其内。每座病房，可容百五十人，常驻医士内外科各一位，并有英、法、德、奥、义诸国内外科眼科产科等专家，为该院特约医生。该院近复与中比庚款委员会合作，向法国购就甫经发明之全部镭锭疗病机，专治各种疝瘤，及一切危难病症，约值二十万金。只镭锭一项，代价驾十万元而上之，在东方允称第一疗养院，因其他各医院尚未有此种设备，该疗病机由留比医学博士葛君担任使用。又自备爱克司光大小各一副，治疗力极强约有三种功用。

（一）诊察人体内部各种病症实况（二）摄影证明病之所在（三）诊治瘰疬肺病等。由 X 电光学专家张友梅博士担任，现在病家求治留院者日众。原有病室供不应求。该院为适应时代需要，造福病家起见，爰特借资添筑最新式钢骨，水泥三层楼，特等病院一所，可容百二十人。内部一切设备，概取现代式的科学化，迩来每逢主日及瞻礼日，邻近教友往院与祭者，日形增多。原有小堂几无容足之地。故又建造耶稣圣心堂一所，可容七八百人，采用罗马式。该院新堂及特等病院建筑，均由陆隐耕先生规划，图样由李文建筑师，会同东亚建筑公司钱少平君设计，建筑由洽兴建筑公司承造，于去年十月廿五日耶稣君王瞻礼。陆先生敦请惠大司牧，举行祝圣主心新堂，及特等病院奠基石典礼。徐家汇姚院长及上海方济堂管账司铎为襄礼，来宾到虹口边院长，土山湾韩院长，暨各会管账司铎等三十余位，以及公教进行会会员，并教友等约共百余人。三时，主教先祝圣心堂基石，继祝圣新病院基石，末恭行大礼降福，典仪隆重，盛极一时。礼毕，款以茶点，摄影尽欢而散。

摘自 1932 年《圣教杂志》

上海发动抗癌战争

中比镭锭研究所位于上海偏僻的地区，除医学专业外其工作几乎不为人所知，它每天都在开展最有价值的工作——癌症治疗和癌症研究。该研究所位于圣心医院，是中国第一个抗癌中心，就在两周前还加入了一些其他的研究这种可怕疾病的中心。

成立圣心医院时，中比镭锭研究所捐出了成立治疗院所需的必要资金（来自庚子赔款）。治疗院成立于1931年，专门从事癌症治疗。1936年初，研究所重组后独立于医院运营，目的是扩大防癌措施的范围。

该研究所的主任希拉底斯（M. A. Hilliadis）曾任职于比利时罗文大学癌症研究所（Institute of Cancer at Louvin University），有五名中国医生在他的带领下工作，他们是唯一接受过抗癌工作培训的中国人。

到此就诊的病人将由每位医生进行检查，以确诊他是否患有癌症，以及患有哪种特殊类型的癌症。确定癌症是否存在的主要方法之一是检查从患者身上取出的微小肿瘤，并通过精心制作的方法对其进行专门制备。研究所实验室中的一种特殊仪器可将肿瘤颗粒切掉千分之一毫米，首先将其浸入石蜡中。然后将其放置在载玻片上，并进行着色处理，癌细胞（如果存在）会在显微镜下很容易显示出来。

同时，研究所每天都在实践成功的治疗措施，给数百名使用这种治疗方法的患者带来了无法估量的好处。在研究所里，有两台最新的X射线设备和一台旧设备。三台设备从上午8点到下午5点不间断地治疗，因为能带来好处的X射线是目前治疗肿瘤的首选方法。设备上装有铜滤光片，以防止对人体有害的柔光穿透。X光室用铅包裹，以防止射线泄露给医院工作人员带来危险。与X光室相邻的是镭治疗科，该科是癌症治疗的第二阶段。该研究所自成立以来已有500例可疑癌症对治疗产生效果，这一事实充分说明了研究所出色的工作。每一个病例都要进行认真的随访，为期五年。有些病例显示没有复发，而另一些病例在一两年后又复发了，他们不得不再到研究所接受进一步治疗。该研究所每年处理700至800例癌症病例。

摘自 1937 年 3 月 31 日《北华捷报》

Shanghai Wages War On Cancer

Situated in somewhat remote part of Shanghai, its work virtually unknown except to the medical profession, the Sino-Belgian Radium Institute carries on day by day a most valuable work—cancer cure and cancer research. The institute, in the grounds of the Sacred Heart Hospital, Yangtszepoo, is the first anti-cancer centre in China, and joined the host of other centres carrying on research into the dread disease only two weeks ago.

When the Sacred Heart Hospital was founded, the Sino-Belgium Radium Institute contributed the money necessary to found a physio-therapeutical department, (drawing it from the Boxer Indemnity Fund), specializing in the treatment of cancer, this being founded in 1931. Early in 1936, the whole institute was completely re-organized, making it independent of the Hospital. The aim being to enlarge the scope of the anti-cancer measures.

The Institute has as its director M. A. Hilliadis, formerly attached to the Institute of Cancer at Louvin University, Belgium, with five Chinese doctors working under him-the only Chinese in the country to be trained in anti-cancer work.

On a cancer suspect being admitted to the institute, he is examined by each doctor on the staff, in order to determine whether or not he has cancer, and if he has, what particular type of cancer it is. One of the principal methods of determining the existence of cancer is by the examination of a minute particle of a tumor taken from the patient, and specially prepared by an elaborate process. A special instrument in the laboratory of the institute cuts off one thousandth part of a millimetre from the particle of tumor, which is first dipped in paraffin. It is then placed on a slide, and subjected to a coloring process which enables the cancerous cells, if they exist, to be picked out with ease under the microscope.

Meanwhile successful curative measures are being practised daily in the institute which are providing of inestimable benefit to hundreds of patients who make use of this treatment. At the institute are two of the most up-to-date X-ray apparatus each developing 250,000 volts, and an older apparatus developing the same power. All three are in constant use from 8am to 5pm each day in the treatment of patients with the beneficial X-ray which is one of the principal methods used in treating disease. Copper filters are fitted to the apparatuses to prevent soft rays, harmful to the human body, from penetrating through. The X-ray room is encased in lead to prevent the rays from escaping and providing dangerous to the hospital staff.

Adjoining the X-ray room is the radium therapy department, which forms the second stage in the treatment of cancer. The radium apparatus consists of four stretchers placed at right angles one above the other, the stretcher next to the top containing 900 milligrams of the precious substance.

The excellent work which the institute has been carrying out since its foundation is well illustrated by the fact that 500 cases of suspected cancer have responded to treatment. Each case dealt with is followed up carefully afterwards for a period of five years. Some show no recurrence of the disease, while in others cancer breaks out again after a year or two, and they have to return for further treatment. From 700 to 800 cancer cases are dealt with by the institute each year.

Excerpt from *the North—China Herald* on March 31, 1937

镭锭治疗院

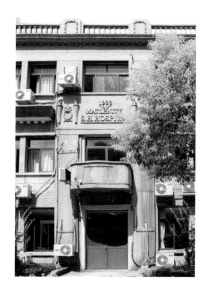

本市林森中路中比镭锭治疗院，原由中比两国以庚款合办，内部设备精良，拥有极多物理治疗器材，为亚洲治癌唯一处所，此次世界大战，该院以中比人士联合保管，幸未遭受损失，去冬并延请吴桓兴博士由英回国主持医务，吴博士为吾国有数之物理治疗专家，先后曾在比英等国各大医院主持医务，久已蜚声海外，最近国防部文职人事司长袁同畴氏，喉患癌疾，不能言语，饮食几濒危殆，即由吴博士施以深部爱克斯光及镭锭之照射，卒获痊愈。

摘自 1947 年 2 月 22 日《文汇报》

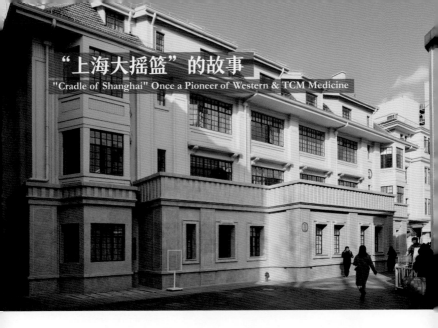

"上海大摇篮"的故事

"Cradle of Shanghai" Once a Pioneer of Western & TCM Medicine

上海第一妇婴保健院（简称"一妇婴"）每年迎接3万名新生儿诞生，被昵称为"上海大摇篮"。但很少有人知道，长乐路536号"一妇婴"西院的米色大楼在1929年开业时是"中西疗养院"，一家尝试融合中西医治疗的实验医院。

周永珍所著的《留法纪事》一书记载，中西疗养院位于上海蒲石路（Rue Bourgeat，今长乐路），因为是中西医结合、治疗效果好而大受欢迎，院内病房常客满。

1934年7月14日，《法文新报》介绍了法商赉安洋行（Leonard, Veyssyre & Kruze）在上海设计建造的众多建筑作品。报纸整版刊登了近60个建筑的黑白照片，琳琅满目，其中就有中西疗养院这座大楼。

百年前的上海，赉安洋行由三位法国建筑师赉安（Alexandra Leonard）、韦西埃（Paul Veyssyre）和克鲁泽（Arthur Kruze）联合经营，洋行的英文名由他们三人的名字组成。

赉安洋行的名字对大众来说也许有点陌生，但他们的建筑

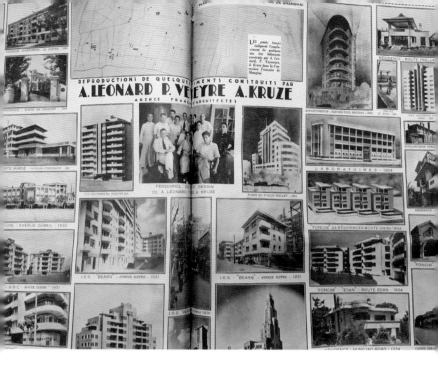

作品，如白色经典的上海花园饭店（原法国球场总会，Cercle Sportif Francais）和巧克力色的上海市妇女用品商店（原培文公寓，Bearn Apartments），都是很眼熟的上海地标建筑。

赛安洋行是一家既高产又注重设计品质的事务所，1925年因为设计法国球场总会取得巨大成功。同济大学郑时龄院士在新版《上海近代建筑风格》中评价，这家法国建筑师事务所对上海的现代建筑和高层公寓建筑设计做出了重要的贡献，其设计和建造活动始于1920年代初，一直持续到1940年代初，是旧法租界、也是上海最活跃和最重要的建筑师事务所，已知保留的作品60多件。

他提到，赛安洋行还承担了旧法租界的许多公共服务设施的设计，作品涵盖多种建筑类型和建筑风格，包括住宅、公寓、办公楼、教堂、修道院、学校、医院、警察局、俱乐部、博物馆等。他们的作品体现出法国的文化品位，对上海旧法租界城市空间的形成影响非常大，在近代上海建筑发展进程中也起了相当大的作用。

赛安曾在巴黎美院学习，韦西埃师从法国建筑大师希达纳（G. P. Chedanne），两人都参加了第一次世界大战，并获得表彰荣誉。1922年，他们在上海相识后合伙创办了赛安洋行，后来第三位合伙人克鲁泽加入其中。

同济大学硕士研究生陈锋在《赛安洋行在上海的建筑作品风格浅析》一文中指出，相对于商业发达的老上海公共租界，旧法租界没有那么多大型商业建筑，而是强调生活，注重环境品质和艺术追求，以居住、文化建筑居多。赛安洋行就是这个时期活跃于旧法租界，并且是影响最大的一个法籍建筑设计公司。

"三位法国建筑师在折中混杂的大上海创造出许多美丽的篇章，他们设计及承建的许多建筑都是当时上海社会变迁的最好例证，其作品涉及各种建筑类型，并且每种类型都做得有声有色。在建筑艺术和风格的探索上，他们以其大量的实践作品使东西方文化以一种特殊方式获得了成功的结合。"陈锋评价。

他将赛安洋行作品分为四个阶段：早期花园住宅设计（1922—1924）、西式复古建筑设计（1925—1928）、装饰艺术风格（Art Deco Style）建筑设计（1928—1932）和现代建筑设计（1933—1936）。中西疗养院这座米色建筑建于1926年，是赛安洋行的西式复古建筑作品之一。

与令赛安洋行一举成名的法国球场总会（今上海花园饭店）相比，中西疗养院这座幽静的医疗建筑相关资料较少。两位海外研究者Spencer Dodington和Charles Largrange在合著的《上海装饰艺术风格大师：保罗·韦西埃的旧法租界建筑》（*Shanghai's Art Deco Master: Paul Veysseyre's Architecture in the French Concession*）一书中，刊登了这座大楼的老照片，注明这座位于蒲石路536号（536 rue Bourgeat）的建筑建于1926

年，为Dr. Lambert的诊所（Clinique Dr. Lambert）。

历史照片显示，这是一座浅色调的古典主义建筑，屋顶覆盖红瓦。外立面装饰有孟莎屋顶、凸窗和外廊。这座钢筋混凝土建筑高达4层，建筑面积2335.2平方米，有花园和暖气设备。

有趣的是，中西疗养院的几位创办人都与法国有缘。根据广州中医药大学郑威的论文《近代中西疗养院研究》，中西疗养院由世界社发起，留法归来的世界社创始人李石曾、外交官褚民谊和法国医生贝熙业（Jean Bussière）等人倡议，"谋中西医术，作实地之试验，以期融会沟通"。

20世纪10年代，世界社由国民党元老李石曾、张静江、吴稚晖等人创办于法国巴黎，是一个传播启蒙思想的非政府组织，通过出版报纸和杂志推动社会变革。李石曾是保守的晚清重臣李鸿藻之子，但他的思想却相当新潮。1902年，李石曾成为"中国留法第一人"。他在法国巴斯德学院用现代化学知识研究大豆之

后，在巴黎创办了豆腐工厂，成为影响深远的勤工俭学留法运动的前奏。

世界社的藏书楼和有着法语特色传统的世界学校位于福开森路393号，今天是武康路393号上海老房子艺术中心。1929年，李石曾提议创办国立北平研究院，下设八个研究所，其中镭学所和药学所于抗战前迁到上海福开森路395号，就在世界社藏书楼的隔壁，现在是上海电影演员剧团。

1929年2月，中西疗养院举办成立典礼，来宾如云。米色大楼前的一张合影显示，李石曾、孙科、蔡元培、吴稚晖、郑毓秀、钱新之、张静江、陆仲安和法国驻华公使等中外名流都出席了庆典。1929年4月，疗养院西医部正式开办，同年7月中医部开诊，分别由西医郎培安和中医陆仲安两位名医主持。

中西疗养院是最早尝试融合中西医治疗的医院之一。这座办院理念前卫的疗养院不仅是试验地，也是一间环境优美、医疗设备先进的医院。除了硬件设备

好，中西疗养院还聘请中外名医坐诊。

1929年7月17日，英文《大陆报》（*The China Press*）刊登一则广告，称瑞士著名外科耳鼻喉科医生嘉腊美（L. P. Calame）将在中西疗养院看诊，治疗时间为每日早上10点到12点半，下午4点到5点半。广告显示是中西疗养院的法文名"Clinique Sino-Etrangere"。1939年10月，儿科专家伍直诲博士自英美考察回国后到中西疗养院开设门诊。1941年12月，中西疗养院聘请张卜熊医师担任外科兼妇产科主任，1943年3月又聘任原香山疗养院院长、上海广仁医院小儿科主任马月青医学博士为肺病科和小儿科主任。马月青还曾担任北平协和医院教师和国立助产学校教授。

而主理中医部的陆仲安（1882—1949）以擅用黄芪而闻名，外号叫"陆黄芪"。他曾经治好胡适、张静江等人的糖尿病，也是孙中山临终抢救团队的成员之一。《上海市静安区文史资料选集》刊登的《中西疗养院创办由来》一文提到，中西疗养院的创办可能还与孙中山先生的遗教有关。孙庆桐在这篇文章里写道，中山先生在卧病期间对陆医生说："我也曾学医行医，感到外国医学固有其特长，然中医治病，亦确有其可贵之处，宜乎中西医学界撷取所长，相互汇通，钩玄提要，融以心得，如是则造福人类者实多矣。"据说陆仲安亲聆教诲后感动至深，遂在上海参与创建中西疗养院。1929年，陆仲安被推选为全国医药团体总联合会执行委员之一。

不过，中西疗养院的筹建不易，经费来源主要为庚子赔款、医院盈利和社会基金。《申报》报道透露，"李石曾君于中法庚子赔款项下，拨出一部分，筹办中西疗养院"。疗养院成立后提供"慈善性质"和"非慈善性质"的医疗服务，其中"非慈善性质"服务是营收的主要来源，而"慈善性质"部分也会获得社会基金的资助。

1929年6月27日，在中西医界的茶话会上，郎培安医生在演讲中介绍"非慈善性质"的优质服务。"即如现在之中西疗养院，组织与普通医院不同，取法最新式设备，使病人住院，一如居家，一切治疗看护等等，无论中外人士来医，靡不尽力，且此间病房，不单由本院医生疗治，且可由病者另请院外任何医生来院医治，惟此非慈善性质，故取费较贵耳。"

因为优质的医疗服务与环境，再加上便利的地段，很多中外政要名流喜欢在中西疗养院治疗或临时居住。疗养院有时还会售卖上等鹿茸等中药材。

中西疗养院的医疗管理制度也很灵活，常根据需要增设新的门诊、医疗设备和专科医师。1934年，疗养院根据求诊者需要增设了小儿科及产科门诊，1947年又增加消化系统诊疗专科，并特聘专家治疗肠胃肝胆脾脏等疾病，还配备了X光机、胃镜、直肠镜等当时最新的检测仪器。

医院也提供一些公益的医疗服务。1949年9月4日《新民晚报》报道，中西疗养院为市民提供防痨服务，设免费X光检验额。"每星期一三五下午四时至五时半，每次暂限五名。凡本市贫苦市民可先来院登记，索取免费证，按号依次检验。"

郑威评价，"中西疗养院虽然经历经济困难、社会各界舆论以及战事的影响，但依然能够坚持开诊，维持疗养院的正常运行。不仅在战时成为伤病医院，为抗战时期的医疗救护工作做出了巨大贡献，同时亦坚持开办施诊部，以普济贫病，虽在抗战期间停办一时，但也颇为难能可贵。中西疗养院首次实现了中西医互相合作，在积极倡导'中西医药合作''中医科学化'的近代社会极具开创意义"。

历史资料显示，中西疗养院不仅尝试结合中西医治疗，还曾探索新疗法。当时，肺结核流行，而预防肺结核的疫苗"皮西其"（卡介苗，Bacillus Calmette Guérin）还未普及应用。1936年，上海雷士德医学研究院（今北京西路1320号上海医药工业研究院）开始自行研发制造卡介苗，1943年便与中西疗养院进行合作，对该院产科的婴孩进行接种。1947年4月11日，

与海市立第一妇婴保健院早产儿医师短期训练班全体合影 1957年1

《申报》报道"本市巴士德研究分院已有该项疫苗发行，此外如蒲石路中西疗养院闻亦已采用该项疫苗有相当时间了"。

1950年11月，上海市第一妇婴保健院迁入中西疗养院原址后，这座米色大楼迎来更多的婴孩，也根据需要不断创新，提供最新的妇产保健医疗服务，如避孕门诊、早产儿寄养室、中医门诊、新生儿研究室、试管婴儿技术和家庭化分娩部等。值得一提的是，历史仿佛轮回，1960年这家西医妇产医院正式引进中医师，并设立中医门诊。如今，"一妇婴"的中西医结合科开展针灸拔罐、熏蒸理疗等多项具有中医特色的传统治疗技术，并与妇科、产科、辅助生殖医学科联动，用传统中医药治疗为患者保驾护航。

2013年，一妇婴位于浦东高科西路的东院落成启用。如今，上海的每4—5个新生儿中，就有一个是在一妇婴浦西和浦东两个院区诞生的。

在过去70多年里，这座米色大楼见证了无数上海家庭迎来新生命的甜蜜时刻。

2020年10月，米色大楼整体大修完工，一年后一妇婴西院区整体修缮竣工。如今，这座百年历史建筑仍旧作为住院部大楼使用，接待孕产妇和妇科患者，一楼是妇科综合病房，三楼是产科普通病房，特需病房位于二楼和顶楼。

楼内环境布置温馨典雅，色调明亮而温暖。近一个世纪以来，这里都是一个新生命与新探索的"大摇篮"。

昨天： 中西疗养院　**今天：** 上海市第一妇婴保健院　**地址：** 长乐路 536 号
建筑风格： 古典主义风格　**设计师：** 赉安洋行（Alexandre Leonard and Paul Veysseyre）

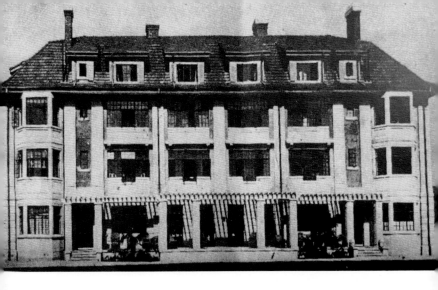

Shanghai First Maternal and Child Health Hospital is nicknamed "the big cradle of Shanghai" as it receives around 30,000 babies every year. But not many people know that the creamy-hued building on 536 Changle Road opened in 1929 as "Clinique Sino-Etrangere", an experimental hospital to include both Western and traditional Chinese medicines.

"The Clinique Sino-Etrangere, or Sino-Foreign Clinic opened on Rue Bourgeat (today's Changle Road) with Dr. P. Lambert as the hospital's Western doctor and Lu Zhong'an as its TCM doctor. The clinic's treatments, combining Western and Chinese medicines, were effective and popular among its patients. It was often fully oc-cupied," said Lu Ming, an expert of Shanghai Medical History from Shanghai No. 4 People's Hospital.

On July 14, 1934, the building was published, among a rainbow of 60 stylish buildings designed by Leonard Veysseyre & Kruze, along with the firm's group photo and a map of the former French concession. The prolific French architectural firm took out a full-page advertisement in Le Journal De Shanghai.

Leonard, Veysseyre & Kruze is an unfamiliar name to many today but the firm's architectural works, included the white, classic Okura Garden Hotel and the grand, chocolate-hued Bearn Apartments on Huaihai Road, are familiar to many in Shanghai.

The firm was co-founded by

two talented French architects, Alexandre Leonard and Paul Veysseyre in Shanghai in the 1920s. When designing the Sino-Foreign clinic in 1926, they had just completed the new Cercle Sportif Francais (today's Okura Garden Hotel) in 1925 which brought huge success. The third partner, Arthur Kruze, joined them in 1934.

According to a new edition of *The Evolution of Shanghai Architecture In Modern Times* by Tongji University professor Zheng Shiling, it was estimated that more than 60 buildings designed by the French firm still exist in Shanghai, including two ward buildings in today's Ruijin Hospital that were previously introduced in this hospital series.

"Leonard, Veysseyre & Kruze was the most important French architectural firm in modern Shanghai, which made a great contribution to the architectural design of modern architecture and tall apartment buildings. Their works showcasing a flavor of French culture had largely influenced the forming of urban spaces in the former Shanghai French Concession," Professor Zheng wrote in his book.

Tongji University graduate researcher Chen Feng revealed in his Master's thesis on the French firm that Alexandre Leonard had studied in the famous L'Ecole des Beau-Arts de Paris and Paul Veysseyre had learned from the maestro G. Chedanne. Both of them joined the fight against Germany in World War I, got injured and received several awards. They met in Shanghai in 1922 and founded the architectural firm.

"Their work achieved great success by demonstrating a new style and perfectly realizing it in architecture. Largely owing to their work, the former French concession had been keeping up with world's architectural trend," scholar Chen said.

Chen classifies their works into four periods: garden residences from 1922 to 1924; Western classic architecture from 1925 to 1928; Art Deco buildings from 1929 to 1932 and modern works from 1933 to 1936. The creamy-hued clinic building was one of the Western classic buildings designed in 1926.

Compared with the firm's more famous works like Cercle Sportif Francais, there was little architectural record of this quiet clinic. Black-and-white historical photos show it's a classical architecture in a light color with, possibly, red roof tiles. The facade is graced

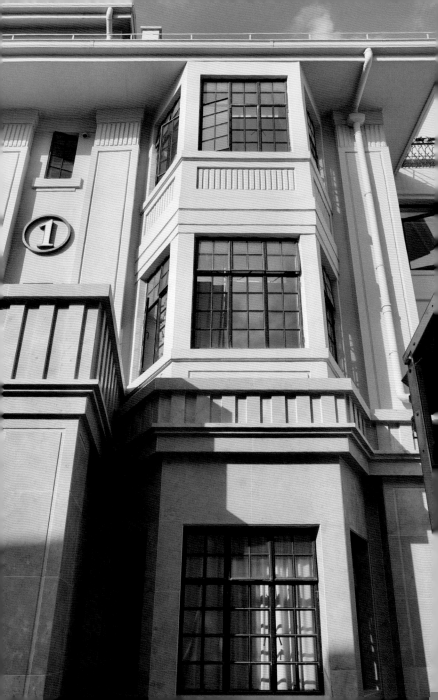

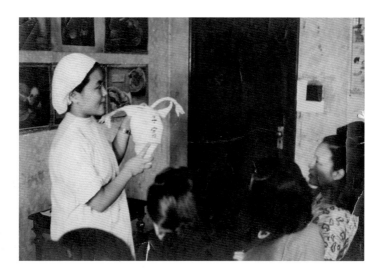

by Mansard windows, protruding windows and verandas.

It's interesting that most founders of the Sino-Foreign Clinic had French connections.

According to Zheng Wei's master thesis on the Sino-Foreign Clinic, the institution was proposed to be founded by Shijie She or the World Society, which was founded by Chinese intellectuals in Paris in the 1910s to promote revolution, science and new culture. The society was famous for its "Work-Study Movement" that sent many young Chinese to study in France starting in 1919. The movement later provided China a considerable number of open-minded talents, including Chinese leaders Zhou Enlai, Deng Xiaoping and Chen Yi. The society's library and school were located at 393 Wukang Road, where British author/playwright George Bernard Shaw visited in 1933.

It was socialist/educator Li Shizeng, the main founder of the World Society, diplomat Chu Minyi and French doctor Jean Bussiere, among others, who established the East-meet-West clinic. The purpose was to make an experiment to permeate Chinese and Western medicines.

"The clinic was the first one to house divisions of both Western and traditional Chinese medicines. The division of Western medicine threw its doors open in April 1929 while its TCM division opened in July of the same year.

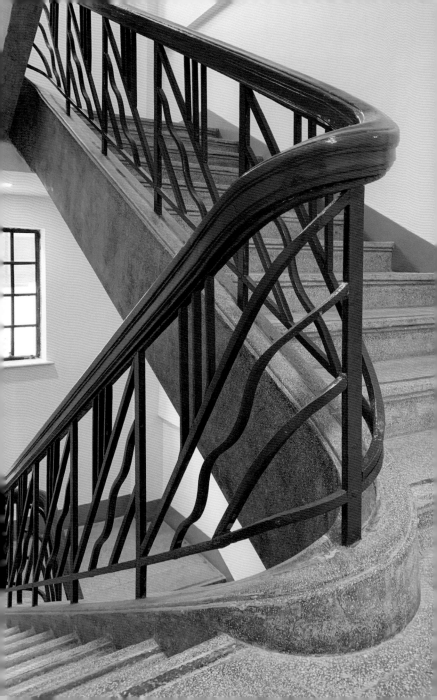

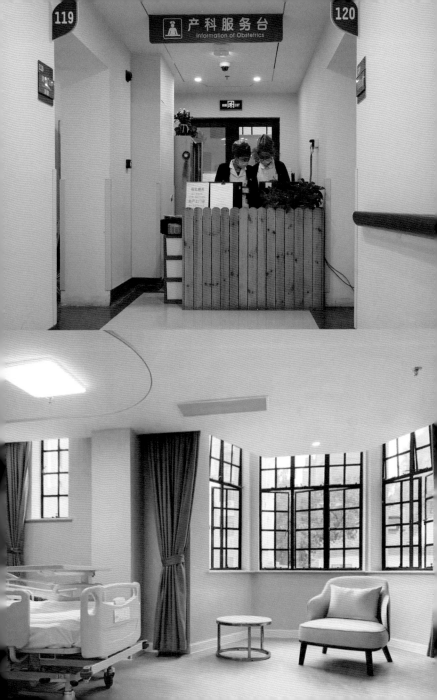

The opening speech noted that it was the first clinic to start the mutual help of the two medicines," Zheng Wei, a researcher from Guangzhou University of Chinese Medicine wrote in the thesis named "Study on Sino-Foreign Clinic in Modern Times."

The clinic was not only experimental, but also featured a nice environment and advanced equipment.

"The environment is quiet, the air is fresh and the clinic is elegant and magnificent, with comfortably decorated wards and excellent facilities. It's very suitable for recuperation. The equipment is advanced, with rooms for solar treatment and X-ray machines," reported Chinese newspaper Shen Pao on December 17, 1929.

In addition, the clinic employed only famous foreign and Chinese experts. Lu Zhong'an (1882—1949), head of its TCM division, was famous for his superb skills using Chinese herb "Huangqi" or Astragalus mongholicus for treating hard diseases. Nicknamed "Lu Huangqi," he was popular among Chinese elites and had cured the diabetes of renowned scholar Hu Shi and Kuomintang senior leader Zhang Jingjiang. He also treated Dr. Sun Yat-sen during his final

days. On July 17, 1929 the clinic invited Swiss surgeon P. Calame, former head of the Ophthalmic Hospital of the Lausanne University to see outpatients.

During World War II, the clinic became one of the hospitals in the city to treat wounded Chinese soldiers.

The funding of the clinic mainly came from the Boxer indemnity, hospital profits and social funds. The clinic treated both "charitable" and "non-charitable" patients. The "non-charitable" part is the main source of operating income for the medical institution.

According to French doctor P. Lambert's speech on a medical gathering on June 27, 1929, the clinic offered the most up-to-date facilities and its considerate nursing service made patients feel at home. Patients could also invite doctors from other hospitals to come over for medical help. So the fees for these "non-charitable" patients were expensive. However the hospital also gave free treatment and medicines to poor patients and contributed to public health work.

Zheng adds that the clinic was operated in a scientific, flexible way to add medical services when needed. On December 28, 1934, the clinic published a notice in the *Shen Pao* newspaper that it would open an outpatient department for obstetrics and pediatrics to answer growing demands.

In August 1947, the clinic added a department of gastroenterology with a new X-ray machine, gastroscope and rectal scope as there were more patients in the city suffering from digestive problems.

"The clinic was founded with a trend of thoughts and exploration to 'make traditional Chinese medicine more scientific'. The clinic had hired a galaxy of famous foreign and Chinese, Western and TCM doctors. Although in the end it did not fulfill the initial purpose to 'permeate Western and Chinese medicines', it did show that the two medicines could support each other. And the clinic often made the first move. For instance, new-born babies were given the Bacille Calmette-Guerin vaccine, produced by the Shanghai Lester Institute of Medical Research in 1943, long before BCG vaccine was widely used in Shanghai," Zheng writes in the thesis.

The creamy-hued building received more new-born babies after Shanghai First Maternal and Child Health Hospital moved here in the 1950s. Today the hospital delivers around 30,000 babies every year in both its Western branch on Changle Road and its Eastern branch in the Pudong New Area. Among every five or six new-born babies in Shanghai, one is born in this hospital. The creamy-hued building has witnessed numerous sweet family moments over the past 70 years.

On October 18, 2020, the building reopened after a restoration. Now it serves as a medical building with an outpatient department on the first floor, VIP wards on the second and top floors and an obstetrics department on the third floor. It is always full of new and expectant moms.

And it's truly a big cradle of new-born babies and ideas.

Yesterday: Sino-Foreign Clinic
Today: Shanghai First Maternal and Child Health Hospital   **Address:** 536 Changle Road
Architectural style: Classic style   **Architect:** Alexandre Leonard and Paul Veysseyre
Tips: The hospital is open for patients only.

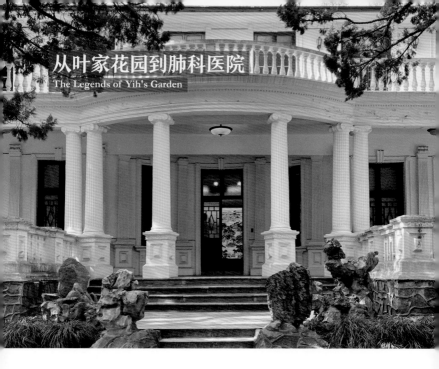

　　1933年6月8日，英文《大陆报》（*The China Press*）刊登新闻，题为《慈善家捐赠医院以治疗遭受病痛和苦难的市民》。新闻称上海著名的江湾叶家花园主人、本地著名商人叶贻铨（叶子衡）在前日进行捐赠。在著名医学教育家颜福庆的建议下，叶子衡将花园捐赠改造为一家肺病疗养院。

　　"这是一项关乎上海市民福祉的重要而值得赞扬的慈善事业。叶先生将在花园里建一家最新式的医院，该医院将特别治疗患有肺结核和神经疾病的病人，以及康复患者。"《大陆报》写道。

　　新闻还介绍，靠近江湾赛马场的叶家花园被公认为是上海最美丽的中式花园。花园占地80余亩，面积广阔，价值约100万美元。捐赠者富商叶子衡先生是著名的慈善家和体育爱好者，还是万国体育会的创始人之一。他的父亲、宁波富商叶澄衷是老一代典型的民族实业家和慈善家。

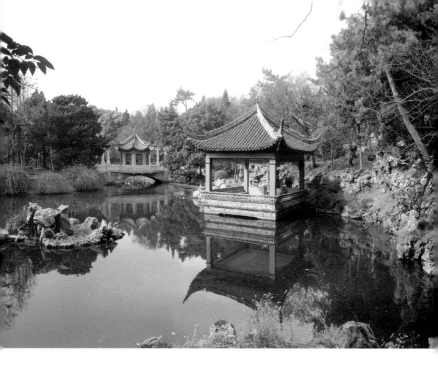

为了纪念父亲，叶子衡将花园里建造的新医院命名为"澄衷医院"。

建于1923年的叶家花园今日犹存，位于政民路507号上海市肺科医院内，占地40000余平方米。这是一座设计精美的海派园林，中西建筑点缀其间，花木葱茏，宁静幽美。静谧的外表下，叶家花园蕴藏的历史丰富多彩，波澜起伏。这个中西合璧的花园仿佛一面巨大的镜子，映射出近代上海许多非同寻常的人生与事迹。

1862年，白手起家来沪打拼的叶澄衷于开了一家小小的五金店，此后他的生意越做越大，涉足钢铁、火柴、蜡烛、棉纱等多个行业，独家代理了美国美孚石油公司的中国业务。他赚到大量财富后积极投身慈善事业，创办了著名的"澄衷蒙学堂"，惠及无数学子，延续至今日。

叶澄衷的七个儿子中，兴建叶家花园的四子叶子衡仪表堂堂、为人豪爽、敢作敢为。当

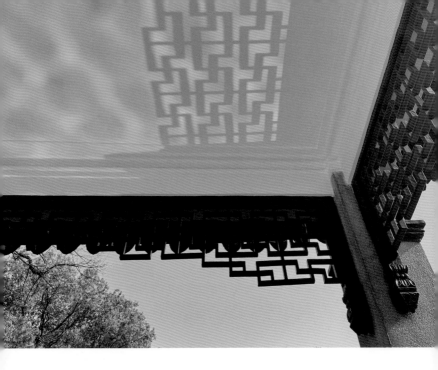

时，他和一批华人精英热爱英式赛马运动，希望和洋人马主一样加入上海跑马总会（Shanghai Race Club），但因为华人身份他两次申请入会都被拒之门外。1908年，年仅27岁的他决心筹建中国人自己的赛马场和赛马会，集资在宝山县江湾购地建跑马场。1909年，这家名为"万国体育会"（International Recreation Club）的英式赛马会开张，兼收华洋会员。江湾跑马场建成后，叶子衡又筹款在跑马场旁边建了一个中式花园，为参加赛马的游客提供赏景休憩的公共场所，就是叶家花园。

1924年2月16日，英文《北华捷报》报道了叶家花园正式的开幕仪式，当天也是万国体育会春节赛马会颁发奖杯的盛典。

"花园要到三月底才是最美的时候，不过虽然昨天天气沉闷，花园还是景致美丽，展示了中国园艺师们出色工作的优势。"报道写道。

根据上海肺科医院院志记

载，叶家花园当年坐落在江湾叶氏路351号，位于今天的杨浦区西北部。整座花园呈东西向的椭圆形，园内奇石罗列，波光岛影，相映成趣。园内有湖，湖中有三个大岛环绕交错。岛与岛、岛与环路，均以亭桥相连。构成全园胜景。花园内设弹子房、舞场、电影场、高尔夫球场等娱乐场所，在夏天晚上也对外开放，时人称夜花园。园中多水杉、桂花、玉兰、雪松、龙柏、樱花、红枫、香樟与竹丛等花木。花园内有湖泊假山、楼台亭阁、喷水池、人造瀑布、彩色路灯等。小溪流水，曲折蜿蜒、空气清新，实为怡性陶情、治病疗养之胜地。

研究医学史的复旦大学高晞教授撰文提到，国立上海医学院创办时条件极差。

"颜福庆认为现代医学院必须有自己的教学医院，就租下红十字会总医院作为教学医院，自己当院长。他每天在吴淞的医学院工作半天，再乘火车赶到市区红十字会总医院指导临床教学。颜福庆为医院制定'病人至上'

的院训，成为平民信赖的医院。沪上工商名人叶澄衷之子叶子衡是颜福庆在圣约翰的校友，颜福庆说服他捐出叶家花园，开设结核病医院，对付当时最致命的痨病，成为医学院的第二所教学医院。" 高晞教授在《颜福庆 一生是为了中国医学现代化》一文中写道。

1933年6月15日，医院正式开幕收治病人。为纪念叶子衡之父，医院命名为"澄衷医院"，又名"澄衷医院国立上海医学院肺病疗养院（亦简称澄衷肺病疗养院）"，院名横匾由慈善家王一亭手书。

澄衷医院开设男女肺科，有专任医师3人、兼任医师4人、护士6人，颜福庆院长兼任首任院长。英文《大陆报》介绍，医院由结核病疗养院、精神和神经疾病医院以及一般疾病康复疗养院组成。这三个部门都很适合这座花园地产的环境，而这些治疗服务也都是大众非常需要的。

根据上海肺科医院院志记载，建院初因缺乏经费与设备，需筹募资金以便购置设备开设病房，颜福庆又发起成立"上海医事事业董事会"，成员有宋子良、郭顺、叶子衡、孔祥熙、吴铁城、刘鸿生、史量才、徐新六、孙科、钱新之等，负责管理"澄衷肺病疗养院"和筹建中的"中山医院"基金。颜福庆还成立了"澄衷医院委员会"，成员除了他本人和叶子衡，还有公共卫生专家李延安、营造商张继光、金融家孙衡甫和钱新之、实业家刘鸿生和担任法租界公董局华董的青帮大佬杜月笙。

建院时因缺乏建设经费，将叶家花园原有旧房、亭阁、车篷甚至马厩作病室，1934年添设医师住所。当时叶家花园很大，一部分作为疗养院使用，剩下的作为花园开放营业，时称"夜花园"。澄衷医院的医疗仪器、设备器材除向卫生部借用部分外，大部分则由美国煤油大王罗氏基金董事会捐赠。设备有X光机、太阳灯、空气注射器等，在当时为新式医疗设备。

1934年4月，中华慈幼协会在澄衷医院内建立克宁汉夫人纪念堂(即慈幼痨病疗养院)专治儿童结核病，以纪念美国驻沪总领事克宁汉之夫人劳特女士（Rhoda Cunningham，原为中华慈幼协会执委)。慈幼痨病疗养院儿科病房于1934年11月落成并收治病人，是中国首创的为儿童设立的肺病疗养机构。

同年，用作特等病房使用的颜氏阁建成，1936年又新建女病房、坎大利氏厅与护士宿舍。历史照片显示，叶家花园里有两座典雅的中式建筑，分别为坎大利爵士茶厅（Sir Elly Kadoorie Tea Pavilion）和坎大利夫人纪念堂（Laura Kadoorie Hall），以纪念坎大利爵士对医院兴建所做的贡献。坎大利爵士又译为嘉道理爵士，是老上海著名的犹太富商。如今，这两座中式建筑仍位于叶家花园内，分别是10号楼和11号楼。

上海肺科医院院志还提到，建院初期因本院位于市郊江湾，当时交通极其不便，故门诊病人较少。当时每周二、四、六下午为普通门诊，周一、五上午为特别门诊及人工气胸门诊。建院初仅设病床40张，病员除由红十

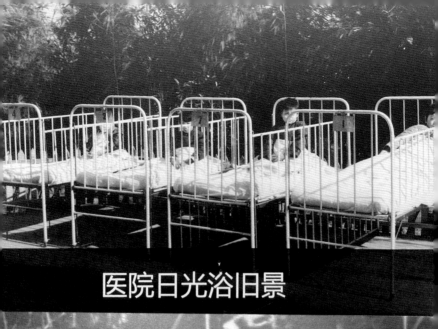

医院日光浴旧景

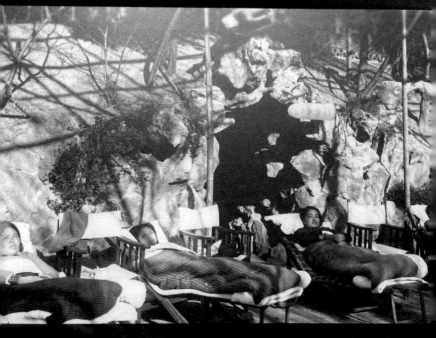

医院室外天然疗养旧景

字第一医院转入外，患者来自八方，以江浙两地居多，并有少数来自马来半岛、南洋及菲律宾群岛。据吴达während《澄衷疗养院报告》一文中记载：1933年6月到1935年10月两年多共收治入院病人476人。医院主要采用的治疗方法有人工气胸、膈神经截除、休息、营养、日光治疗与紫外线照射、防痨教育和训练、新鲜空气与康复。

医院设立蒙养园(幼稚园)，在户外为小孩授课。医院还请人每周讲授防治结核病的常识，在病室中设问事箱，悬挂图画标语，告知病者调养和避免传染他人的种种方法。医院对收治的骨结核病人施行日光疗法及紫外线照射法，对肺结核患者试用全身照射法等疗法，疗效都令人满意。

1937年抗战爆发后，改为澄衷疗养院的叶家花园历尽沧桑，波折不断。医院在抗战初期遭到日军炮火严重破坏，爱国将领张治中将军曾坚持在叶家花园水塔上督战。上海沦陷后，医院被日军占据后用作侵华头目岗村宁次

等人的住地。1940年，日军又将医院交给日本恒产株式会社管理，并一度把花园对外开放，改名为"敷岛园"，后因经营不善而关闭重新改作日本特务机关。由此，医院陷于敌手被迫停办达九年之久。

1947年4月8日，《文汇报》刊登新闻，题为《肺痨可怕 上海现有十六万病人每半小时有一人死亡》，提到"至于计划中之江湾叶家花园设立之疗养院亦拟于最短期内开幕"。当年复院后，澄衷医院与当时的肺病中心诊所、红十字会第一医院肺病科、中山医院肺病科，同属四防痨机构之一，但更侧重于治疗。

2020年成为互联网医院，以"互联网+医疗"为特色，已发展成为一家集医疗、教学、科研于一体的现代化三级甲等专科医院。除传统优势的结核科、职业病科外，胸外科、呼吸科、肿瘤科等呼吸系统疾病诊疗及相关学科也发展迅速，其中如肺移植、肺部肿瘤外科及微创外科、肺癌诊疗、肺血管病诊疗、耐多药结核病诊疗等取得了一批国内领先

的成就。

叶家花园的主楼是一座名为延爽馆的"小白楼"，建于1920年，位于园内最大岛屿的中央，占地504平方米。这是一幢两层高的西式建筑，背山面水，底层东、南、西三面为敞柱环廊，前为平台，二楼前半部亦为平台。登上平台，可眺望全园秀色。2011年2月，延爽馆被评为"杨浦区历史文物保护建筑"。近年经过设计改造后，延爽馆成为上海市肺科医院院史馆。

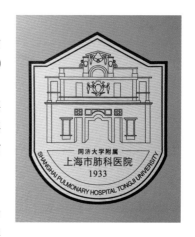

医院现占地面积10.1万平方米，建筑面积12.6万平方米。虽然上海肺科医院的规模比昔日扩大很多，但叶家花园仍是医院的重要组成部分。如今，椭圆形的花园由三个岛屿环绕而成，以亭桥相连，湖泊环绕，园中有树有花，景色迷人。虽然几经战乱变迁，景观已有改变，但仍然可以领略昔日海上名园的风采。

如今，自叶澄衷1862年开设五金小店已近一个半世纪之遥，他的慈善精神与许多中外人士的仁心匠心汇聚在美丽的叶家花园。在新时代里，叶家花园不仅得以留存，还得到科学的保护修缮，成为珍贵的海派建筑与园林瑰宝。而澄衷医院也发展为一家与昔日文脉相连的大型专科医院——上海肺科医院。这家以叶家花园为中心的新型现代医院环境宜人，疗愈无数病痛，为抗击新冠疫情做出贡献。这个上海故事，如此真实而动人。

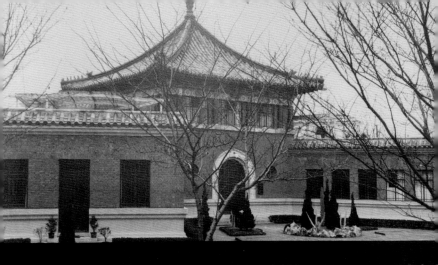

坎大利夫人纪念堂旧景(现11号楼)

The China Press published a report titled "Philanthropic Benefactor Donates Hospital to Care for City's Suffering" on June 8, 1933. Local businessman T. U. Yih (Ye Ziheng) donated the Yih's Garden to build a sanatorium.

"An important and praiseworthy piece of philanthropy for the welfare of citizens in Shanghai was revealed here yesterday in the donation of the famous Yih's Garden in Kiangwan by its owner. Mr T. U. Yih, prominent local businessman, for the purpose of an up-to-date hospital which will soon be erected in the garden to take special care of invalids suffering from tuberculosis and nerve

diseases as well as convalescents recovering from illness," the 1933 report said.

According to the newspaper, the garden near the Kiangwan Racecourse was recognized as the most beautiful Chinese garden in Shanghai. Occupying a spacious ground of more than 80 mow (53,360 square meters), the garden was worth about 1 million dollars.

The donor, Ye Ziheng was a well-known businessman/philanthropist and sports enthusiast, being one of the founders of the International Recreation Club which operated the former Kiangwan Racecourse. Ye inherited wealth from his father, Yih Ching-chong

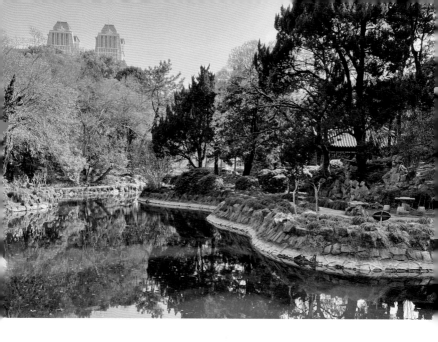

(Ye Chengzhong), a legendary Chinese tycoon from Ningpo who was noted in his day as a typical Chinese merchant with his word of promise more reliable than a written contract. The new hospital to be built in Yih's garden was named Ching Chong Medical Hospital in memory of the father.

Today, the century-old Yih's Garden is concealed in the depth of Shanghai Pulmonary Hospital on Zhengmin Road in north Shanghai's Yangpu District. Covering an area of around 40,000 square meters now, it's a stylish garden graced by Chinese and Western buildings, lake and bridges, flowers and green plants. The

history behind the tranquil garden is eventful. This East-meet-West garden is like a huge mirror that reflected incredible lives and stories of modern Shanghai.

According to the book *The Century-Old Famous Factories and Stores in Shanghai*, Ye Chengzhong, who was born to a poor family in Ningbo of Zhejiang Province, had a humble beginning in Shanghai by selling food to foreign sailors on a small boat.

In 1862 an American businessman hired Ye's boat for a ride but left behind a briefcase full of cash and valuables. Ye Chengzhong waited for a long time for the owner to return for the briefcase,

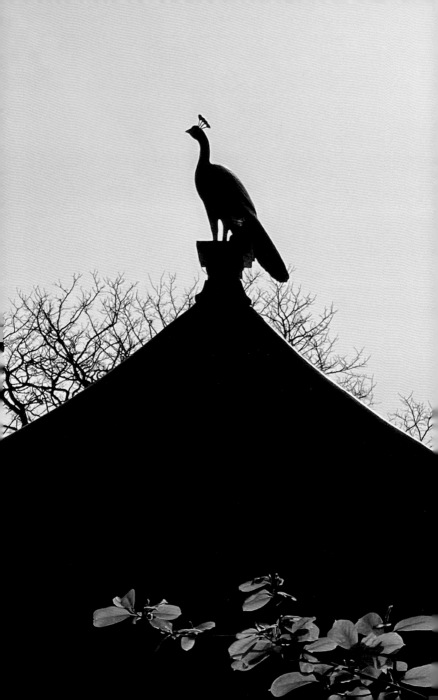

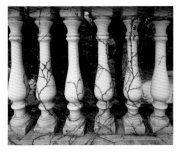
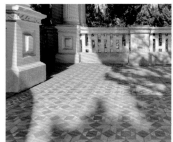

who was greatly touched by the young man's honesty and helped him open the city's first hardware shop. As Ye's hardware business boomed, he further expanded into areas of finance, industry and shipping before he died in 1899. The growing of Ye's business empire also echoed with the development of the Bund at the early stage.

As the fourth son of Ye Chengzhong, Ye Ziheng was well-educated and enamored of horse racing. But Shanghai Race Club denied his application to join as a member due to his Chinese identity. So the young man raised funds and bought an 800,000-square-meter farm in Jiangwan Town of north Shanghai to build a racecourse in 1908, which allowed the Chinese to be club members. The foreign-owned Shanghai Recreation Fund became a major shareholder.

Near the racecourse, Ye built the breathtakingly beautiful Yih's Garden in 1923 for the members to rest and relax. In 1933, Ye agreed to donate the garden to open a pulmonary sanatorium at the advice of famous medical educator Ye Fuqing, who said patients suffering from pulmonary tuberculosis needed a place for healing.

According to the 1933 report, the new hospital was composed of three units, namely, a tuberculosis sanitarium, a mental and nerve disease hospital and a convalescent home for general cases. The garden property was "admirably fitted" for all the three units of which the community was in great need. The hospital also served as a teaching hospital for Shanghai Medical College.

Although Ye's family had already left Shanghai, the garden is well preserved and still used by a pulmonary hospital. It was such a large and breathtakingly quiet garden with few visitors, a bit unreal in densely populated Shanghai.

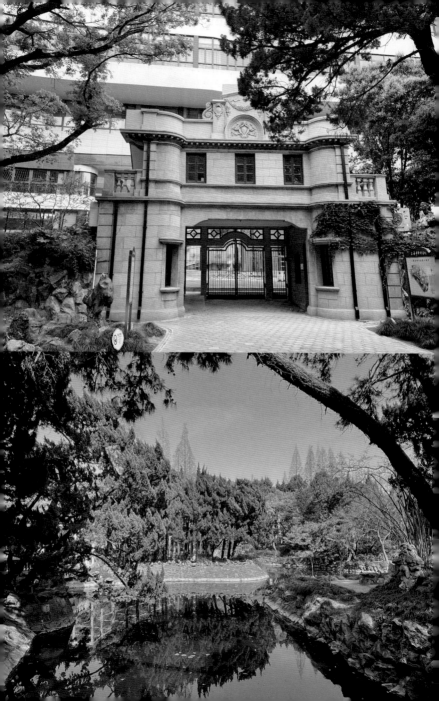

A mirror-like green lake was the centerpiece, which was dotted with small islands, a nice bridge and pavilions of all styles. Although full of Oriental ambience, the garden appeared to be designed in a simpler, cleaner style. In cloudy, chilly days, this oasis presented a Zen mood.

It was interesting wandering in the garden and sample Ye Chengzhong's life stories. Without a good heart from the start, the Ye's family may never have the opportunity to build a nice garden like this. In the depth of the garden stands a white classic western building, highlighted by an array of huge Ionic columns. The floors of the building were graced by beautiful mosaic tiles featuring different colors and patterns.

During the Sino-Japanese War, the garden was occupied by Japanese military forces and returned to Shanghai Medical College after the war ended in 1945.

After 1949, the hospital endured changes and developed to be Shanghai Pulmonary Hospital, a modern hospital integrating medical treatment, teaching and scientific research. In addition to its traditional advantages of tuberculosis and occupational diseases, the diagnosis and treatment of respiratory system diseases such as thoracic surgery, respiratory department and oncology of the hospital have also developed rapidly, including lung transplantation, lung tumor surgery and minimally invasive surgery, lung cancer diagnosis and pulmonary vascular treatment.

In recent years, the hospital restored Yih's Garden to its former glory. The white building was renovated to be a small museum to exhibit the history of the garden and hospital. After wars, turmoil and changes throughout the past century, the legendary garden remains in good shape. And as the wish of the Ye family, it is still used for pulmonary patients for a good breath.

Address: inside the Shanghai Pulmonary Hospital on 506 Zhengmin Road, Yangpu District.
Built in: 1923
Tips: You can walk into the garden. Enjoy a good breath and the tranquility.

江湾叶家花园捐充之

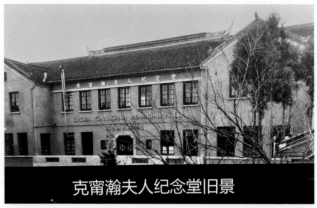

克甯瀚夫人纪念堂旧景

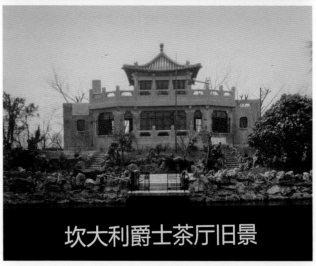

坎大利爵士茶厅旧景

　　江湾叶家花园，风景清幽，空气新鲜，宜于养病，经该援助——叶子衡先生捐充疗养院后，内部组织计分肺病、精神病及普通病三部分，定名为澄衷医院，以纪念园主之封翁叶澄衷先生。先设肺病疗养部，各项器械设备大致完全，并由美煤油大王罗氏基金董事会捐赠爱克司光镜，以便检查。精神病疗养部，特聘奥国专家医师主持其事，俟其到沪即可开办。至普通病疗养部，专收慢性勿药诸症，其性质与普通医院有别，因普通医院仅收急性及亚急性病症，一经治愈，即令出院，以便收纳其他病人。因都市人口繁盛，疾病盛时，各大医院往往供不应求，故疗养之设，一俟落成即可开办，其肺病疗养部，定于今日（十五日）开幕，收纳病人四十名，闻该院既为各界人士所赞助，自当组织董事会，以便管理，已在组织中，不日即可成立。"

摘自 1933 年第九期的《卫生杂志》

慈善家捐赠医院

迄今为止，还没有一家专门用于治疗肺结核病人的疗养院。一般而言，普通医院并非治疗肺部疾病的理想场所。对于肺结核患者来说，他们有特殊的需求，例如新鲜的空气、良好的环境和充足的阳光，而普通医院不容易具备这些条件。位于乡村地区的叶家花园却是结核病疗养院的理想地。

目前已经对疗养院的第一单元病房进行翻新并配备有40张病床，其中至少20张病床将免费提供给贫困患者。洛克菲勒基金会已经捐赠了1500两白银，用于购置一套X射线设备。而其他必要的设备（如透热疗法、气胸等）由卫生部和国立上海医学院等机构出借。

花园中众多的凉亭和建筑物现已变成病房，每个建筑自成一个单元，配有卧室、浴室、卫生间，都享有优美的风景。现在正在推进翻新工程，计划6月15日开始，第一个科室将接待所有类型的结核病患者，包括肺结核、颗粒状结核和骨结核。

摘自 1933 年 6 月 8 日《大陆报》

Philanthropic benefactor donates hospital to care for city's suffering

Up to present, there is not a single sanitarium specially devoted to the treatment of tuberculosis patients and generally the ordinary hospitals are not the ideal places for curing lung diseases. For sufferers from tuberculosis have their special needs, such as fresh air, good environment, and plenty of sunshine, which the ordinary hospitals do not find it easy to provide. The Yih's Garden, being in the rural district is therefore an ideal place for a tuberculosis sanitarium.

Steps have already been taken to renovate and equip the first unit of the sanitarium with 40 beds, 20 of which at least will be free for poor patients. The Rockefeller Foundation has already donated a sum of Tls 1,500 for the purchase of a set of X-ray apparatus, while other necessary equipment such as diathermy, pneumothorax, etc., have been loaned by such organizations as the National Health Administration and the National Medical College of Shanghai.

The numerous pavilions and buildings in the garden have now been turned into wards, each forming a unit by itself and equipped with bedroom, bath, toilet and commanding fine views. Renovation work is now being pushed and it is scheduled that this first unit will be ready to receive all types of tubercular patients, including pulmonary, granular and bone tuberculosis, on June 15.

Excerpt from *The China Press* on June 8, 1933

本市肺结核病防治院新厦落成 医疗设备完善已开始收容中度肺病患者

在江湾叶家花园的幽美环境里，市立肺结核病防治院新厦已经落成，并已开始收容病人。这是本市第一个专治肺病的设备完善的医院。它的前身是澄衷肺结核病防治院，本来只可容纳一百张病床，设备方面也很差，如开刀房、化验室、药房间都很小，特别是开刀间，只能动小手术，如遇需要进行肺截除术、切肋骨的严重肺病患者，都要转送上海医学院外科学院动手术。这次人民政府花了一百多亿元，建成适合于病人疗养的新厦，病床扩充到三百五十张，医疗器械设备也增加了许多，如大小X光机就有六架，大小手术室共有五间，同时又添聘肺科和胸腔外科专家多人，今后任何大手术都可以在院内进行了。

市立肺结核病防治院所收容的病人，是以享受公费医疗的国家工作人员和劳保工人为主。由于病床的限制，该院现阶段只能收容一些中度的急需住院治疗的肺病患者，一般住院疗养期间是三个月到六个月。因为严重的肺病人往往要住院疗养两三年才能痊愈，这在病床周转上就有困难，所以暂且不收。至于初期的肺病人，经医生诊断后，可以回家休养，市立肺结核病防治院经常派出公共卫生护士，到病人家里进行访问和指导。

住院的病人，每天除了接受医生护士的指导进行治疗外，生活是恬静的、舒适的。在每个散发着油漆和杉木混合香味的房间里，病人们有的倚枕欣赏画报和收音机中播送出来的令人神往的音乐，有的正在抚弄着琴弦。经过医生允许可以起床散步的病人，不仅有宽敞的休息室让他们做读报等集体活动，还可以漫步在池边林下，享受那和煦的阳光和清新的空气。那些别致的小亭子里，陈列着乐器和图书，让这些满怀着希望的病人更好地消磨养病的时日。

摘自 1953 年 1 月 15 日《文汇报》

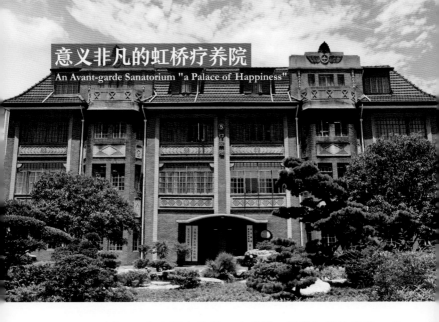

意义非凡的虹桥疗养院
An Avant-garde Sanatorium "a Palace of Happiness"

　　2019年，由中国文物学会、中国建筑学会联合主办的"第四批中国20世纪建筑遗产项目"公布。上海新增了七处国家级建筑遗产，其中一处就是上海虹桥疗养院。

　　这座历史建筑深藏于上海市淮海中路966号徐汇区中心医院内，其实它是著名的上海虹桥疗养院新址，而疗养院初建时的大楼也是列入中国建筑史的佳作。

　　上海医学史专家陆明提到，虹桥疗养院由丁惠康创办于1934年。医院原先位于上海虹桥路，是一所可容纳百余张病床的肺病

疗养院，后增加精神病科。疗养院的主楼是一幢四层阶梯状疗养式建筑，病房全部朝南，具有隔音条件，医疗设备为当时最新型。医院曾为上海医学院实习医院，1938年迁到霞飞路（今淮海中路）。

　　上海市徐汇区中心医院档案显示，医院创始人丁惠康于1904年出生于江苏无锡一个书香门第的医学之家。他的父亲丁福保（1863-1952）曾担任京师大学堂教授，作为全国医科考试优秀内科医士特派赴日本学习考察医学，回国后开办医学书局，编辑

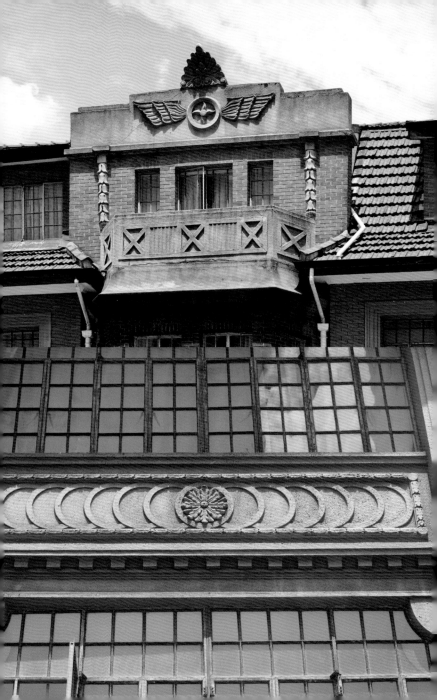

并发行医学业书目百余种。

1927年，丁惠康毕业于上海同济大学医科。当时正是结核病传播猖獗的年代，根据北平第一医学事务所1926—1931年的统计，肺结核是中国最致命的传染病。丁惠康的几位直系家属都因肺结核病丧失了生命，他下决心以防痨治痨作为自己的终身事业。

1928年，在父亲的支持下，丁惠康在大西路（今延安西路）2号创办了上海市肺病疗养院。1932年在此基础上，丁氏父子共同筹资30万元在虹桥路201号建造上海虹桥疗养院，于1934年6月17日隆重开业，中外宾客云集，上海市长吴铁城亲自为这座现代化的疗养院剪彩。

虹桥路201号

1934年6月20日，英文《北华捷报》（*The North-China Herald*）报道透露，吴铁城市长参观虹桥疗养院后"对出色的设备表现出明显的兴趣，对该院的设计表示赞同，这令每个患者都可以享受隐私"。

虹桥疗养院的开业典礼有中外宾客一千余人参加，轰动一时。疗养院的建筑设计一流：阶梯式楼房，每间病房均为向阳，有大幅玻璃窗，阳光可直晒到每张病床。病区内均有暖气，地板采用橡皮铺设，柔软舒适，降低噪音并可防滑。手术室的无影灯、冷气和病区其他设备都是当时最新型的。国立上海医学院院长颜福庆参观医院后对丁惠康说："我9次去过美国，国内各大医院足迹遍布，尚未见过比虹桥疗养院更好的医院。"丁惠康听之大为兴奋。

丁惠康之子丁大海在一次采访中回忆，他本人就在虹桥疗养院出生，当时医院吸引了众多名医，时常爆满。他说，父亲认为德国有当时世界上最先进的医院模式，所以请留德归来的中国建筑师奚福泉设计虹桥疗养院。

曾在德国德累斯顿工业大学学习建筑的奚福泉设计水平高超，患者在虹桥疗养院可以享受阳光、新鲜空气，同时保留个人隐私。这座现代、实用的钢筋混凝土建筑成为上海建筑史乃至中国建筑史上的标志性作品。

"奚福泉的作品受德国现代主义建筑影响，以现代建筑见长，注重功能，造型简洁。虹桥疗养院作为医疗建筑兼具实用、卫生、坚固、美观。"同济大学建筑系副教授刘刊评价道。

他研究发现，建筑师考虑到肺病患者接受阳光的重要性，设计将病房布置于南侧，手术室、X光室、太阳灯室和诊疗室等都位于北侧。每户前设阳台，层层退台方便病人随时接受阳光。阳台正好能放下2米长的病床，阳台还有雨棚，可以确保上层的人看不到下层的人，保护了病人隐私。

疗养院的顶层还有消遣娱乐用房，音乐室为病人提供钢琴、无线电，图书馆里有杂志和书籍可供借阅。在设计虹桥疗养院时，奚福泉受到德国建筑师理查德·多克尔（Richard Docker）的启发，后者于1926年在德国斯图加特用同样的退台式剖面概念设计过医院建筑。

"虹桥疗养院的建筑形式追随内部功能，没有任何与结构无关的装饰。这座建筑一建成便被看作是一座上海最具代表性的现代主义建筑。可惜在抗日战争中，大部分建筑被炸毁，仅留下入口部分，但也几乎不能辨识。"刘刊在《儋石之储：中国第一代建筑师奚福泉（1902—1983）》里写道。

同济大学伍江教授也认为奚福泉在设计虹桥疗养院时，不是从美观和装饰方面来设计，而是从建筑的功能方面来设计。

"需要太阳就有大玻璃，需要朝南就做台阶式，在上海近代建筑史上，这是少有的一幢真正按照现代主义思想理念去设计的一座现代建筑，而不仅仅是现代风格的建筑。所以它在中国近代建筑史上的地位很高。"伍江教授评价。

1935年，丁惠康赴德国、奥地利、瑞士三国考察，调研医疗制度和防痨工作，将考察收获编撰成《实验肺痨学》《各国肺痨统计》等书出版。丁惠康出国期间，颜福庆代理虹桥疗养院院长，并将疗养院作为国立上海医学院第二实习医院。

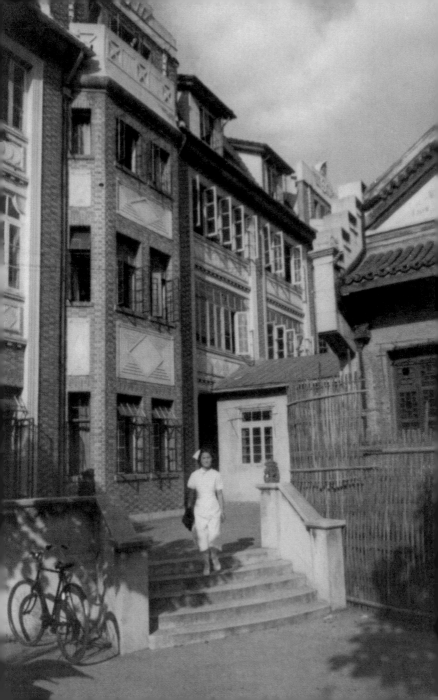

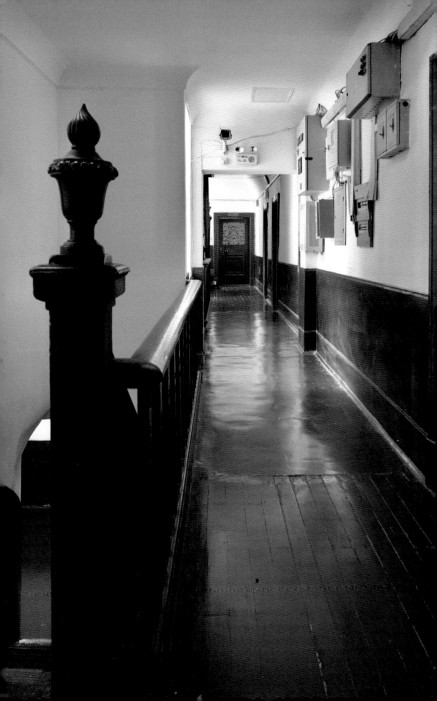

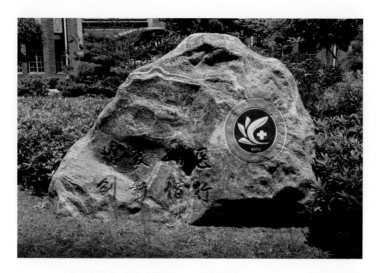

1936年丁惠康考察回国后兼任上医教授，继续坚持防痨事业，控制结核病的传播。他建议创设中国防痨协会，又利用新建成的五洲大药房（西藏路北京路口）举行大规模防痨宣传活动，展出肺结核病理标本、结核病胸片、显微镜下的结核菌等实物来教育市民，使参观者受益匪浅。他还亲自编写《肺病疗养法》《肺痨的预防》等宣传资料免费赠阅，制作各种防痨标语和幻灯片，同时还为近万人次免费做X光检查。

丁氏父子是中国防痨运动的先驱，为中国的防痨事业做出了积极贡献。在1937年再版的《肺病指南》，丁福保将虹桥疗养院形容为"幸福之宫"，"不仅为抵抗病魔之劲军，实为接近一切大自然之无上乐园，设计方面，于实用卫生，处处顾到，尤合于国人之习惯"。

不过就在那一年，虹桥疗养院因为抗战爆发而暂停营业。

淮海中路966号

1937年"八·一三"事变后，日军战火将这座"幸福之宫"毁于一旦。丁惠康将病人转移至永嘉路404号。1938年，他租借霞飞路990号住宅（今淮海中路966号）重新开办新虹桥疗养院，就是今天徐汇区中心医院的院址。

这座花园洋房占地10亩，建于20世纪20年代，原为一位英国侨民住宅，后来转卖给海上名绅叶鸿英。与虹桥疗养院现代感十足的老大楼相比，这座新院却是一座古典风格的建筑。清水砖墙的外立面装饰有大山花、凸窗和许多图案，顶部采用法国孟莎式屋顶。

伍江教授评价这是法租界里一座比较大规模的建筑，"不是完全传统的西方式样，看出来有英国风格，出现好多比较现代化的装饰，是混杂的风格"。

陈恒、张颖禾在《上海虹桥疗养院简史》一文中提到，虹桥疗养院迁址后规模已大幅缩小，床位减少至二三十张，租到占地14亩的霞飞路990号房产后床位恢复到六七十张。虹桥疗养院除了收治肺结核病人还配合中国防痨协会开展团体X线胸部检查业务，定期发布检查结果，提示结核病问题的严重性，引起社会广泛重视。

新虹桥疗养院花木葱翠，环境幽静，除原有肺科外，又增设内科、外科、妇科、儿科、骨科等科室。疗养院像以前一样聘用上海一流专家主持各科业务，如精神科粟宗华、心脏科董承琅、黄铭新、骨科屠开元、外科任廷桂、儿科宋杰、肺科刘德启、放射科陈惊伯、眼科郭秉宽以及林元英、黎相斌、夏其昌、林兆耆等知名专家。这些专家在虹桥疗养院挂牌诊治及亲自手术，大大提升了医院的知名度。1949年初民盟领导人张澜和罗隆基曾在此"养病"，后被成功营救。

1956年，虹桥疗养院成为一家公立医院，后来历经几次更名，1961年成为上海市徐汇区中心医院。2020年，医院成为上海首家获得互联网医院牌照的公立医院，成为一家提供远程医疗服务的云医院，为患者带来福音。

昨天： 新虹桥疗养院　**今天：** 上海市徐汇区中心医院　**地址：** 淮海中路 966 号
建造年代： 20 世纪 20 年代

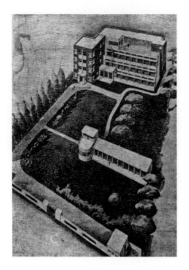

The classic building in Shanghai Xuhui Hospital was listed as an important monument of 20th century architectural heritage by the Chinese Society of Cultural Heritage.

Hidden deep in the hospital compound on 996 Huaihai Road, the building once served as a new site of the famous Hongqiao Sanatorium.

Known as "Hongjiao Sanatorium" in the 1930s, the original site on Hongqiao Road was also significant in the history of Shanghai architecture.

"The sanatorium founded in 1934, on Hongqiao Road by Dr. Ding Huikang was a 100-bed hospital for patients who suffered from tuberculosis," said medical historian Lu Min from Shanghai No. 4 People's Hospital. "The main building was a four-story structure that had south facing wards which were all soundproofed".

"The sanatorium, which boasted to have the latest medical equipment of its time, moved to Huaihai Road after the Japanese invaded China in 1937," he said.

Xuhui Hospital archives reveal Ding was born into a family of intellectuals from Wuxi of Jiangsu Province, in 1904. His father Ding Fubao, who had studied medicine in Japan, published hundreds of medical books.

Ding Huikang graduated from Tongji Medical College in 1927, a time when TB was an epidemic in China. After several of Ding's family died from the disease, the young medical graduate was determined to devote his life to relieve the pains of TB patients.

In 1928, he opened Shanghai Sanatorium for Lung Disease on No. 2 Great Western Road (today's Yan'an Road W.) with support from his father. While based at the hospital, the Dings raised funds to open Shanghai Hongqiao Sanatorium on 202 Hongqiao Road on June 17, 1934. The opening ceremony invited some

1,000 foreign and Chinese guests, including Shanghai mayor Wu Tiecheng.

The old sanatorium

A report in *the North-China Herald* on June 20, 1934, revealed the mayor inspected the building and displayed "evident interest in the splendid equipment provided and commenting with approval upon the planning of the institution which has made it possible for every patient to enjoy privacy".

Patients could enjoy privacy, sunlight and fresh air thanks to the excellent design work of Chinese architect Fonzien G. Ede (Xi Fuquan), who had studied architecture in Germany. The modern, functional steel-and-concrete structure became a signature work in Shanghai architectural history.

"Xi Fuquan's work was influenced by German modernism architecture that values function and features simply-cut forms. As medical architecture, it's practical, hygienic, solid and beautiful," Liu Kan, an architectural scholar from Tongji University said.

Liu's research found that the architect attached great importance to sunlight in treating patients with lung problems. He arranged all the wards on the south side of the hospital and the oper-

ation room, X-ray room and clinic rooms on the north side. The wards were equipped with balconies. made it easier for patients to enjoy the sunlight at any time of the day. The top floor featured a music room with a piano and a library for patients to enjoy. Xi was inspired by German architect Richard Docker, who had designed a similar medical building in Stuttgart of Germany in 1926.

"The form of Hongqiao Sanatorium follows the requirements of its interior functions. There were no decorations unrelated to the structure. The building was regarded as the most representative of modernism architecture in Shanghai after its completion," Liu said.

Tongji University vice president Wu Jiang also agreed the architect designed the building to be functional, instead of an unfunctional aesthetically beautiful construction.

"He designed large windows and the terraced structure to introduce more sunlight. It was not only a modern-style building, it was a rare building in modern Shanghai architectural history that was truly designed according to the conception of modernism. So it had a very high status even in modern Chinese architectural history. It's a pity the building was demolished during the Chinese War of Resistance against Japanese Aggression," Wu said.

In 1935, Ding Huikang went to Germany, Austria and Switzerland to investigate the medical system and anti-tuberculosis work. He compiled the survey data into books like *Experimental Tuberculosis* and *Statistics of Tuberculosis in Various Countries*. During his inspection abroad, Dr. Yan Fuqing acted as the dean of Hongqiao Sanatorium, which served as the second practice hospital of Shanghai Medical College.

In 1936, Ding returned to China to be an active advocator and promoter of China's anti-tuberculosis movement. In the large-scale anti-tuberculosis publicity campaign he conducted, Ding exhibited TB pathological specimens and bacteria under a microscope to introduce to the disease to the public, which was fatal among Chinese.

Ding also compiled various free publicity materials, launched a city-wide free X-ray physical examination activity and treated poor patients free of charge.

In his book *The Guide of Lung Diseases*, Ding Huikang called this sanatorium "a palace of happiness".

"This sanatorium is not only a strong army to fight with the evils of diseases, it's an ultimate paradise close to great nature. In terms of design, it's functional, hygienic, considerate and adapts to Chinese habits," Ding wrote in the 1937 book.

However in the same year, the hospital was forced to cease operation because of World War II. The sanatorium moved to 404 Route Herve de Sieyes (today's Yongjia Road) and later to 990 Avenue Joffre (today's Huaihai Road M.), which is the compound of Xuhui Hospital today.

The new sanatorium

The garden villa that served for the new Hongqiao Sanatorium was built for a British resident in the 1920s and sold to Chinese merchant Ye Hongying afterwards. Ding rented the building from Ye to relocate the sanatorium in 1938.

Compared with the simply-cut modern building on Hongqiao Road, the sanatorium's new home is a more classic architectural building with three floors. The facade is graced by two patterned gables, Mansard windows, large windows, protruding windows and a rainbow of decorative patterns.

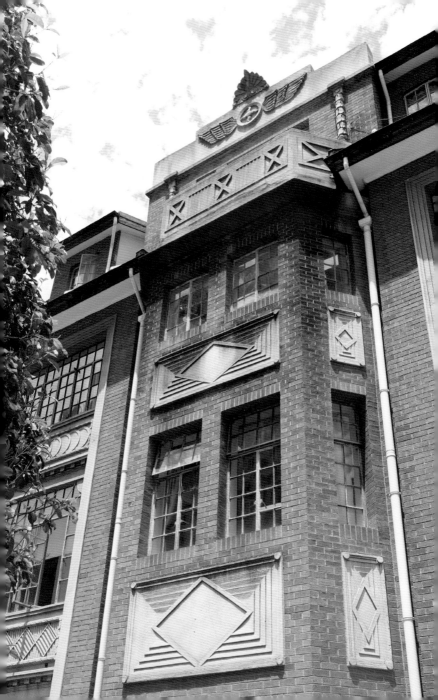

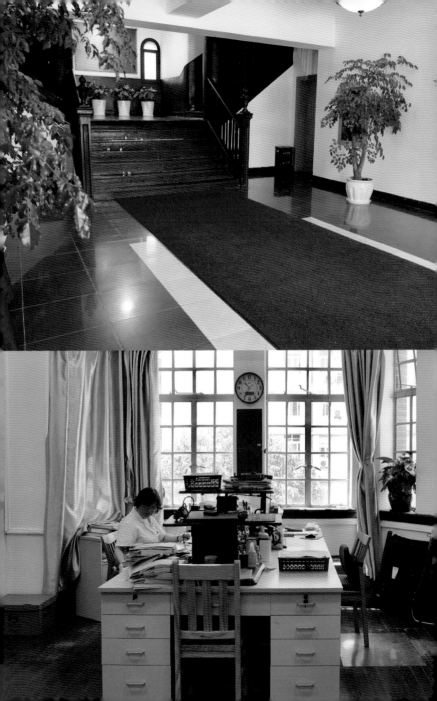

"It was a building of a comparatively large scale in the former French concession. The building was not in a traditional Western style. It reveals a British or mixed style. There are more modern decorations on this building," Wu said.

In their co-authored article, "A Short History of Shanghai Hongqiao Sanatorium," Chen Heng and Zhang Yinghe wrote that the new sanatorium saw a shrinking scale at first with only 20 to 30 beds. Later on the number of beds increased to 60 to 70. In addition to treating TB patients, the sanatorium also conducted group X-ray examinations and released examination results regularly to raise the awareness of the disease.

Covering an area of 66,700 square meters, the new sanatorium is fronted with a quiet garden of lush flowers and trees. In addition to the original pulmonary department, there were additional departments for internal medicine, surgery, gynecology, pediatrics and orthopedics. The sanatorium employed the city's top medical experts to preside over the treatments of various subjects and the hospital won plaudits for its work.

The sanatorium became a public hospital in 1956, renamed Hongqiao Hospital in 1957 and renamed again to be Huaihai Hospital in 1958. In 1961, it became Shanghai Xuhui District Central Hospital.

A hospital attached to Shanghai Zhongshan Hospital today, it was granted the city's first Internet hospital license for a public hospital to be a "cloud hospital" with online inquiries and appointments. During the COVID-19 outbreak, the former sanatorium building served as a 24-hour consulting platform to answer calls from patients who had a fever and suspected symptoms.

Yesterday: a new site of Hongqiao Sanatorium   **Today:** Shanghai Xuhui Hospital
Address: 966 Huaihai Road M.   **Built in:** the 1920s   **Architectural style:** British style

新疗养院提供远离疾病的避风港

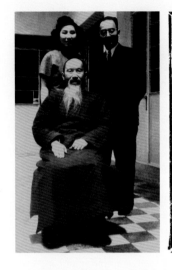

　　供应茶水和点心时，招待会上的所有人都度过了愉快的时光。现场来宾们被带领参观了这座宏伟的疗养院大楼的不同区域。

　　新疗养院代表了上海迄今为止最新、最先进的医疗机构。疗养院远离城市的喧嚣，周围环绕着虹桥路的小农场和菜园，是病人和那些想要安宁和休憩的人的天堂。

　　大约一年半前，新疗养院的建筑设计最初是来自德国留学回国的奚福泉博士构思。该建筑包括卫生和供暖设施的总成本约为 13万美元，加上室内陈设和医疗设备，该项目的总成本约为20万美元。

摘自 1934 年 6 月 18 日《大陆报》

New sanatorium provides safe haven from disease

A delightful time was had by all present at the reception when tea and other refreshments were served. Guests present were led in an inspection of the different parts of the imposing sanatorium building.

The new sanatorium represents the latest and most up-to-date medical institutions Shanghai has yet seen. Situated far from the hustle and bustle of the city and surrounded by small farms and vegetable gardens on Hungjiao Road, the sanatorium will be haven for the ill and for those who want peace and rest.

Architectural design for the new sanatorium was first conceived about 1 year and half ago by Dr. Fonzien G. Ede, a returning student from Germany. The total cost of the building, with sanitation and heating facilities, is approximately US$130,000 while the interior furnishings and medical equipment bring the total cost of the project to approximately US$200,000.

Excerpt from *The China Press* on June 18, 1934

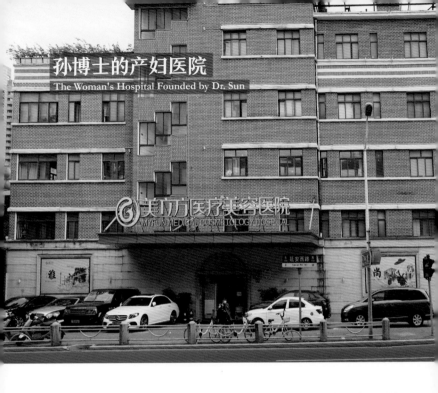

孙博士的产妇医院
The Woman's Hospital Founded by Dr. Sun

1935年，美国约翰霍普金斯大学医学博士孙克基在上海开办了上海妇孺医院。这家产妇医院英文名叫"Woman's Hospital"，仅有11张床位。孙博士是唯一的医生，但他的精湛医术很快为产妇医院赢得声誉。

如今，孙博士的产妇医院已发展为有相当规模的上海市长宁区妇幼保健院。昔日产妇医院的建筑犹存，这座位于延安西路934号的红砖小楼由同样留美归来的中国建筑师庄俊设计，是被列入上海建筑史的经典之作。

孙克基和庄俊虽然专业不同，但他们的人生道路有相似之处。

孙克基(1892—1968)是湖南湘潭人，1922年获美国约翰霍普金斯大学医学博士学位，毕业后留校担任助教及住院医师。他曾在妇产科期刊发表《人类子宫肌肉的自然收缩规律》和《骨盆狭窄及处理》等论文，还赴英、法、德、奥等国深造，在瑞典肿瘤医院进修妇科肿瘤镭锭疗法。1926年孙克基回国，在湖南湘雅医学院任教，又先后担任武昌同仁医院妇产科主任和苏州阊门妇女医院院长，1928年担任上海医学院妇产科教授及中国红十字会总医院妇产科主任。1935年，他创办中国首家妇产科专科医院——上海妇孺医院，并担任院长。

设计妇孺医院的庄俊（1888—1990）是中国最早的建筑界留学生之一，曾在美国伊利诺大学和哥伦比亚大学研究生院学习。1925年，庄俊在上海开设了私人事务所，成为最早在上海开业的中国建筑师之一。1927年，庄俊与范文照、吕彦直等共同发起成立了上海建筑师学会，1928年改称中国建筑师学会，庄俊担任第一任会长。

根据同济大学伍江教授的研究，庄俊早期的作品为西方复古风格，如1928年建成的金城银行（今江西中路200号交通银行）。四年后他设计了位于南京路的大陆商场（又名慈淑大楼），建筑风格发生了重大转变，建筑形象趋于简洁，复古装饰被彻底摒弃，立面上采用了大量装饰艺术派风格的图案。1935年，他设计的孙克基妇产科医院已成为"国际式"，此时他已推崇"能普及而又切实用"的现代建筑。

这座现代风格的医院建筑高达6层，为钢筋混凝土框架结构，建筑面积为3128平方米。红砖立面被白色线条分割，底层、走廊和楼梯均铺设彩色马赛克地砖。

同济大学郑时龄院士在新版《上海近代建筑风格》中写道，这家产妇医院完全从使用功能出发进行布局。

"底层中央门厅两侧一边是门诊、检查化验及药房等，左边则是厨房、餐室、洗衣、锅炉等辅助用房；二三层全部为病房；四层一侧也是病房，另一侧则为手术、分娩、消毒及婴儿室等。底层外墙采用芝麻石饰面，二层以上贴泰山面砖，立面的处理强调水平向。建筑造型完全摒弃装饰而表现出简洁实用的'国际

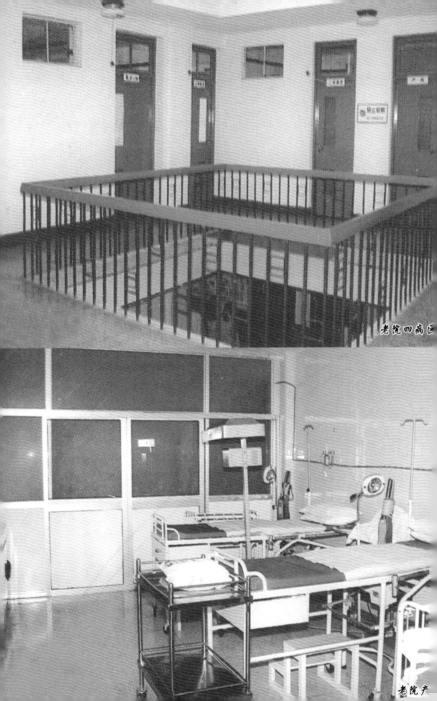

老院四病区

老院产

式'风格。"郑院士写道。

他认为，从1928年的金城银行到1932年的慈淑大楼，再到1935年的孙克基产妇医院，庄俊完成从新古典主义到现代建筑的转变，也只有七八年的时间。

另一位学者曹汝平则认为，孙克基产妇医院是一个里程碑式的建筑作品，"它标志着庄俊设计师事务所正式迈入现代主义建筑设计的大门"。

"孙克基产妇医院的建筑外部造型上，已经具备了许多现代主义设计的'极简'元素；内部的走道隔墙采用空心砖砌筑，以达到良好的隔音目的；病房的地面则铺设树胶块毡，这就从墙体构造和材料两方面降低了噪声干扰。如此处理，自然让人联想到'形式追随功能'（Form Follows Function）的口号式宣言。"曹汝平在《庄俊建筑师事务所的设计美学观探微》一文中写道。

他评价，庄俊设计的产妇医院与留德归来的建筑师奚福泉设计的上海虹桥疗养院（已拆除），都是现代主义设计在中国落地后产生的一批成果。

"这批公共建筑的出现，既是西方现代主义设计在中国的回响，同时也为'海派建筑'增添了经济、适用、卫生、简洁、不求奢华的清新格调。从社会功能上，这一设计观体现出的，正是可贵的对人民大众的社会关怀。"他评价道。

除了现代设计，孙博士的产妇医院使用了当时最先进的医疗设备，其中多数是孙克基自费从美国购置带回的。

长宁区妇幼保健院档案显示，孙博士为医院制定了一套严格的管理规定。他的医术高超，手术精巧，术后求"不发热、不输血、不使用抗生素"，减少病人痛苦及经济负担。正因如此，红色小楼开业伊始就是一家忙碌的产妇医院。

1935年2月6日的《北华捷报》（the North-China Herald）刊登简讯，波尔夫妇（Mr. and Mrs. G. V. Ball）的女儿于1月29日在大西路（今延安西路）妇孺医院出生，此时距医院正式开业仅一个多星期。医院

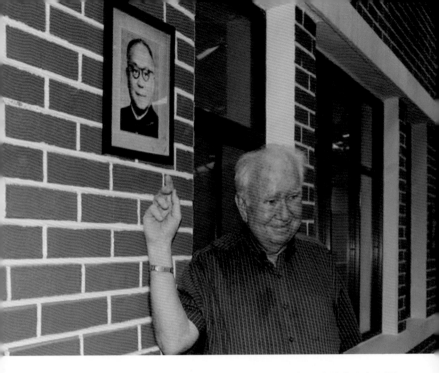

的病人还包括陈毅夫人张茜和宋子文夫人等社会名流。

2014年，美国著名植物学家、美国科学院院士、中科院外籍院士雷文（Peter Raven）造访了红色小楼。他在2021年出版的自传*Driven by Nature*中写道，1936年6月13日一个闷热的夜晚他出生于这家产妇医院，由孙克基博士亲自接生，后来一家人与孙博士成了好朋友。雷文家族档案中至今仍保存着几张珍贵的照片，微笑的孙博士或抱着还是男婴的雷文，或站在产妇医院简洁现代的大门前。

孙博士讲究礼仪规范，曾要求医院的医务人员在白大褂里也要穿西装打领带。如今，长妇婴延续了这项传统，每周一为全院"着装日"，医院工作人员要打领带或系丝巾。

创办产妇医院后，孙博士持续地钻研学习专业知识。他很早就已进行镭锭放射治疗子宫颈癌手术，后来从国外带回大批医疗器械和镭锭、巴氏染色法染料、

RH标准血清，在国内推广巴氏染色法普查宫颈癌，使用RH血清诊断母子RH血型不符的新生儿溶血症。1947年，他再度赴美国、瑞典、丹麦及法国讲学考察，在美国妇产科年会上宣读重要论文。

由于孙克基在妇产科领域采取先进的治疗手段，加上他重视医德医风建设，他创办的产妇医院在上海医学界享有盛名。

1956年，孙克基自费五万元人民币将住院部大楼整修一新，连同院内一切设备无偿献给国家。他自己仍担任院长，亲自示范手术带教青年医生，还举办了上海市妇产科主治医师进修班，为中华人民共和国培养了很多杰出的产科医生。

1949年后，设计孙克基产妇医院的庄俊也到国营设计机构工作，担任上海华东建筑设计院总工程师，同样培养了一批优秀的建筑师。

1985年9月22日，《解放日报》刊文报道200多位建筑师集会祝贺庄俊从事设计、教学工作七十周年。建筑学会赠送给庄俊一枚镌刻"建筑泰斗"的印章。

而这位泰斗也以长寿而闻名，1990年去世时享年102岁。

不过，人生轨迹曾经相似的孙博士没有如此幸运。由于"左"的影响，1958年，孙克基被错误批判为上海医学界四大"白旗"之一，"文革"后又遭迫害，于1968年2月12日含冤去世。十一届三中全会后，孙博士得到平反，1986年长宁区有关部门举行了孙克基医师诞辰九十四周年纪念会。

值得欣慰的是，孙博士的产妇医院历经多次更名与合并，发展为上海重点产科医院之一，1993年更名为现在的"上海市长宁区妇幼保健院"。医院一直在庄俊设计的红砖小楼运营，直到2002年。

方文莉院长介绍，2003年，长妇婴是全国首家实施水中分娩的医院，被国际水中分娩协会列为永久会员单位，如今已有一万多个成功案例。

2002年，长妇婴从延安路红砖小楼迁到武夷路，昔日的小楼现由一家医美机构使用。由于医

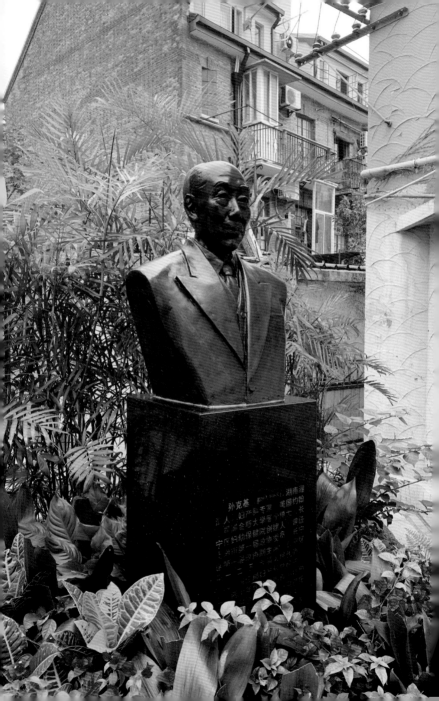

孙克基 (1895-1957)，湖南湘
人，妇产科专家，美国约翰
斯·霍普金斯大学医学博士。曾任
宁区妇幼保健院创建人、主任
州市第一届妇协会委员、妇科
妇第一届妇协副主任

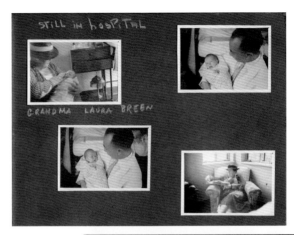

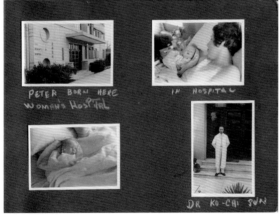

院业务增长的需求，长妇婴对武夷路院区进行扩建，过渡时期医院临时在愚园路运行。

虽是临时办公，医院仍把创始人孙克基的雕塑安放于门前醒目位置。这座雕塑正如老照片上抱着新生儿的孙博士，整洁精干，穿西服、打领带。

昨天：上海妇孺医院　**今天：**美立方　**地址：**延安西路 934 号　**建筑风格：**国际式
建筑师：庄俊　**参观指南：**可在延安路欣赏建筑简洁现代的立面

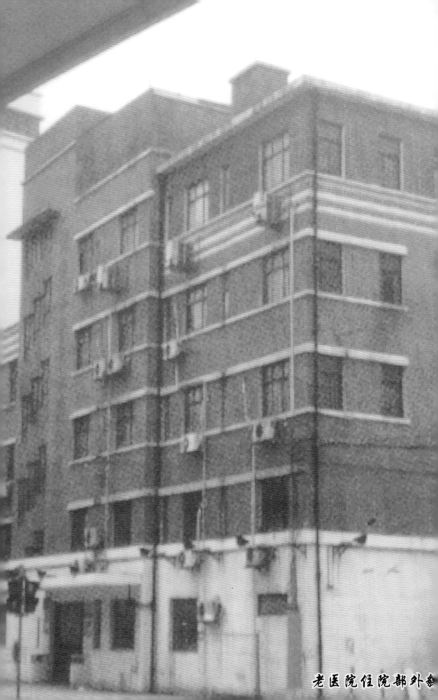

老医院住院部外观

Two of Shanghai's most distinguished figures joined hands in the early 20th century to construct a pioneering hospital dedicated to women. The idea of such a hospital was inspired by the death of one of their mothers. It is a fitting legacy to both men that the hospital still survives today.

Situated on 934 Yan'an Road W., the red-brick building was a collaboration between a Chinese doctor and a Chinese architect, both of whom where dedicated to bringing modernity to Shanghai in the 1930s.

The "Woman's Hospital," designed by architect Zhuang Jun for Sun Keji, a gynecology and obstetrics doctor, established a medical center for the welfare of women.

"Our hospital has been caring for women and children since its founding year of 1935," says Fang Wenli, director of the hospital, which was the first to conduct a water birth in Shanghai.

Hospital archives reveal it was founded as the "Woman's Hospital" by Dr Sun Keji at 105 Great Western Road, today's 934 Yan'an Road W. The hospital officially opened on January 17, 1935 and Dr Sun was its first director.

Born in Hunan Province in 1892, Dr. Sun went to study gynecology and obstetrics in the John Hopkins University in the United States in 1922. He chose this major because his mother died while giving birth to him.

Talented and hard-working, Sun became one of the favorite students of Dr. John Whitridge Williams, famed founder of academic obstetrics in the United States. Williams wrote the first obstetric book, the Williams Obstetrics textbook. After graduation, Dr. Sun could have remained and practised in the US but he decided to return to his motherland, a country which lacked doctors for women.

He taught at the Hsiang-Ya Medical College in Changsha of Hunan Province and Shanghai Medical College from 1926. He also headed the gynecology and obstetrics department of the Chinese Red Cross General Hospital, which is Huashan Hospital today.

In 1935, he obtained a site on the Great Western Road and commissioned Zhuang Jun to design a new private hospital for women.

Zhuang Jun and Dr. Sun's experiences mirrored each other, only in different fields.

Born in 1888, Zhuang went to study architecture at Illinois and Columbia universities in the US and established his own design studio in Shanghai in 1925. Among the Chinese architects active in old Shanghai, Zhuang was the first to study overseas and the first to return home to practice architectural design in China. In 1928 he founded the Society of Chinese architects to unite Chinese designers in a competitive market with foreign architects.

According to a study of Tongji University vice president Wu Jiang, Zhuang initially preferred a Western classical style, such as his noteworthy work, the Kincheng Bank (today's Bank of Communications on 200 Jiangxi Road M.). His skills allowed him to compete with first-class Western architects of the same period. But his later work, the Continental Emporium on Nanjing Road, marked a change of style, on which Zhuang thoroughly abandoned classical decoration, adapted Art Deco patterns and opted for a simple-cut appearance.

Zhuang's later work, the "Woman's Hospital" for Sun Keji, showcased a more modern "international style".

Covering an area of 3,128 square meters, the new hospital was a steel-and-concrete structure of six stories. The red-brick facade is divided by white horizontal lines. The building is adorned by steel gates and windows. The ground floor, the corridor and the staircases were paved with colorful mosaic tiles. The rooms were decorated with dados made of ceramic tiles.

In the new edition of *The Evolution of Shanghai Architecture in Modern Times*, Tongji University professor Zheng Shiling noted that the layout of the hospital is completely based on the emphasis of functions.

The central lobby on the ground floor is flanked by outpatient clinics, clinical lab and dispensary on one side and auxiliary rooms such as the kitchen, dining room, laundry, and boiler on the other side. The second and third floors are all wards. The fourth floor had wards as well as rooms for surgery, childbirth, disinfection and babies.

The outer wall of the ground floor is decorated with sesame stone while the upper floors are covered with Taishan bricks.

"The architectural form completely abandons decoration and presents a simple and practical international style. From the Kincheng Bank in 1928 to the Cishu Building (Continental Emporium) in 1932, to the Sun Keji Woman's Hospital in 1935, it took only seven or eight years for

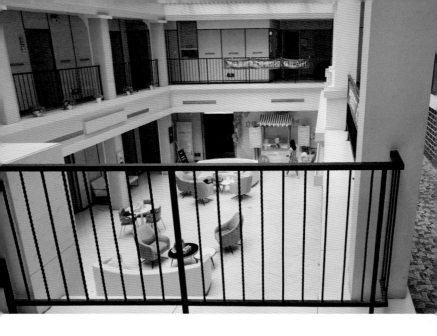

Zhuang Jun to complete the transition from neoclassical to modern architecture," Zheng's review noted.

Another scholar named Cao Ruping regarded the hospital "a milestone architectural work" and added that "Zhuang's firm officially entered the gateway of modern architectural design".

According to Cao's research, Zhuang published an article to expound on modernist architectural design of "Chinese architects" in September 1935, the same year of the hospital's opening.

"The outlook of the woman's hospital has many of the simplest elements of modernism design. Inside, the partition walls of the corridors are built with hollow bricks and the floors of the wards are paved with rubber mats for good sound insulation. The architect's treatment reminds of 'form follows function', a principle of modern architecture," Cao wrote in his article named "On the Design Aesthetics Concept of Zhuangjun Architects".

"Both the 'Woman's Hospital' by Zhuang Jun and the Hongqiao Sanatorium by Xi Fuquan are fruits of modernism design arriving in China. These public buildings are not only echoes of Western modernist design in China, but also add a fresh touch of eco-

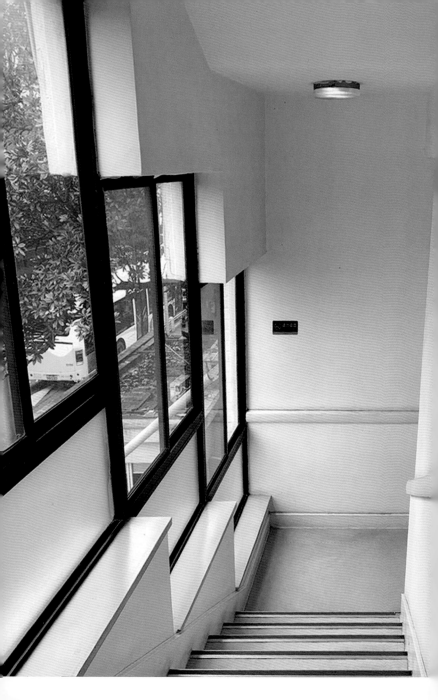

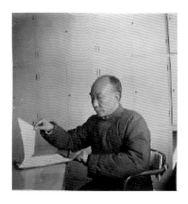

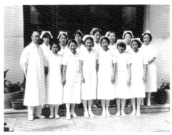

nomic, functional, hygienic and simple-cut to Shanghai buildings," Cao reviewed.

In addition to modern design, the hospital was well equipped with state-of-the-art medical equipment, some of which were purchased in the US by Dr. Sun.

The hospital started with only 11 beds and 20 medical workers, including 11 nurses, while Dr. Sun was the only doctor.

Hospital archives reveal that Dr. Sun made a set of strict regulations to manage the hospital. He was also reputed for his exquisite medical skills. His surgery was so refined and scientific that he reduced damages to minimum. He was renowned for operating without fever, blood transfusion and antibiotics.

The red-brick hospital was busy and well received from the beginning.

According to *the North-China Herald* on February 6, 1935, a daughter of Mr and Mrs G. V. Ball was born in the Woman's Hospital on Great Western Road on January 29, 1935, only more than a week after the official founding.

Among the hospital's famous patients were Zhang Qian, wife of Chen Yi, Shanghai's first mayor after 1949 and the wife of T. V. Soong, minister of finance of the Kuomintang government. During a special visit to the red-brick building in 2014, famous American botanist Peter Ravan said he was delivered by Dr. Sun in 1936 in this hospital.

"He required medical staff to wear a suit and ties inside a doctor's white overall. Our hospital inherited this tradition and designated Monday as our 'dressing day' for wearing ties and scarves," said Ai Min, director of administrative office of the hospital.

After founding the private hospital, Dr. Sun continued to study medicine tirelessly. In 1947, he went to the US, Sweden, Denmark and France to give lectures and inspected other hospitals and studied gynecological tumor radium therapy at a Swedish Cancer Hospital.

And he brought home a large number of medical equipment, radium ingots, reagents and serum. He promoted pap staining in China to screen for cervical cancer and used serum to diagnose hemolysis of newborns with inconsistent mother and child RH Blood System types.

After 1949, Dr. Sun became an obstetrics and gynecology consultant of the Shanghai Municipal Health Bureau. In 1956, he renovated the red-brick hospital and dedicated it to the government. Dr. Sun still served as director of the new public hospital where he enjoyed a reputation for his high rigorous academic style and superb medical skills. He had unique insight into the diagnosis of infertility and the pathological development of cervical cancer. He also trained a number of physicians and laid the foundation for the development of obstetrics and gynecology.

While Dr. Sun dedicated his private hospital to China, Zhuang Jun, who designed his hospital, became chief engineer of the state-owned East China Architectural Design Firm after 1949. Zhuang also trained a number of young architects.

A news report in *Jiefang Daily* on September 22, 1985, revealed more than 200 architects gathered to celebrate Zhuang's 70 years' career in architectural design and education. He was given a stamp engraved with "architectural maestro" by the Architectural Society of Shanghai. Zhuang was also famous for his longevity, and he managed to live to a grand old age of 102.

Compared with the architectural maestro, Dr. Sun was less fortunate. He died in 1968 during the "Cultural Revolution" (1966—1976), but his medical legacy lives on.

After several mergers and name changes, the "Woman's Hospital" got its present name C. N. Maternity & Infant Health Hospital in 1993 and operated in the red-brick building until 2002. Today it's one of Shanghai's leading maternity hospitals.

"Our hospital was the first to conduct a water birth in Shanghai to alleviate birth pains and now we have more than 10,000 successful cases," said director Fang.

In 2002, the hospital moved

from the red-brick building on Yan'an Road to Wuyi Road. Today the building is used by the Myfun Medical Cosmetology Hospital.

During the expansion and renovation of the Wuyi Road compound, the C. N. Maternity & Infant Health Hospital temporarily operated in a smaller place on Yuyuan Road.

But every time the hospital moved it took the statue of Dr. Sun Keji with it, attired in a suit and a tie.

Yesterday: The Woman's Hospital (Dr. Sun's)　**Today:** Myfun Medical Cosmetology Hospital
Address: 934 Yan'an Road W.　**Architectural style:** Modern style　**Architect:** Zhuang Jun
Tips: The facade can be admired on Yan'an Road.

长宁区妇幼保健院见闻

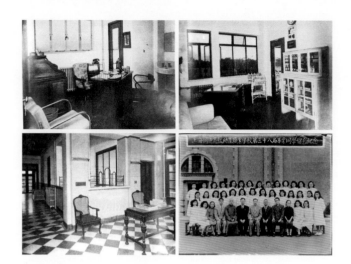

　　如今，在本市的各家产院，几乎都能见到"母婴同室"房。最近，笔者在全国三优（优生优育优教）试点单位——长宁区妇幼保健院采访，亲眼见到这家医院正在硬件和软件两个方面，积极为提高母乳喂养的比例创造条件。这家由著名妇产科专家孙克基博士创办的医院，经过修缮，如今的硬件称得上全市一流。一间间母婴同室房雅致幽静，各种规格的房间满足不同层次产妇的需要。一二等房配有空调、彩电、电话、沙发及进口配套床。丈夫可日夜在内陪伴自己的妻子和孩子，充满一派温馨的家庭气氛；三等房和普通房除床位较多、家属不能日夜陪伴外，与一二等房享受同样的优质服务。护士小姐笑容可掬地为每一位产妇洗脸、擦身、洗脚、喂饭，指导正确的母乳喂养方法，搀扶上厕所，为婴儿换尿布，还一遍又一遍地巡视察看，生怕产妇熟睡后，在一旁小床上躺着的婴儿会发生吐奶等现象，这一切服务都是免费的。在这样的环境中，原先对母乳喂养有畏惧和厌烦心态的年轻妈妈们，都显得心平气和、精神爽朗。

　　目前，从本市各区和外省市慕名到这家医院登记生产的孕妇络绎不绝，医护人员们说，我们将一如既往尽心尽职，因为我们的服务关系着两代人的健康。

摘自 1993 年 12 月 29 日《解放日报》

我国建筑界泰斗庄俊昨庆百岁华诞

　　昨天，上海欧美同学会给被誉为我国建筑界泰斗的庄俊举行了百岁寿庆活动，庄俊的87岁的学生介绍了庄老先生在建筑界"三个全国第一"的业绩。

　　祝寿活动在庄俊居住处举行。这所住宅是他当年亲手设计的。装饰简朴的客厅，被红烛、花篮和大蛋糕点缀得满室生辉。坐在轮椅上的庄俊虽然刚从医院回家，却仍显得神采奕奕。

　　追随庄俊多年的学生、原民用建筑设计院院长陈植，昨天向大家介绍他的老师的三个全国第一：1914年在美国获建筑工程学士学位，是我国第一个接受西方建筑教育的建筑师；1924年，在上海开设了庄俊建筑师事务所，成为中国第一个挂牌营业的建筑师；1950年，庄老第一个放弃经营25年之久的事务所，联合50多名同行来到北京，被交通部华北建筑工程公司任命为首都第一个国营建筑单位的总工程师。

　　庄老从事建筑设计70多年来，门下究竟有多少弟子？陈植说：徒子徒孙不计其数。这句话赢得满堂笑声。

摘自 1987 年 10 月 18 日《文汇报》

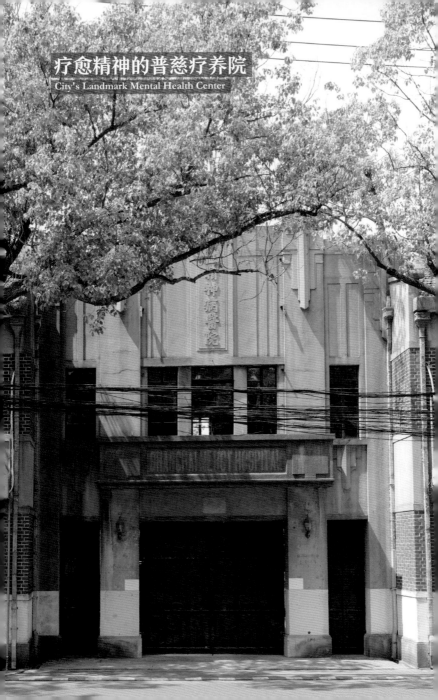

疗愈精神的普慈疗养院
City's Landmark Mental Health Center

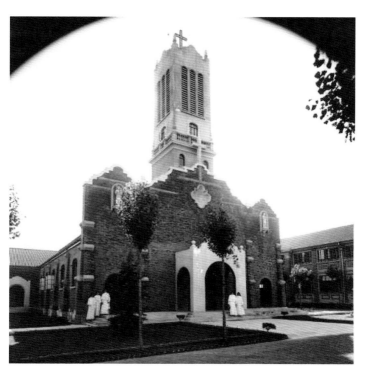

上海精神卫生中心的前身——普慈疗养院（Shanghai Mercy Hospital for Nervous Diseases）建于1935年，曾是远东最大、设备最完善的精神科专科医院之一。乡村田园风的院区今日犹存，一座座红砖历史建筑点缀其间，环境幽美。

同济大学建筑系钱宗灏教授介绍，普慈疗养院是由近代中国知名实业家、慈善家、天主教人士陆伯鸿集资创办并担任首任院长，收治精神疾病患者，设有300至400张床位，日常院务由天主教神职人员负责管理。疗养院原址现在是上海市精神卫生中心闵行院区，每一栋建筑依照原先的设计正常使用，是上海市文物保护单位。

普慈疗养院开张之际，1935年7月3日英文《北华捷报》（the North-China Herald）报道称，"中国在其长长的现代化医疗机构名单中又增加了一家。这次是专门为观察和治疗神经系统疾病而建造的医院"。

此前，陆伯鸿开办过收治精神病人的新普育堂。但他发现精神病人多而疯癫部的床位少，很多病患流落街头遭受歧视，因此决心建设一座更大、更专业的精神病治疗机构。1934年，他以教会的名义向社会募资购地百亩建造普慈疗养院，1935年启用。疗养院位于沪闵公路北桥与颛桥之间，总建筑面积约3万平方米。除了8幢病房，另有3幢院务职员用房、水塔和一座小教堂。

1935 年 6 月 29 日，普慈疗养院举行了隆重典礼，庆祝正式开业。大约1000 名政府官员、医疗界领袖和中外天主教传教士出席，陆伯鸿亲自主持仪式。

报道提到，当天的天空呈铅灰色，看起来肯定下雨，但巧的是雨水到仪式结束才落下。很多尊贵的客人前来参观疗养院建筑，并在其中一个俯瞰花园的露台上参加茶会。

普慈疗养院的八栋建筑占地约66.7万平方米，可入住600名患者。此外，还有几座用于治疗的建筑、实验室、行政办公室和宿舍。疗养院由Messrs. Yao Tze-ti 事务所在精神病学专家的指导下建造，拥有先进的精神疾病治疗设备，设有理疗科、水疗科、职业治疗科等。医院的一部分专门用于上海国立医学院教学使用。

"这些建筑由红砖和混凝土建成，带有红瓦屋顶，舒适地矗立于宜人的乡村背景中。它们彼此间隔一定的距离，中间是花园，精心种植着富有装饰效果的灌木和花卉。昨天，这些房子都以许多颜色的旗帜装点，花园里也喜庆地挂满了彩旗。"1935年6月30日英文《大陆报》（The China Press）报道写到。

开幕当天，宾客涌入建筑内部，欣赏到了许多不同寻常的建筑特色。来宾们对每层楼都带有阳光明媚的长阳台印象深刻，对很多宽敞的单人间也感兴趣。

"这家机构在中国是一种创新，因为以前没有这样规模的精神病院。它将治疗与研究相结合，很大一部分将用于深入研究，这将在国立上海医学院的指导下运作。"《大陆报》报道。

1935年的报道还提到陆伯鸿的努力，称他为打造一流精神病院的梦想无私地付出努力。开幕典礼时，他表现出"平静而谦虚的喜悦，朴素地表达了满足和自豪"。

上海宗教史专家、复旦大学教授李天纲认为，陆伯鸿是上海近代史上的重要人物。

"他出生于南市的一个天主教家庭，家族受徐光启的影响而皈依天主教。陆伯鸿擅长与法国人做生意，创办了多个公司、宗教机构和慈善项目。"李天纲说。

陆伯鸿曾任闸北水电公司、上海华商电气公司、大通仁记航业公司、和兴码头堆栈公司、新和兴铁厂、浦东电气公司、上海内地自来水公司董事长或董事，1927年当选上海法租界最早的5位华人董事之一。

意大利建筑历史学者卢卡·彭切里尼（Luca Poncellini）在《邬达克》一书中写道，陆伯鸿运营着一个庞大的慈善捐赠网络，同时还在上海的商业活动中发挥着关键作用。

"陆伯鸿天生有种本事，能在上海经济与政治生活的利益网络中如鱼得水，这些网络部分是公开的，部分则是秘密的，隐藏在操控这个城市的秘密群体背后。"他评价道。

根据钱宗灏教授的研究，在旧址大门面东，保存有原门诊楼、第三至第十病房楼和一栋原为教堂的10栋历史建筑。建筑砖混结构，风格统一，清水红砖外墙夹饰水刷石毛条块，墙垛之间开钢窗。院区花园西南角有一座刻有中英文题记的墓碑，那是外籍传教士、上海普慈疗养院白景明院长的墓葬。

在1935年的开幕典礼上，有人指出上海很重视公共卫生问题，但对神经和精神疾病的关注太少。上海有许多新医院，但却没有专门治疗精神病患者的医院。上海普慈疗养院将会尽力满足这一需求。

奥地利籍精神病专家韩芬(Dr. Fanny G. Halpern)在典礼上

的发言提到，许多神经和精神疾病不得不在私人家中治疗，必须要改变环境了。她指出，只要提供足够的设备，许多病例是可以治愈的，而预防性精神病学应该是这个项目的主要内容。

韩芬曾在享有精神病学盛名的维也纳大学医学院学习。维大名师如云，有以《梦的解析》为精神分析学奠基的弗洛伊德（Sigmund Freud，1856—1939）、获诺贝尔医学奖的精神病学专家尧雷格（Julius Wagner-Jauregg，1857—1940）等。韩芬是尧雷格的得意门生，毕业后在母校任教，1933年应邀来华，先后在国立上海医学院（上海医科大学前身，后并入复旦大学）和上海圣约翰大学任教，是上海精神病学的先驱。她培育了很多精神病学人才，同时还在红十字会总院（今华山医院）、中山医院、公济医院（今上海市第一人民医院）、同仁医院、仁济医院等上海各大医院兼职担任神经科主任。

普慈疗养院的建立，是上海精神病学史上的创举，疗养院筹建过程中得到这位世界顶尖级精神病专家的大力支持。韩芬教授任普慈疗养院医务主任，医术精湛，富有才干。许步曾所著的《寻访犹太人：犹太文化精英在上海》一书提到，在中华医学会于1935年广州举行的会议上，韩芬的论文从医学、社会、法律的角度提出了中国精神病学存在的问题和解决方案。与会者专门成立了一个委员会来研究这些问题，如需要在中国建立精神病学机构，将其从收容疯人的病院类型转变成现代化的医疗精神；实行预防精神疾病和促进心理卫生的措施等。委员会由来自中国各地的专家组成，以颜福庆为主席，韩芬为干事，这是中国精神病学历史上的重要大事。

普慈疗养院开张后，在《申报》刊登广告，称医院聘请中外专家医护人员担任诊治护理，专治"文痴武痴、神经衰弱、精神萎顿、产后成疯、杨梅疯症、各种疯病、新法戒烟、用脑过度、疗治休养"。

1937年抗战爆发后，普慈疗养院设立了伤兵医院和难民所。

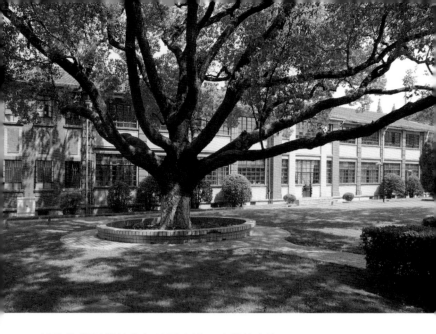

医院的德国籍神父与日军交涉周旋，最终确保了医院的正常运行。战后医院又获得联合国善后救济总署和中国天主教福利会的资助。国共内战中，国民党军队撤离上海之前炸毁了医院的水塔和教堂钟楼。

1952年，普慈疗养院由上海市军管会接管，更名为上海市立精神病院，由著名精神病学家粟宗华担任院长。后来，私立虹桥疗养院的精神科、中国疯人医院、复生医院、清心医院和上海精神病疗养院等私立精神病疗养院和疗养院的精神科先后并入市立精神病院。

经过80多年的发展，昔日普慈疗养院已发展为中国最大的精神卫生医疗机构——上海精神卫生中心，担负着全市精神卫生的医疗、教学、科研、预防、康复、心理咨询与治疗和对外学术交流等任务，是全国规模最大、业务种类最全、领衔学科最多的精神卫生机构。2006年5月，上海市精神卫生中心成为上海交通大学医学院附属医院，总部位于宛平路，旧址为闵行院区。

与昔日作为上海国立医学院教学医院一样，上海精神卫生中

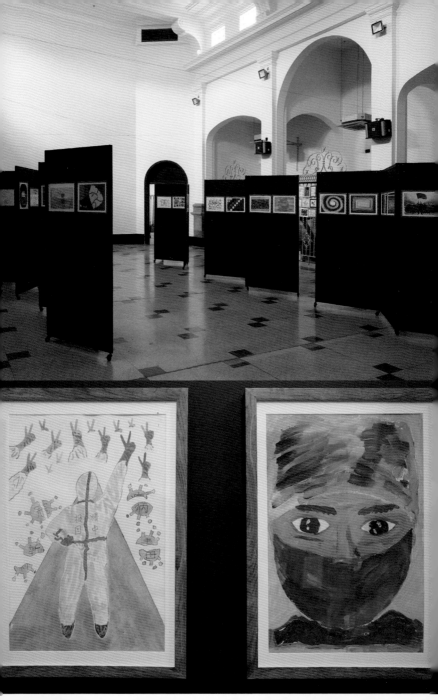

心也是上海交通大学医学院和复旦大学上海医学院等多家医学院的教学医院，同时也是上海师范大学、华东师范大学的心理学教学研究与实践基地。作为WHO精神卫生研究与培训合作中心之一，中心与世界各国的精神医学界进行学术交流与科研合作。

如今，昔日普慈疗养院的建筑遗存大多保留完好，院区草木繁盛，相当静美。闵行院区收治1400多名需要长期住院的患者，如阿尔茨海默症病人。与建院初期相比，治疗精神疾病的药物和方法越来越多。在历史悠久的红砖教堂里，病情较稳定的患者通过绘画、阅读和冥想来治疗。教堂里会展示患者创作的艺术作品。

新冠疫情爆发后，上海精神卫生中心担负着全社会的心理工作，为整个社会缓解焦虑情绪，普及心理健康。1935年普慈疗养院开幕时，媒体曾经称赞，"这是一个致力于人道主义的仪式，标志着一个美好的开端"。

昨天： 普慈疗养院　**今天：** 上海市精神卫生中心闵行分院
地址： 闵行区颛桥镇沪闵路 3210 号　**建造年代：** 1935 年　**建筑风格：** 现代风格
建筑师： Yao Tze-ti Architect Co.　**参观指南：** 在沪闵路可以欣赏到医院大门的历史立面

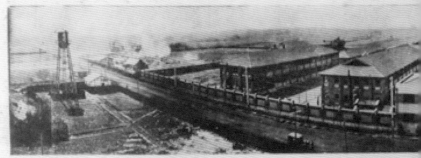

VUE GÉNÉRALE DE
慈 全 院

Shanghai Mental Health Center celebrated its 85th anniversary on September 6,2020 with a grand ceremony that mirrored its opening in 1935.

Established as Shanghai Mercy Hospital for Nervous Diseases, the center was then known as the largest mental hospital in the Far East.

"The hospital was founded to treat patients with mental illness by Lu Bohong (Lo Pa-hong), a well-known Chinese industrialist, philanthropist and Catholic who was the first director. Now the former site serves as the Minhang hospital of Shanghai Mental Health Center. Most buildings are well preserved and used according to the original design. It is a historical and cultural heritage site protected at the municipal level," said Tongji University professor Qian Zonghao, an expert of Shanghai architectural history.

When the hospital opened in 1935, *the North-China Herald* reported that "China has added on more modern health institution to her already lengthening list".

"This time, it is a specially built hospital for the observation and treatment of nervous diseases," the paper reported on July 3, 1935.

The institution celebrated its official opening with a grand ceremony on June 29, 1935. Around 1,000 persons, representing civic officials, leaders in various medical fields, missionaries of Catholic orders and both foreign and Chinese, assembled outside the hospital. Lu Bohong presided over the ceremony.

A leaden sky promised rain for the occasion, but it happened that "this promise was not fulfilled un-

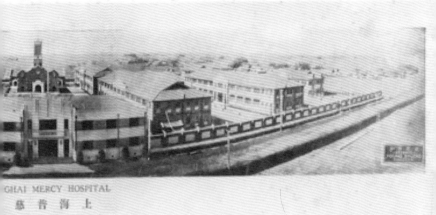

GHAI MERCY HOSPITAL
慈普海上

til the ceremonies were well over". Many distinguished guests came to see the buildings and attend a reception of tea on one of the terraces overlooking the garden.

The hospital's eight buildings occupied about 667,000 square meters of land to offer accommodation to 600 patients. In addition, there were several buildings for therapeutic purposes, laboratories, administration offices and dormitories. The hospital was built by Messrs. Yao Tze-ti Architect Co. under the supervision of experts for psychiatry. It had state-of-the-art equipment for the treatment of mental diseases, with departments for physiotherapy, hydrotherapy and occupational-therapy etc. A part of the hospital was devoted to teaching for the National Medical College of Shanghai.

"The buildings themselves are of red brick and concrete, with red-tile roofs and sit comfortably against the background of the pleasant countryside. They are spaced at some distance from each other. In between there are gardens carefully planted with decorative shrubs and flowers. Yesterday the buildings were decorated with flags of many colors, and the gardens were festive with bunting," *The China Press* reported on June 30, 1935.

During the opening day, guests surged through the interiors of the structure, admired the many unusual features and were impressed with the long and sunny verandas that lined the buildings on every story. They were also interested in the spaciousness of the numerous private rooms.

"This institution is something

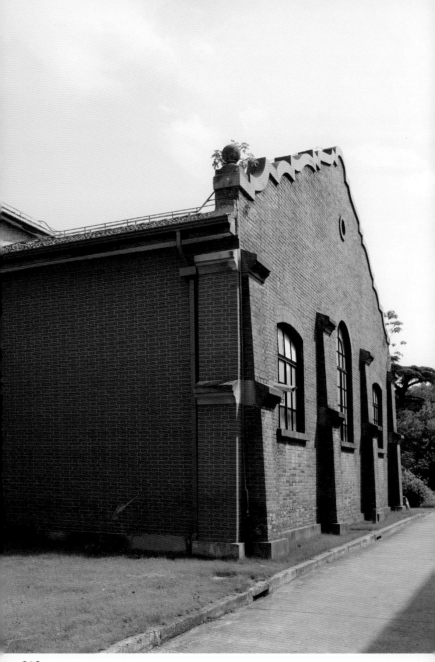

of an innovation in China, for at no previous time has there been a mental hospital built in this scale. It combines treatment with research. A large section has been reserved for intensive study. This will be operated under the direction of the National Medical College," the newspaper reported.

The 1935 report also introduced the efforts of Lu who had "worked unselfishly for his dream of a first class institution of this sort".

"His quiet and modest pleasure at what he saw yesterday spoke plainly of his satisfaction and pride," the newspaper said.

Fudan University professor Li Tiangang has called Lu "a famous figure in the modern history of Shanghai".

"Lu's family was influenced by Xu Guangqi, a Ming Dynasty (1368—1644) minister whom Xujiahui was named after, to convert to Christianity. Adept at doing businesses with the French, Lu founded a galaxy of companies, religious institutions and philanthropic projects," Li said.

According to Professor Qian's research, a rainbow of 10 original buildings including the former outpatient building, No. 3 to No. 10 wards and a chapel are still preserved today.

"The buildings are all brick-concrete structures in a uniformed style. The red-brick external walls are graced by granitic plaster sticks. Steel windows are opened between the wall stacks," he said.

During the 1935 ceremony, it was pointed out that much attention had been paid to the problem of public health in Shanghai, but that far too little consideration had been given to nervous and mental diseases. There had been many new hospitals but there had been none, especially for the treatment of psychopathic cases. The Shanghai Mercy Hospital for Nervous Diseases would do much to satisfy this need.

Dr. Fanny G. Halpern, medical director of Shanghai Mercy Hospital, said many nervous and mental cases had to be treated in private homes when a change of environment would seem almost a necessity. She pointed out that many cases were curable, provided adequate facilities were offered. She added that preventative psychiatry should be a major part of its program.

Graduated from medical school at the University of Vienna, Dr. Halpern had worked with Nobel laureate psychiatrist Julius Wagner-Jauregg and several other no-

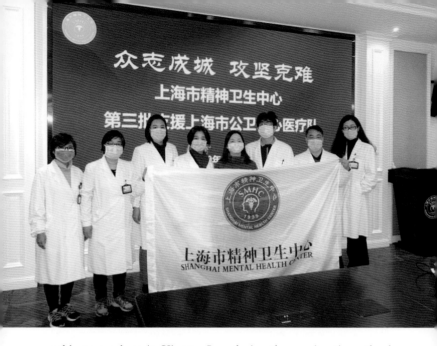

table researchers in Vienna. In 1933, she was invited by Dr. Yan Fuqing, the president of the National Medical College of Shanghai, to work as a professor of psychiatry and neurology. She had made contributions in the field of mental hygiene in Shanghai through teaching students and treating patients in a rainbow of big Shanghai hospitals. The Mercy Hospital received a great support from this top expert of mental hygiene.

"After the war broke out in 1937, a hospital for wounded soldiers and a refugee center was established here, which continued to operate in a normal way

during the warring times thanks to a German priest of the hospital who negotiated with the Japanese army. After the war, the hospital received funding from the United Nations Relief and Rehabilitation Administration and the Chinese Catholic Welfare Association. But during the civil war, the water tower and bell tower of the chapel here were blown up by the Kuomintang troops," Qian added.

After 1949, Shanghai Military Management Committee took over the hospital in 1952 and renamed it Shanghai Municipal Mental Hospital. Famous Chinese psychiatrist Su Zonghua was in charge of the hospital which merged with the city's other private mental hospitals.

After 85 years' development, the hospital has become China's largest medical institution of mental health that incorporated medical care, medical education, scientific research, preventative psychiatry, therapy and psychiatric consulting. In 2006, it became a hospital attached to the Shanghai Jiao Tong University Medical College.

Today, Shanghai Mental Health Center is headquartered on Wanping Road S. The former site serves as its Minhang Hospital.

The Minhang hospital received patients who needed to stay for a longer period of time, such as those who suffered from Alzheimer's dementia. With the most cutting-edge medical facilities and technologies, the hospital treats some 1,400 patients now.

Compared with the 1930s, there has been more medicines and treatments for mental diseases. In the former red-brick chapel, the center offers therapies from painting and reading to meditation for patients who are in a more stable condition. Artworks created by these patients grace the interiors of the chapel. Some artworks vividly showed medical workers' fight with the COVID-19 virus.

And in the center's 85 years' celebration, Shi Jianrong, deputy Party secretary of Shanghai Jiao Tong University Medical College, specially praised Shanghai Medical Health Center's contribution.

"After the outbreak of the COVID-19 epidemic, it is responsible for the mental health of Shanghai's residents, alleviating anxiety for the whole society, and popularizing the knowledge of mental health," she said.

Back to 1935, the opening ceremony of this institution was admired as a notable event for "it was an occasion dedicated to humanitarianism. It marked an excellent beginning".

Yesterday: Shanghai Mercy Hospital for Nervous Diseases
Today: Shanghai Mental Health Center, Minhang Hospital   **Address:** 3210 Humin Road
Built in: 1935   **Architectural style:** Modern style
Architect: Messrs. Yao Tze-ti Architect Co.
Tips: The facade of the hospital entrance can be admired on Humin Road.

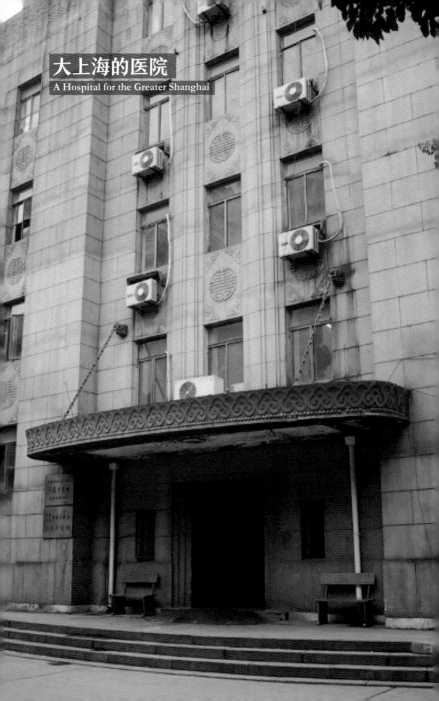

大上海的医院

A Hospital for the Greater Shanghai

1929年，上海发布了历史第一个城市规划方案："大上海计划"，拟在江湾建造由九座公共建筑组成的新城。建筑师董大酉（Dayu Doon）设计的市府大楼、市立图书馆和市立博物馆均为大屋顶的中国古典复兴风格，但他却为市立医院采用了简洁的现代风格。

20世纪30年代，这些"大上海计划"的建筑纷纷落成，大多幸存至今，坐落于城市东北角的杨浦区（原江湾区）。昔日的上海市立医院现为长海医院"中心楼"。大楼于1935年建成，1936年竣工，1937年投入使用，医院附近还建了一座上海市立卫生试验所。

1935年1月3日，英文《大陆报》（The China Press）报道了市立医院和卫生试验所的奠基仪式。

"上海市政府公共建筑的扩建又迈出了一步，新的市立医院和卫生试验所是未来上海医学中心首批兴建的建筑，周二由大上海特别市市长吴铁城奠基。"《大陆报》报道。

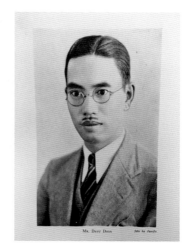

MR. DAYU DOON   foto by Junshi

市立医院兴建中的1935年，董大酉在"大上海 大视野"（Greater Shanghai Greater Vision）一文中提到，当时的上海由公共租界、法租界和华界组成，这三个区域在没有任何先行规划的情况下自由生长，导致这座城市的"现状"无法满足时代的发展要求。于是，"大上海计划"启动，拟建设一批具有现代便利设施的中式建筑作为新的市政中心。

"20世纪20年代开始，民国政府提倡复兴中国传统文化，要求董大酉将这些政治性的建筑设计为西式结构，但要加入中国传

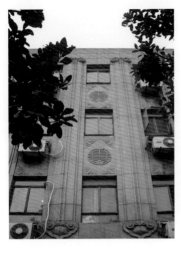
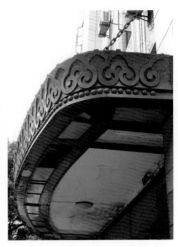

统元素。"研究中国近代建筑师的同济大学钱锋教授说。

董大酉设计的旧上海特别市府大楼（现上海体育学院行政楼）是一座钢筋混凝土建筑，却宛若一座清代宫殿，覆盖着琉璃瓦大屋顶，入口是壮观的大红木门，外墙装饰有精美的传统图案。市立图书馆（现杨浦区图书馆）和市立博物馆（现长海医院影像楼）也都是这种被学界称为"中国古典复兴"的风格。

钱锋教授提到，董大酉的自宅是一座有着平顶和水平栏杆的双层住宅，风格极其现代。而上海市立医院也是一座风格"极其

现代"的建筑，与其他"大上海计划"建筑的画风不同。

根据《大陆报》报道，市立医院工程原计划是建设一个"扇形布置"的医疗中心建筑群，包含2所内科病院、2所外科病院、1所妇产科、1所儿科、1个门诊部及五官科病院、1间护士学校及宿舍和1座行政楼及医学院。

"扇形布置"方案最终脱颖而出，是因为放射状分布的建筑能最大限度地获得空气和阳光。行政楼位于扇形建筑群的中心，两侧是分别是门诊部和护士学校及宿舍。从行政楼辐射出6个不同的单元，所有病房都设置在这

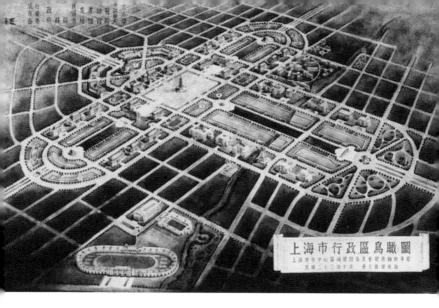

6个单元中。每个病房单元的长边大致面向东或向西，南侧保留给日间休息室（day room）。建筑物之间的梯形区域是供康复期病人使用的花园。服务区位于地块的西南上风角，可以消除烟雾等污染物对医院的侵扰。

由于缺乏资金，先建造9座建筑中的行政楼及医学院。1937年1月4日，行政楼作为一家综合医院——上海市立医院，开业门诊。

市立医院大楼是一座钢筋混凝土结构，外墙为人造石，长264英尺，宽52英尺，占地11,400平方英尺，建筑面积48,600平方英尺。建筑中部高达五层，两翼为四层，配备两部大型电梯，有150到200张床位。

浅灰色外立面设计为简洁明快的现代风格，但装饰有祥云和如意等中式纹样。门厅地砖上是红十字和拆分的繁体字"卫生"组成的纹饰，十分切题，引人注目。同期建造的上海市立卫生试验所的外墙也雕刻着"卫生"纹饰，而地砖纹饰是显微镜，也很呼应试验所研制疫苗的功能。

"建筑外观是设计的直接表达，设计方案与市府在新城建造的其他建筑物的气质相符合。

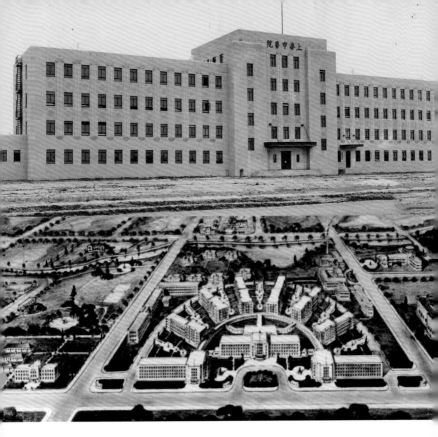

典型的中式风格不适合医院建筑，因为成本较高，而且浪费空间。"建筑师董大酉在"New Shanghai"（新上海）一文中解释市立医院的设计思路。

《大陆报》报道也提到，建筑师虽然选择了现代风格，但发现可以使用中式装饰赋予现代建筑中国特色，同时满足现代医院的所有要求。

"建筑内部简单而庄重。所用建材与世界上最好的医院使用的材料一致，用最少的空间浪费来进行规划，并为所有必要的工程新应用提供足够空间，确保经济的舒适的供暖。"董大酉在文章里介绍。

建筑学者许乙弘在《Art Deco的源与流》一书中评价，随着摩登风格在上海的迅速兴起，董大酉开始将中国古典主义风格与某些Art Deco（装饰艺术派）的手法结合起来。1934年建造的博物馆和图书馆虽然延续了复古主义风格，但墙面比较简洁，浮雕装饰趋于几何。一年后建成的上海市体育场（江湾体育场）、上海市体育馆（江湾体育馆）和上海市游泳池（江湾游泳池）中，他采用充满现代感的摩登风格，同时保留中国古典的元素作为装饰题材。此后，董大酉设计的飞机楼、市立医院和卫生试验所都是典型的Art Deco风格，他的摩登设计手法也愈发娴熟。

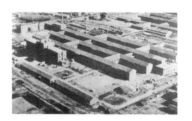

市立医院的设计科学，设备先进。内部隔断多为木板条，走廊沿线的墙壁使用空心瓷砖。木板条隔板可以很容易地拆除和重新布置，而不会对地板、墙壁或天花板造成太大损坏。病房地面使用沥青砖，大堂、手术室和其他杂物间的地面则铺设水磨石。

医院各层功能布置紧凑。地下室是锅炉、电气和机械设备房。一楼设有入口大厅、行政办公室、X光室和门诊部。入口大厅周围是接待室、问讯处和电梯大堂，还有急诊和药房等。

二楼为外科和手术室，男子病房和女子病房分别设在东西翼，均有杂物间、服务厨房、床单室、护士站、浴室和厕所等配套设施。普通病房配有5至10张床位，此外还提供单间和半双人房。靠近电梯大厅有1间教室、1间小实验室和1间带宽敞阳台的日间休息室。考虑到经济因素，手术室成对布置，均朝北。手术室的墙壁和地板根据外科医生的要求，分别用青灰色瓷砖和同色水磨石铺设。

三楼设有儿童小间病房和隔离病房、产科病房、婴儿房、早产儿保育室等。四楼是男女内科。五楼是厨房，煤炭和食材通过电梯从地下室运上来，烹饪好的食物通过两台升降机送至不同楼层的服务厨房和备餐室。

整个建筑虽然规划紧凑，但

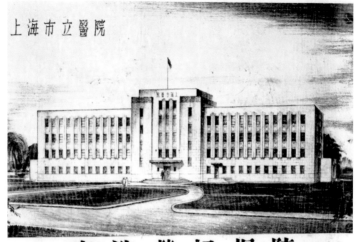
为所有基本功能都提供了足够的空间。建筑平面布局的流线合理，能以最少的路线提供方便高效的服务。

市立医院工程的原计划是将综合医院发展为融研究、教学和治疗为一体的现代医疗机构，但1937年"八·一三"淞沪会战的爆发永远打断了"大上海计划"。最终，"扇形医院

302

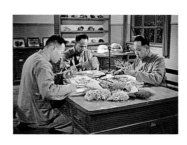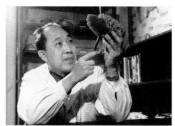

建筑群"只建成了9座建筑的一座——市立医院大楼。侵华日军将市立医院扩建为日本陆军病院，成为抗战期间日军收治伤病员最大的中转场所。1945年日本投降后，国民党政府接管日本陆军病院，成立联勤第二总医院，1946年又在此建国防医学院。

1949年5月上海解放后，华东军区接管原联勤第二总医院和国防医学院，组建华东军区人民医学院附属医院，就是今天长海医院的前身。1949年后，大楼曾作为病房和机关办公使用，1956年按原有建筑风格加建一层，如今为肾脏病诊疗单元。被誉为"中国肝胆外科之父"的吴孟超院士等多位医界泰斗都在这座历史丰厚的大楼里工作过。

回望历史，"大上海计划"是一个理念先进的科学规划，描绘了一个新的大都市蓝图，包括道路系统、港口铁路和行政、商业和居住区域。在杨浦区的很多地方，都有"大上海计划"留下的印记。

如今，昔日的市立医院大楼矗立在长海医院偌大的院区中，与院里其他几座"大上海"建筑——市立博物馆（影像楼）、飞机楼（校史馆）、卫生试验所（卫勤楼）交相辉映。简洁的立面上，窗间墙壁强调竖向线条，祥云如意点缀其间，默默诉说着"大上海"建筑师的匠心。

昨天：上海市立医院　**今天**：长海医院"中心楼"　**建造年代**：1936
建筑风格：现代主义风格　**建筑师**：董大西
参观指南：大楼对住院病人开放。也可以参观董大西的其他作品：中国古典复兴风格的原上海市立图书馆（现杨浦区图书馆）和武康路40号西班牙式别墅。

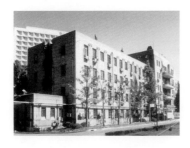

Shanghai released its first-ever urban planning scheme, "the Greater Shanghai Plan" in 1929 to build a new Civic Center of nine proposed buildings. Chief architect Dong Dayou (Dayu Doon) designed the city hall, the city library and museum all in Chinese renaissance style with overhanging roofs, but he chose a simply-cut modern style for the city hospital.

Today, all the above mentioned Civic Center buildings survived in northeast Shanghai's Yangpu District, formerly Kiangwan District. The once city hospital is now used as Building No. 21 of Changhai Hospital. It was built in 1935, completed in 1936 and put into use in 1937. A pathological research laboratory was constructed nearby at the same time.

On January 3, 1935, the municipal hospital and the health laboratory were called "latest additions to Kiangwan Civic Center" by English newspaper *The China Press*.

"Making another step in the expansion of public buildings of the Shanghai City Government, the new Municipal Hospital and Health Laboratory, first units of a future Chinese Medical Center of Shanghai, were dedicated at the Civic Center Tuesday by General Wu Tiechen, mayor of Greater Shanghai," *The China Press* reported.

According to architect Dong Dayou's 1935 article "Greater Shanghai-Greater Vision", Shanghai was then composed of the International Settlement, the French Concession and the Chinese controlled areas. The three areas had been allowed to grow by themselves without any preconceived scheme. As a result, Shanghai was unable to meet the demands of the times in the 1920s. So "the Greater Shanghai Plan" was launched to build a new Civic Center featuring a group of Chinese-style buildings with modern conveniences. Dong, a renowned Chinese architect and a graduate from the University of Minnesota in the USA, was appointed chief architect.

"During the 1920s, Chinese government began to call upon Chinese to revive traditional culture. Dong was required to design these political buildings in Western structure but add tradition-

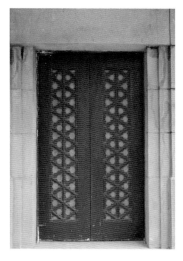
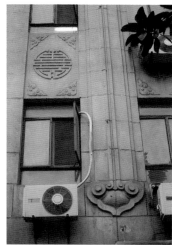

al Chinese elements," says Tongji University professor Qian Feng, who has been researching on China's first generation of modern architects.

Dong's version of Shanghai City Hall is reminiscent of a Chinese emperor's palace with overhanging roofs, upturned eaves, huge scarlet wooden gates and exquisitely painted traditional patterns on its exterior. But the general structure is concrete and steel. He designed the City Library (now Yangpu District Library) and the City Museum (now Changhai Hospital's Screening Building) in this style namely "Chinese renaissance".

"It's interesting that Dong's own residence, a two-story house with flat roof and horizontal railings, is utterly modern and contrasts with 'Chinese renaissance' buildings that he was famous for," Professor Qian adds.

The city hospital is also an utterly modern building which looks different from a galaxy of big-roofed "Greater Shanghai Plan" buildings.

According to *The China Press*, the initial plan was to construct a medical center of "fan-shaped" hospital buildings: two medical units, two surgical units, one for gynecology and obstetrics, one for pediatrics, one for out-patients to include ear, nose, throat and eye departments, one for nurses' school and home etc. The plan was co-worked by the architects of the City Planning Commission and officials of Bureau of Public Health.

In 1934, the "Fan-shaped" plan was chosen from various schemes for giving maximum amount of air and sunshine to all sides of the radiating buildings. The administration building was located in the center flanked by out-patient department and nurses' school and home. From the administration building radiated the six various units mentioned above. All wards were contained in the six radiating units. Every ward unit had its longer sides facing approximately east and west with the south side reserved by day rooms.

The plan was human-oriented. Gardens were designed in the trapezold-shaped areas between buildings where the convalescent patients could walk or be wheeled around. The service quarters were located at the southwest corner of the lot. As the prevailing wind traveled from the southeast or northwest direction, smoke nuisance could be eliminated. Noise and smells were also avoided by the distance. Beside the nine principle buildings, residential and service quarters were well provided.

But owing to a lack of fund, the administration and medical school building was the first unit to build. It served as a general hospital after opening for outpatients on January 4, 1937.

The hospital building was of reinforced concrete construction with artificial stone exterior wall. It measured 264 feet long and 52 feet wide, occupying an area of 11,400 square feet and with a floor area of 48,600 square feet. The central portion had five floors and the two wings had four, being equipped with two large elevators. It accommodated 150 to 200 beds.

"The exterior is a straight-forward expression of the plan so designed that it conforms in character with the number of other buildings erected by the City Government at the Civic Center. Typical Chinese style is not suitable for hospital buildings because of the higher cost as well as waste of space." architect Dong explained his design in an article titled "New Shanghai."

Although Dong opted for modern style, he found it possible to use Chinese decoration on a modern building so as to give a Chinese character and at the same time to embody all the requirements of a modern hospital.

"The interior is simple and dignified. The material used are in line with those used in the best

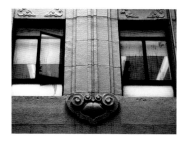

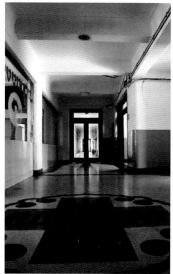

hospitals of the world. The building is planned with the least waste of space and provided adequate space for all essential new application of the well-known engineering principle which assures economical and comfortable heating," Dong introduced in the article.

The hospital was scientifically designed and advanced equipped. Interior partitions were mostly of wood laths, the walls along the corridors were of hollow tiles. Wood laths partitions were used because they could be removed and rearranged easily in the future without much damage to floor, walls or ceiling. Asphalt tiles were used for floors in wards, while terrazzo was used for the floors of main lobby, operating rooms and other utility rooms.

The basement floor contained rooms for boilers, electric switches and mechanical equipment. The ground floor featured the entrance hall, the administrative office, X-ray and Private Patients Department and Out-patients Department. Surrounding this hall were the reception room, visitors' room information desk and elevator lobbies. The pharmacy examining emergency, treatment and administration facilities were immediately adjacent.

The first floor was devoted to surgical department and operation units, with male patients' wards on the east wing and female patients' wards on the west wing. Each section had its own various utility rooms essential to the hospital management and equipment such as serving kitchen, linen room, nurses' stations, baths and toilets etc. General wards were planned to contain 5 to 10 beds. Private and semi-private room were also provided. Adjacent to the elevator lobbies were a class room, a small laboratory and a day room with a spacious sun balcony exposed the south. Special attention had been given to the construction of the operation rooms, which for economy of use were arranged in pairs, all facing north. Walls of the operation rooms were finished with greenish gray tile with terrazzo floors the same color as desired by many surgeons.

The second floor housed cubicle wards and isolation suits for children, maternity wards, the infants' room, the incubator room for prematures and other accessary rooms. The third floor featured medial department for men and women. The fourth floor was a tower-like terminal feature used for kitchen and its accessory rooms. Coal and raw materials were delivered up from the basement in a lift. Cooked food was distributed to the serving kitchens at different floors through two electric dumb waiters.

The whole building, although compactly planned, was provided with adequate space for all essential functions. And these were located and arranged for convenient and efficient service with a minimum of travel.

It was proposed to establish a modern medical institution by gradual expansion of general hospital and medical school facilities into a community of closely related institutions each covering a specialized division of the medical field; namely, research, teaching and healing.

It's a pity that the "Greater Shanghai Plan" was halted as Sino-Japanese War broke out in 1937. Only the hospital building, the center of the "fan-shaped" group of nine buildings, and the health lab were finally built. The city hospital was used by the Japanese as an army hospital during World War II and was taken over by the Kuomintang army after 1945.

Today, the façade is adorned with simplified Ironic Columns to emphasize vertical lines. Chinese characters and patterns with auspicious meanings were used to grace the walls.

Tongji University professor Liu Gang notes that the "Greater Shanghai Plan" had been a very scientific one which painted a blueprint of a new metropolitan including road system, port and railroad plans and different regions for administration, commercial activities and residence.

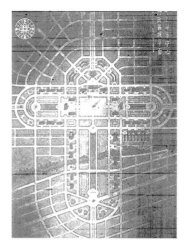
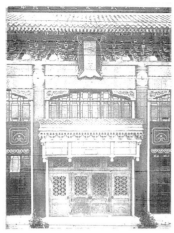
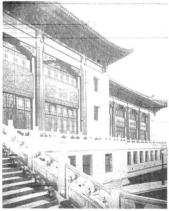
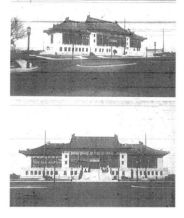

Now traces of the plan including the modern, advanced hospital building are still visible in some parts of the Yangpu District.

Yesterday: Shanghai Municipal Hospital
Today: Building No. 21 of Changhai Hospital   Built in: 1935
Architectural Style: Modern Style   Architect: Dong Dayou (Dayu Doon)
Tips: The building now used as Central Building of Changhai Hospital is open for hospital patients. You can visit Dong Dayou's other works, the former City Library (now Yangpu District Library) in Chinese Renaissance style and a Spanish-style villa at No. 40 Wukang Road.

上海市立卫生试验所（现长海医院卫勤楼）

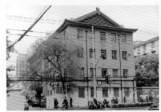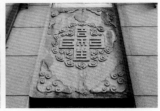

　　在市立医院医疗中心附近征地十亩，建立病理研究室。该建筑建筑面积约为 20,000 平方英尺，结构为钢筋混凝土结构，风格与市立医院大楼相似。

　　主入口在北面，可通往主要街道。入口大厅位于中心，直接与贯穿建筑的走廊相连。大厅周围是通往上层的主楼梯、信息办公室、候诊室、接待室和医生更衣室、商务办公室，所长办公室和图书馆位于东翼，西翼为材料室、清洁室和蒸汽消毒室等。

　　二三楼的布局与底层相似。疫苗、天花疫苗和狂犬病疫苗实验室位于二楼东翼，同层西翼为细菌学研究室、培养室和解剖室。包装间和男女洗手间与楼梯厅相邻。三楼为化学实验室、天平室、药物室、病理研究室。这一层还有一间博物馆和演讲室。四楼是储藏间。

　　该建筑配备了煤气、压缩空气、真空、直流和交流电、高压、高压蒸汽和电冰箱。此外，还为装实验用动物的卫生箱提供了 3 个独立的小房间，通风特别好。

　　市立医院和卫生试验所的平面图由大上海市中心区域建设委员会的董大酉和王华彬设计，并得到了卫生局官员的确认。Loh Keng Kee 是总承包商。建筑于 1935 年元旦奠基，计划于 1935 年 9 月底竣工。

摘自 1935 年 1 月 3 日《大陆报》

Research Laboratory to be built

Adjacent to the Municipal Medical Center, ten mows of land are acquired for this purpose, of establishing a Pathological Research Laboratory. The site is bounded by Chun Yuan Road on the west and Fu Ting Outer Road on the north.

The building has an overall dimension of 134 ft. by 49 ft with total floor area of about 20,000 square feet. Its approximate volume is 220,000 cubic feet. The whole structure is of reinforced concrete with a style similar to that of the hospital building.

The main entrance is on the north, accessible to the main street. The entrance hall is located at the center and connects directly with a corridor extending the length of the structure. Surrounding this hall are the main stairways to upper floors, information office, waiting room, reception room and doctors' lockers room, business offices, Directors' office and library occupy the east wing and medium rooms, materials room, cleaning room and rooms for steam and dry heat sterilization occupy the west wing.

The arrangement of the first and second floor is similar to that of the ground floor. Laboratories for vaccine, small pox vaccine, and rabies vaccine are located on east wing for the first floor while the west wing of the same floor is allotted to rooms for bacteriological research, incubator, and dissecting. Packing room and toilets for men and women are adjacent to the stairs hall.

The second floor is assigned by chemistry laboratories, rooms for balance, materia medica, and pathological research. A museum and a lecture room complete the arrangement of this floor.

The third floor is a tower-like terminal feature, used for storage purposes.

The building is equipped with gas, compressed air, vaccum, direct and alternating current, high voltage, high pressure steam, and electrically operated refrigerators. Besides 3 separate smaller houses especially well ventilated are provided for the hygienic case of animals used in experimentations.

Plan for the Hospital and Research Laboratory buildings are prepared by Messrs. Dayu Doon and H. P. Wang, of the City Planning Commission of Greater Shanghai with corroboration of officials of Bureau of Public Health. Messrs. Loh Keng Kee are the general contractors. The foundation-stone will be laid on New Year's Day, 1935 and the building is scheduled to be completed by the end of September, 1935.

Excerpt from *The China Press* on January 3, 1935

上海市立博物馆（现长海医院影像楼）

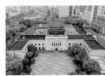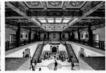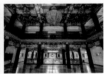

经过两年的紧张筹备，大上海市立博物馆在新市中心展出的丰富艺术品让中国丰富多彩的过去焕发光彩，该博物馆将于周日向公众开放。

作为上海首个市立博物馆，该机构不仅将进一步巩固上海作为中国门户的地位，而且还将作为一个文化中心，让外国游客可以在此首次接触到中华民族古代的工艺美术。

博物馆座落于一栋由董大酉先生设计的中式风格的建筑内，拥有超过2万件藏品，包括无价的瓷器、古代青铜器和中国古代画家的珍贵杰作。

市立博物馆馆长、著名考古学家胡肇春昨天向《大陆报》记者解释了博物馆的组织结构和展品选择。他介绍，这座建筑的建造成本为30万元，大约5万元用于购买各种展品。

从大门进来是设有售票亭的前厅，再向里走就进入了一个大厅，天花板装饰得五彩缤纷。大外是博物馆的主展厅。

大厅的四周由朱红梁柱环绕，上方有回廊，高高的殿堂正中有一尊巨大的金色佛像。

佛像的两侧是四块巨大的石碑，上面刻有明代上海最著名的艺术家Lu Shen (疑为陆深)先生的雕刻。墙上挂着12幅精美的露香园顾绣。

正殿旁的走廊里陈列着展现上海百年变迁的文献和艺术品。其中一件展品是旧会审公廨的照片，一名囚犯正在向外国陪审员叩头。

展出的其他陈列包括很多明清名窑出品的瓷器。

摘自 1937 年 1 月 8 日《大陆报》

City Museum Opens Sunday at Kiangwan

China's colorful past is revived in all its glorious hues and rich variety by the wealth of art objects on display at the City Museum of Greater Shanghai at the Civic Center which will be opened to the general public Sunday following two years' of intensive preparation.

Having the distinction of being the first institution of its kind ever to be projected by the city, the museum will not only further the claim of Shanghai as the gateway of China, but also act as a cultural center where visitors from foreign lands may get their first contact with the nation's art and crafts of the yester-years.

Housed in a building in the Chinese style of architecture and designed by Mr. Dayu Doon, the museum boasts a collection of over 20,000 pieces, including priceless porcelains, ancient bronzes and valuable masterpieces of China's historical painters.

Mr. Hu Chao-chun, Director of the Museum and a well-known archaeologist in his own right, explained to a China Press reporter yesterday the various plans which resulted in the organization of the museum and the selection of the display articles. The building, he said, was erected at a cost of $300,000, while some $50,000 was expended in buying the various articles on display.

A visitor coming through the main door will find himself in a front foyer with the ticket booth. As he walks in, he enters a large hall, with a ceiling decorated in a splash of many colors. Beyond the hall is the main exhibition room of the museum.

With big red pillars all around and with a corridor above, the high-ceilinged hall has a large god statue of a Buddha in the middle, standing on a diaz of two or three feet high.

On two sides of the statue are four massive stone tablets with carvings by Shanghai's foremost artist, the late Mr. Lu Shen, who lived during the Ming dynasty. On the walls hang 12 exquisite embroidered pictures of the famous Lu Hsiang Yuan.

In the corridor beside the main hall are displayed the documents and art objects representing the changes of Shanghai during the past century. One of these displays is in the form of a picture of the old Mixed Court, showing a prisoner kowtowing to a foreign assessor.

Other articles on exhibition include a host of porcelain aware of the famous Ming and Ching kilns.

Excerpt from *The China Press* on January 8, 1937

中国航空协会会所（飞机楼，现为第二军医大学校史馆）

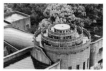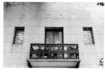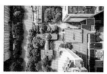

昨天下午2点，在江湾市中心中国航空协会举行了令人印象深刻的新楼落成仪式，1000多位政界与民间领袖出席，有来宾人数六七倍之多的热心航空事业的观众参观了举办航空展的新大楼。

从远处俯瞰新大楼，它就像一架最新型的巨大飞机。两架真正的中国航空协会飞行俱乐部的飞机在落成仪式上洒下传单。

仪式在新大楼二楼举行。主席团成员主要为著名的政府和民间领导人，其中包括大上海市长吴铁城、临时参议会议长王晓籁、原外交部长王正廷、中汇银行总经理杜月笙...

在王晓籁先生的开幕致辞中，新大楼的落成，被誉为中国航空发展的一大步。

中国航空协会总干事姚锡九先生在汇报大楼建设情况时表示，工程于1934年7月18日开工，今年3月20日竣工。建筑的总成本估计为11万4700元。董大酉先生负责大楼的设计。他表示，有了现在这座大楼，中国航空协会将能为刚成立的飞行俱乐部继续开展航空人员培训工作。

王正廷博士强调，在当今世界，航空是缩短空间和时间的最有效的手段，他列举了蒋介石委员长最近通过这种交通工具，在很短的时间内跨省旅行到另一个城市。他敦促所有中国人都应该加入航空协会学习和练习飞行，以便在外国侵略时可以为保护自己的祖国而做出贡献。

吴市长表示，新航空大楼的落成，或许令每一个中国公民开始重新认识国家防空建设的重要性。市长最后提到了正在上海进行的募捐活动，筹集足够的资金购买10架飞机，以在蒋介石委员长50周岁生日庆祝之际捐赠给政府。

　　昨天开幕的新大楼全天向公众开放，展出了与航空有关的各种设计、地图、图表，吸引了大约 7,000 名观众。

摘自 1936 年 5 月 6 日《大陆报》

Civic Center Aviation Home is Dedicated

More than 1,000 people including local government and civic leaders were present at the impressive ceremony marking the dedication of the new building at Kiangwan Civic Center of the China National Aviation Associaition held at 2 o'clock yesterday afternoon while six or seven times that number of air-minded Shanghailanders inspected the new building in which was held an aviation exhibition during the day.

Over the newly-dedicated building which, from a distance, looks like a huge airplane of the post up-to-date type, were two real airplanes of the Flying Club of the C. N. A. A. showering down leaflets and handbills while the dedication ceremony was on.

The ceremony was held on the second floor of the new building. Prominent government and civic leaders forming the presidium included Mayor Wu Te-chen of the Municipality of Greater Shanghai, Mr Wang Hsiao-lai, Chairman of the Provisional Board of the City Counsellors, Dr. C. T. Wang, formerly Minister of Foreign Affairs, Mr. Tu Tueh-sen, President of General Manager of the Chung Wai Bank...

The dedication of the new building was hailed as another long stride of progress toward national aviation through aviation development in an opening speech given by Mr. Wang Hsiao-lai.

Reporting the construction of the building, Mr. Yao His-chin stated the work was commenced on July 18, 1924, and was completed on March 20 this year. The total cost of the construction was estimated at $114,700. Mr. Dayu Doon was responsible for the design of the building. With the dedication of the now building, Mr. Yao said that the China National Aviation Association will be able to carry on the work for the training of aviation personnel for the recently inaugurated Flying Club.

Dr. C. T. Wang emphasized that aviation is the most effective means of shortening the space and time indispensable in the present-day world, citing the fact that Generalissimo Chiang Kai-shek was able to travel as he did recently from one city to another through several provinces within a short time only through this means of transportation. He urged that all Chinese should enroll in the membership of the C.N.A.A. for the privilege of studying and practicing flying so that in time of foreign aggression they may contribute to the protection of their fatherland.

Mayor Wu said that the dedication of the new aviation building may be the beginning for every Chinese citizen of a new awakening to the importance of upbuilding of the air defense of this country. The mayor finally mentioned the campaign now proceeding in Shanghai for raising funds enough for the purchase of 10 airplanes to be donated to the government on the occasion of the celebration of the 50th birthday anniversary of Generalissimo Chiang Kai-shek.

The new building in which was opened beginning yesterday an exhibition of all kinds of designs, maps, charts having a bearing on aeronautics was thrown open to the public throughout the day, drawing approximately 7,000 spectators.

Excerpt from *The China Press* on May 6, 1936

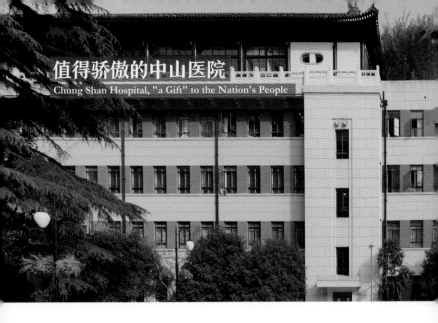

值得骄傲的中山医院

Chung Shan Hospital, "a Gift" to the Nation's People

1937年4月1日，中国人自己创办的第一家大型西医院——中山医院正式开业。医院的建筑设计为中国古典复兴风格，中西合璧，引人注目。

研究中国近代医学史的中山医院杨震教授认为，全中国名叫"中山医院"的医院不少，但上海中山医院是"根正苗红"的。1931年，孙中山之子孙科、孔祥熙、宋子文、颜福庆等名流联合发起建立一所公立医院，为纪念国父孙中山而命名为"中山医院"。

在1937年中山医院开幕典礼上，孔祥熙夫人宋霭龄剪断彩带，推开医院的大门，孔祥熙则发表演讲回顾了医院创办的历程。

"中山医院开业也许是令这座国际大都市的公民感到自豪的另一个原因。长期以来，人们一直难过地感到缺乏足够的医院设施。300多万人口却只有5000张病床可供使用，对于这座城市的病人和其他需要医疗照顾的人来说，是一个不幸的状况。"孔祥熙说。

根据1937年4月7日英文《北华捷报》（the North-China Herald）报道，孔祥熙透露中山医院项目是为纪念孙中山先生的精神，于1930年首次提出。此后，

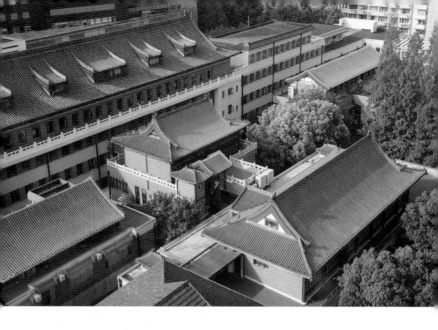

美国洛克菲勒基金会捐赠了位于劳神父路（Rue Pere Froc，今合肥路）的一块地产。在颜福庆医生"干练而充满活力的指导下"，医院的募款活动相当成功，捐款总额达到了55万4850美元。杨震提到，虽说是建立一家大型公立医院，但中山医院的建设经费全部来自社会慈善募集，创办者用了整整五年集齐了建院经费。

1935年春，医院筹委会购买一块6.67万平方米的地皮，就是中山医院位于枫林路的现址。建造工程立即展开，医院还订购了当时最现代化的医疗器械。

1936年冬，一个中国古典复兴风格的医学建筑群在新址落成。中山医院与同期兴建的上海国立医学院近在咫尺。两家医学机构后来相互合作，成为融医学教育与实践为一体的上海医事中心。

国立上海医学院可容纳300名学生，原址在海格路（Avenue Haig，今华山路），靠近上医的教学医院——中国红十字会总院（今华山医院）。与中山医院比邻的医学楼新楼由隆昌建筑公司设计，采用现代建筑加传统大屋顶的设计手法。主体建筑简洁悦目，大楼的两端设计有中式凉亭，中央部

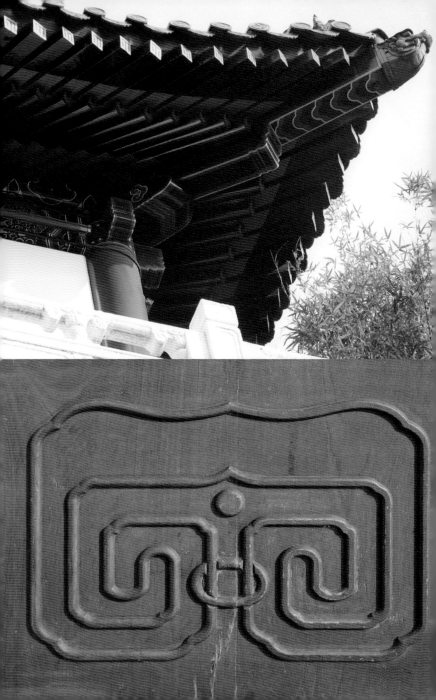

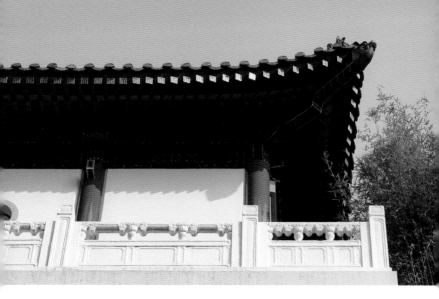

分高达四层，覆盖着琉璃瓦。

1936年，这个项目被英文《大陆报》25周年银禧版（*The China Press*, Silver Jubilee Edition）誉为"一件献给中国的礼物"。当时恰逢民国成立25周年，中山医院和医学院的落成带有纪念之意。英文报纸还刊登了这个宏伟的中式医学建筑群的草图。

"参观施工现场的人都会对中山医院的体量与宏伟印象深刻。项目即将完工，将可容纳 500 张病床。中式建筑的特征明显。主楼的长度超过400英尺，呈现中式城墙的外观，两侧平台延伸至五楼和主屋顶。五层楼高的中央部分饰有优雅的绿色瓷砖，形成宝塔般的日光室。整体外墙铺设人造石和红砖，采用主要为钢筋混凝土的防火材料建成。虽然设计简洁又体量庞大，但在许多地方都有中式的精美细节。"1936年的报道描述。

设计这座国风医院的是有影响力的中国建筑设计事务所——基泰工程司，由建筑师关颂声、朱彬、杨廷宝和土木工程师杨宽麟组成，1920年创办于天津。基泰工程司在全国多个城市都有作品，在上海还设计了南京路大新公司（今上海第一百货）和九江路大陆银行大楼。

同济大学建筑系钱宗灏教授

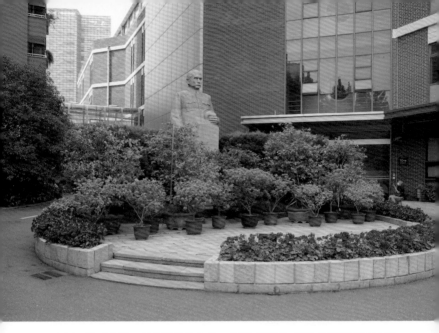

介绍，除了宝塔，以木结构为主的传统中国建筑一般不超过两层。但从20世纪20年代起，政府倡导复兴中国传统文化，当时的中国建筑师用西方建筑学知识来设计带有中国元素的多层和高层建筑，建筑学界称之为"中国古典复兴风格"。

同济大学郑时龄院士在新版《上海近代建筑风格》中介绍，中国的民族主义建筑在1930年代进入高潮，中国近代第一代建筑师们借鉴西洋古典建筑的设计理念和美学思想，用中国传统建筑的元素来创建中国现代建筑文化。设计中山医院的基泰工程司就设计了不少这种风格的。关颂声自美国留学回国后，用了十多年时间，悉心研究中国古典建筑，收集大量书籍和图样，仿制了几十座古建筑模型。而中山医院的图纸上有基泰工程司建筑师朱彬的签字。

"这是一幢建筑面积约4万平方米、钢筋混凝土结构、4层现代医疗建筑，中部5层十三开间。大楼是按医疗及护理的功能设计，但又具有中国建筑传统样式。屋顶采用仿清式，但两翼则比较简洁。目前在平顶上加建房屋，经重新装修后的外墙仍保留红砖清水墙与粉刷相间的做法，但是已不同于原有的色彩。"郑院士在新版《上海近代建筑风格》一书中评价。

1936年的英文报道透露，由于一些对洛克菲勒基金会捐赠地产选址的异议，最早的计划中止，原来的建筑方案被重新研究设计。

"从建筑师新的设计方案可以明显看出，所采用的建筑类型更加中国化，因此也更适合一家国立机构。新址占地超过66,700平方米，位于枫林桥，紧邻当时的外交部驻上海办事处，基地四边都有道路。建院工程在上海国立医学院院长、中国红十字会第一医院院长、中华医学会医学教育委员会主席颜福庆医生那干练而不懈的领导下，突飞猛进。他是这项伟大事业的推动者之一，将担任上海医事中心的秘书长。" 报道写到。

杨震介绍，1937年上海中山医院建成开业时，被誉为远东最先进的公立医院，设施设备和规模都远超当时大多数综合型医院，条件好得惊人。X光机是西门子最新的放射诊断机和治疗机，超大电梯可以容下一个病床推车，冬天暖气夏天空调，还拥有全上海唯一的高压蒸汽消毒设备。

"所以，蒋介石在'西安事变'后首选在上海中山医院休养体检。20世纪50年代，中山医院模仿苏联模式曾被改为'上海医学院外科学院'。因此可以理解，为何今日的中山医院有着极为强大的各类手术服务能力，这是有历史底蕴的。"他说。

如今，这座医院建筑保存完好并保留昔日的功能，由复旦大学中山医院用于诊疗。大楼的风貌宛若昔日，简洁现代的立面装饰着浓郁的中国传统元素，如黄色琉璃瓦、带云纹的木门、深红色立柱和图案精美的横梁。而身世不凡的中山医院已经发展为中国最大的综合型医院之一，这件"礼物"凝聚很多努力与期望，幸运地延续至今。

昨天·中山纪念医院　**今天**·复旦大学附属中山医院　**地址：**枫林路 180 号
建筑风格：中国古典复兴风格
建筑师：基泰工程司（Messrs. Kwan, Chu & Yang Architects and Engineers）
参观指南：请欣赏中国传统建筑元素与现代建筑的巧妙结合。

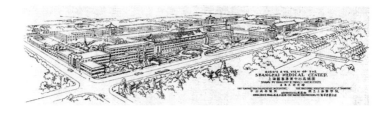

Madam H. H. Kung, wife of the Chinese minister of finance, cut the ribbon and pushed open the front gates of the Chung Shan Memorial Hospital on April 1, 1937. It was one of the first, and largest Western hospitals founded by Chinese, and the medical institution still operates today under its modern name, Zhongshan Hospital, with Chinese-style architecture.

"There are many Zhongshan Hospitals named after Dr. Sun Yat-sen in China but Shanghai Zhongshan Hospital is the most authentic one. It's a public hospital proposed by a group of prominent Chinese, including Sun Ke, son of Dr. Sun Yat-sen, minister H. H. Kung, financier T. V. Soong (Song Ziwen) and medical educator F. C. Yen (Yan Fuqing)," said Professor Yang Zheng, from Shanghai Zhongshan Hospital, who is also a medial historian and collector of Chinese medical archives.

During the 1937 opening ceremony, Kung, chairman of the institution, traced its history.

"The opening of the Chung Shan Hospital may be considered an additional reason for civic pride in this great cosmopolitan city. The sad lack of adequate hospital facilities has long been felt. That there should be only 5,000 hospital beds available for a population of over 3 million people has been an unfortunate situation for the city's sick men and others who need medical attention," Kung said.

The North-China Herald on April 7, 1937 revealed that Kung said the plan was first proposed in 1930 as a fitting memory to the work and spirit of Dr. Sun.

The trustees of the Rockfeller Foundation donated an estate of 86,710 square meters on Rue Pere Froc (now Hefei Road). The financial campaign "under the able and energetic direction of Dr F. C. Yen" proved a success and contributions soon reached a total of US$554,850.

"All construction funds came

from charitable donations. Please note that although it was a large public hospital, the funds were all collected from the society. The predecessors spent a full five years to gather the funds for the construction of Zhongshan Hospital," Yang said.

In the spring of 1935, a new piece of land covering 66,700 square meters was bought, where the hospital stands now on Fenglin Road. Construction started immediately and no effort was spared to supply the hospital with the most modern medical instruments available at the time.

In the winter of 1936, a group of medical buildings, representing a modern adaptation of Chinese architecture, was completed on the new site. The hospital and the National Medical College of Shanghai were situated close together to cooperate with each other and serve as the Shanghai Medical Center for learning and practice.

The college, with an accommodation for 300 students, had been situated on Avenue Haig (today's Huashan Road) near its teaching hospital, the First Hospital of the Red Cross Society of China (today's Huashan Hospital). In this new construction, the main building of the college was a U-shaped edifice in a simple but pleasing Chinese style, the two ends being balanced by two Chinese pavilions. The four-story central section was roofed with glazed tiles from Beijing.

In 1936, this whole project was called "a gift to China befitting so auspicious an occasion as the 25th anniversary of the founding of the republic" on the Silver Jubilee Edition of *The China Press*. The newspaper published a big drawing of this grand architectural complex of medical buildings in a Chinese style.

"No visitor to the scene of the construction can fail to be impressed by the bulk and magnificence of the Chung Shan Memorial Hospital, which is fast nearing completion and which will accommodate 500 beds. The Chinese architectural characteristics are evident. The main building, over 400 feet in length, takes on the appearance of a Chinese city wall with terraces stepping up from both sides to the fifth floor and the main roof level. The central portion of five stories is crowned with a graceful sweep of beautiful green tiles forming a pagoda-like solarium. Entirely constructed with fire-proof material, mostly reinforced concrete, the general facade is in artificial stone and red

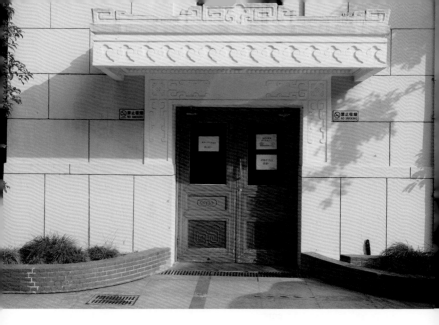

brick, which though simple and massive, has touches of fine Chinese details in many parts," the 1936 newspaper reported.

"With the exception of pagodas, ancient Chinese buildings, most of which were made of wood, seldom have more than two floors. But starting from the late 1920s, the Chinese government began to call upon Chinese to revive traditional culture. Chinese architects applied their Western knowledge to design taller buildings with traditional elements. We call it 'Chinese Renaissance Style,'" said Tongji University professor Qian Zonghao.

According to the newspaper,

an objection to the location of the Rockefeller Foudation-donated site halted the preliminary plans. The delay enabled the original building plans to be thoroughly re-studied.

"From the architects' new designs, it is evident that the type of architecture adopted is distinctly more Chinese and, therefore, more befitting to an institution which was a national enterprise. Covering an area of more than 66,700 square meters, the new site is situated at Feng Ling Chiao, close to the then Shanghai Office of the Ministry of Foreign Affairs. It occupies an area of over 100 mow of land with road frontage on all four sides," the 1936 report said.

And no sooner had this site been acquired than building operation begun. They had since been "progressing by leaps and bounds under the able and untiring direction of Dr. F. C. Yen, director of the National Medical College of Shanghai, superintendent of the First Hospital of the Red Cross Society of China and chairman of the Council on Medical Education of the Chinese Medical Society, who is one of the prime movers of the gigantic undertaking and who will be the General Secretary of the Shanghai Medical Center".

"In 1937, Shanghai Chung Shan Memorial Hospital was established and opened, with facilities and scale far exceeding that of most general hospitals at that time. The equipment was amazingly good. Its X-ray machine was the latest product from Siemens and it had the only high-pressure steam sterilization equipment in Shanghai. The super-large elevator could accommodate a patient's bed and there was special elevator for delivering meals. There were winter heating and summer air-conditioning. Even Kuomintang leader Chiang Kai-shek chose to recuperate at the hospital after he was injured in a hasty escape during the Xi'an Incident," Yang

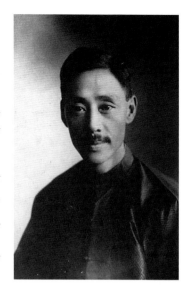

said.

"In the 1950s, Zhongshan Hospital learned from the former Soviet Union model to develop a department of surgery for the Shanghai Medical College. So that's why Zhongshan Hospital has been extremely capable of various surgical services. This has historical roots," he added.

Today, the well-preserved construction functions as Building No. 3 of Zhongshan Hospital. The grand building features a modern simply cut facade with strong Chinese characters, including yellow glazed tiles, wooden doors with cloud patterns, scarlet columns and richly adorned tradi-

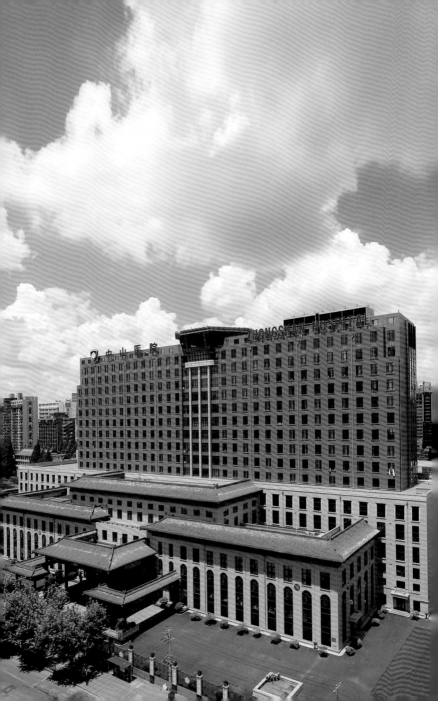

tional beams.

The architect of the building was a big Chinese firm Messrs. Kwan, Chu & Yang Architects and Engineers, which also designed the Sun Department Store on Nanjing Road and the Continental Bank on Jiujiang Road.

The Zhongshan Hospital has grown to be one of China's largest and most comprehensive hospitals. The well-preserved historical buildings and newly built modern constructions are all connected through glass galleries for convenient transportation.

In 2020, the institution sent medical teams to aid hospitals in Wuhan for treating COVID-19 patients. One of the doctors sent to Wuhan, 27-year-old Liu Kai, and an 87-year-old COVID-19 patient witnessed a spectacular sunset on their way back from a CT scan in Wuhan. Liu stood next to his bedridden patient to watch the sunset and the shot was snapped by a fellow hospital volunteer.

The photo, showing the back of the young doctor, while the patient points to the sun, triggered netizens' empathy and warmth. Shanghai Zhongshan Hospital posted this sunset photo in the historical compound among a sea of golden glazed tiles.

Yesterday: Chung Shan Memorial Hospital   **Today:** Zhongshan Hospital, Fudan University
Address: 180 Fenglin Road   **Architectural style:** Chinese renaissance style
Architect: Messrs. Kwan, Chu & Yang Architects and Engineers
Tips: Please note the artful combination of traditional Chinese architectural elements and modern functions.

中山医院弘扬孙中山精神

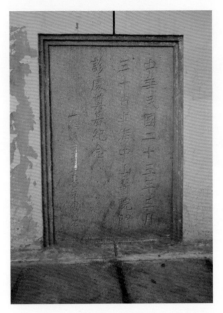

　　这家医院以孙中山先生命名，他的职业生涯就是从医生开始的，后来转向政治。因此，孙先生不仅是人民的医生，也是中华民族的医生。他的民生主义旨在促进人民的身体健康并改善他们的经济状况。因此，我们应该在上海拥有一座设备齐全的现代化医院，以纪念这位伟大的中国医生和中华民国之父的精神。社会服务精神是这项事业的标志。来自全国各地和各行各业的馈赠使这些机构的建立成为可能。无论是在医院还是在医学院，都聚集了一批工作人员，他们被专业服务的最高理想而非个人利益而所打动。

　　　　　　　　　　摘自 1937 年 4 月 7 日《北华捷报》刊登的孔祥熙致辞

Chung Shan Hospital dedicated to the spirit of Dr Sun Yat-sen

The hospital bears the name of Dr. Sun, who starting his career as a medical doctor, and turned his attention to politics in his later life. Dr. Sun was thus not only a doctor among his people but a doctor of the Chinese nation. His principle of the People's Livelihood aims at promoting the physical well-being of the people as much as at ameliorating their economic condition. It is thus most fitting that we should have in Shanghai a modern and well-equipped hospital dedicated to the memory of the great Chinese doctor and the spirit of the Father of the Chinese Republic. A spirit of social service marks the entire enterprise. Gifts, large and small, coming from all parts of the country and all walks of life, have made the institutions possible. Both in the hospitals and the medical college, a staff of workers has been gathered who are moved by the highest ideals of professional service rather than by hopes of personal gain.

Excerpt from Dr. H. H. Kung's speech in *the North-China Herald*
on April 7, 1937

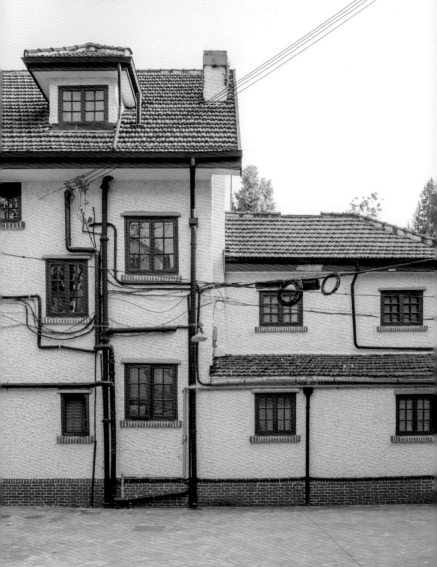

2009年初冬，武康路综合整治工程接近尾声。徐汇区政府在武康路40号举行了简短仪式，挂上"颜福庆旧居"的铭牌。

40号院落由4座不同风格的西式别墅围合，宽敞静谧，近年荣获"星级弄堂"的美誉。20世纪40年代，曾创办上海医学院和中山医院的著名医学教育家颜福庆在4号小楼居住。

颜氏旧居是武康路一带常见的英国乡村风格住宅。砖木结构的小楼建于1923年，红瓦斜屋顶，姜黄水泥拉毛墙。装饰不多，但窗框有精致的红砖饰带，与黄墙对比鲜明。

朝院落的北立面镶嵌着十几个木窗，大小不一、高低错落，既满足采光需要，又让简洁的立面丰富耐看。

在上海黄金的20世纪二三十年代，颜福庆的医学事业也如此丰富精彩。他游说政界和金融界的实权人物，辛苦筹款终于建起了集医学院、医院和研究院于一身的医事中心。这是第一个中国人自己的医事中心，将临床实践与教学科研有机结合，达到欧美医学院同类水平。他还说服圣约翰校友、沪上工商名人叶澄衷之子叶子衡捐出自己的花园，设结核病医院。此外，他又创办了中华医学会，沪上英文报刊都时常报道他的讲话和活动。

1928年11月7日，颜福庆一张精瘦癯铄的照片登上美国报纸《密勒氏评论》"Who's who in China"栏目，这是专门向西人介绍华人名流的专栏。

"颜福庆博士1882年7月18日出生于上海，1903年毕业于圣约翰大学医学院。大学毕业后他去南非当矿医，后赴美深造，1909年获得耶鲁大学学位。他又前往英国利物浦大学从事研究，并获得博士学位。"报道对他的医学事业高度评价，认为颜福庆"不仅仅是卓越的医生和医学教育家，还做了大量关于公共卫生和慈善方面的工作。为提升中国医学教育水平和医疗水准，他甘于奉献"。

颜福庆出生于上海的一个牧师家庭，8岁父亲因病去世后他被过继给伯父颜永京。颜永京曾留学美国，是教会学校圣约翰书院的创办人及首任院长。他希望长子颜惠庆学医，但颜惠庆后来成为政治家

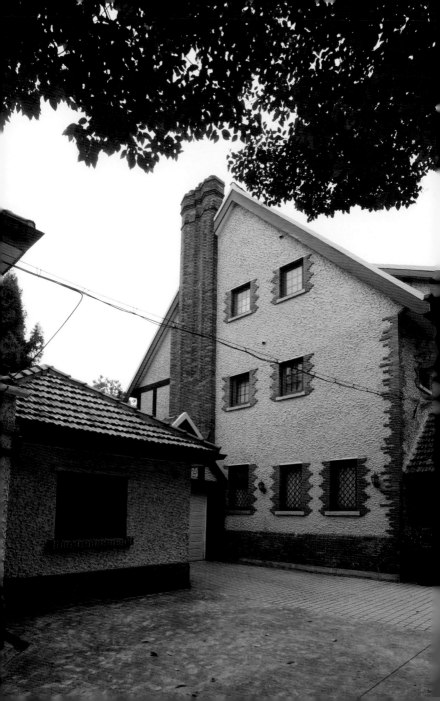

和外交官，这个心愿在颜福庆身上却实现了。

1903年，颜福庆从圣约翰大学医学院毕业后，报名赴南非为劳动环境险恶的华人矿工治病。1906年，他赴美深造，1909年成为首位获得耶鲁医学博士的亚洲人。

颜福庆毕业后应雅礼会（由耶鲁同学会组成的致力发展中国医学与教育的非营利组织）邀请，赴长沙雅礼医院工作，1914年创办湘雅医学专门学校，担任校长。同年，他与伍连德共同倡议，在上海成立中华医学会。1927年后，他回到上海，想创办一所中国人自己的医学院，实现医学现代化的理想，因为"医学为民族强弱之根基，人类存在之关键"。

复旦大学历史系高晞教授撰文提到，上海医学院初创时办学条件极差。

"颜福庆认为现代医学院必须有自己的教学医院，就租下红十字会总医院作为教学医院，自己当院长。他每天在吴淞的医学院工作半天，再乘火车赶到市区红十字会总医院指导临床教学。颜福庆为医院制定'病人至上'的院训，成为平民信赖的医院。沪上工商名人叶澄衷之子叶子衡是颜福庆在圣约翰的校友，颜福庆说服他捐出叶家花园，开设结核病医院，对付当时最致命的痨病，成为医学院的第二所教学医院。"高晞《颜福庆 一生为了中国医学现代化》一文中写到。

叶家花园捐赠后，颜福庆游说政界和金融界的实权人物，辛苦筹款终于建起了集医学院、医院和研究院于一体的医事中心。据高晞教授采访颜福庆的孙子颜志渊回忆："1949年前有些有轨电车，好像是分几等了，他是坐在最后一等，手拿个算盘，还拿个包，还有个账本。他没穿华丽的衣服，他要省每个铜板，所以得了个雅号，叫犹太人。"

1937年，颜福庆终于用筹来的100万两银元建起了他心中的医事中心，设上海医学院、药学院、护士学校、公共卫生学院和中山医院等教学医院。4月1日，国立上海医学院、上海中山医院中国古典复兴风格的新院舍落成典礼举行。这是第一个中国人自己的医事中心，将临床实践与教学科研有机结合，达到欧美医学院同类水平。

《颜福庆传》提到，购买上海医学院和中山医院地基的费用由美国洛氏基金会捐助，教育部16万元拨款用于建筑医学院院舍，中山医院的建筑及设备费80万元来自各界募捐。

据说江湾长大的颜福庆虽然思维西式，但一生讲一口上海土话。他认为"医学为民族强弱之根基，人类存在之关键"，要为公众利益为目的去学医，而不是赚钱。

颜氏旧居现在是一家公司用房，虽然处于保护状态，但并未对公众开放。铁门紧锁，围墙上有高高的竹篱，但仍可以看到故居有偌大的花园。几棵参天大树比武康路行道树还要高大茂盛。

复旦大学李天纲教授研究颜福庆堂哥颜惠庆的日记发现，颜福庆可能1937年到1950年都居住在福开森路24号住所（今武康路40弄）。他认为，颜福庆旧居在武康路上初看不是亮点，但是按旧主人一生造福于上海人来看，这幢普通民宅的价值和意义，超过了他的邻居黄兴、唐绍仪、陈果夫、陈立夫。

"颜福庆是我们这座城市不能忘记的恩人，'颜氏三杰'（惠庆、福庆、德庆）都对中国的新式事业做出了重要贡献。颜惠庆（1877—1950）是外交家、慈善家、北洋政府总理；颜德庆（1878—1940）是著名工程师，中国铁路事业先驱。颜福庆则是一生从事医学事业，他给上海留下的是中山医院、华山医院和上海医学院。忽然想到，颜福庆可以与马相伯相提并论，后者给上海留下了震旦大学、复旦大学。马相伯是百年树人，颜福庆是治病救人，都是积善积德的事业。"他在题为《颜福庆在武康路》文中写到。

1970年，颜福庆去世。这一生中，他培养出了一大批中国医学的优秀人才，提出建立的公共卫生防疫系统，将医学的关注点从疾病转向人群和社区。他创办的医事中心成为今天的上海医科大学和中山医院，澄衷医院发展为上海市肺科医院。这些凝聚他心血智慧的医学事业，延续至今。

说上海土话的洋博士颜福庆

辛勤种下的种子，仿佛已长成他武康路旧居前的大树，特别地高大和葱茏，仍在荫泽和护佑这座城市的人们。

昨天：颜福庆旧居　**今天：**公司用房　**地址：**武康路 40 弄 4 号　**建造年代：**1923 年
参观指南：星级弄堂里的 1 号和 4 号都住过中国近代史有影响力的人物，这个院落值得细细品味。

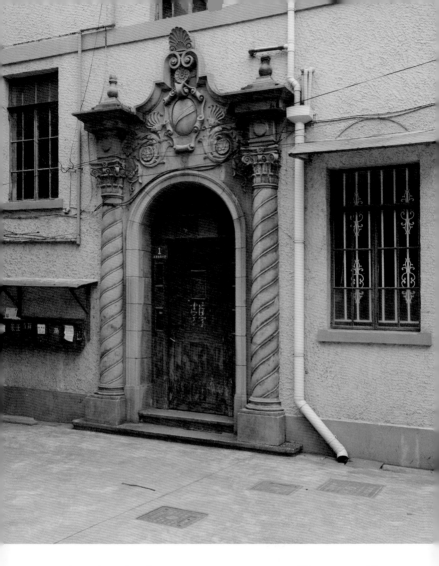

As Wukang Road's rejuvenation project was nearing completion in the early winter of 2009, the Xuhui district government held a simple ceremony to hang the name plate of "Former Residence of Yan Fuqing (or F. C. Yen)" on the wall of 40 Wukang Road.

Awarded as a "star-rate lane", the ample, tranquil compound on

No. 40 houses four western villas in different architectural styles. Dr. Yan Fuqing, the famous medical educator and founder of both Shanghai Medical College and Zhongshan Hospital had lived in building No. 4 of this compound in the 1940s.

Yan's residence is modeled after a British country villa, a style commonly seen in the Wukang Road neighborhood. Built in 1923, the villa features ginger-hued stucco walls holding up a steeply sloping, red-tile roof. Ornaments are used with great restraint but the window frames are laced with delicate red-brick strips which contrast with the yellow walls.

Facing the yard, the northern façade is mosaicked with more than 10 wooden windows at different heights and sizes, which not only introduced ample sunlight into the house but also enrich the otherwise simple façade.

Back in the golden 1920s to 1930s, Dr. Yan also lived such an enriched life as he lobbied prominent politicians and financiers to establish a medical center comprising a medical school, a hospital and a medical academy all in one institution. This was China's first medical center to organically combine a medical practice with education and reached the standards of its European and American counterparts.

He also persuaded Ye Ziheng, a classmate from St. John's and son of Shanghai tycoon Ye Chengzhong, to donate his garden as a tuberculosis hospital. Yan was one of the founders of the National Medical Association of China.

On November 7, 1928, he was introduced by the column "Who's who in China" of *The China Weekly Review.*

"Dr. F. C. Yen was born in Shanghai on July 18, 1882 and graduated from St. John's Medical School in 1903. After college, he traveled to South Africa while serving as a medical officer in the China Labor Corps from 1903—1904. From South Africa he went America for further study and graduated from Yale University with an M. D. cum laude in 1909. From America Dr. Yen went to England where he conducted research at the University of Liverpool and secured the degree of D. T. M."

The newspaper sang high praise of Dr. Yan, who was "not only prominent as a doctor and a medical educator, but also worked to promote public health and other philanthropic work. He is a devoted worker in promoting medical education and in and in raising

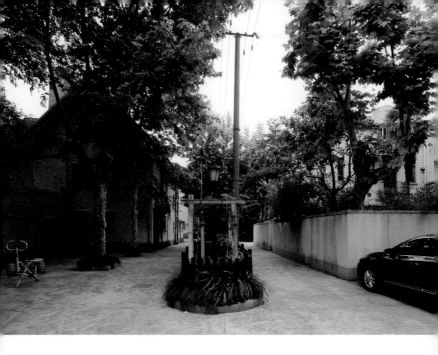

the standard of medical practice in China".

Yan's residence is now used by a company and not open to the public. The iron gate is always locked but a spacious garden behind is still visible. Several trees in the garden are even taller and more flourishing than avenue trees along Wukang Road.

Having grown up in the Jiangwan area, Dr. Yan had a western mind but always spoke local Shanghai dialect. Throughout his life he held the belief that "medical science is fundamental for nation's development and human's living". The purpose for medi-

cal study, he always maintained, should be for public interest, not for profit.

According to Fudan University professor Li Tiangang's research, Dr. Yan used to live in this residence at 24 Route Ferguson (today's 40, Wukang Road) possibly from 1937 to 1950. The professor reviewed that the residence was not eye-catching at the first glance, but its value in terms of the owner's contribution to Shanghai surpassed other celebrity homes along Wukang Road, such as the residences of revolutionist Huang Xing, politicians Tang Shaoyi, Chen Guofu and

Chen Lifu.

Dr. Yan had helped to train a large group of excellent medical practitioners for China before he passed away in 1970. The medical center he founded developed into the Shanghai Medical University and Shanghai Zhongshan Hospital. The former became the medical school of Fudan University. Ye's garden docated at his advice is now the Shanghai Pulmonary Hospital. The public health and epidemic prevention system proposed by him has continued until today, which turned medical focus from disease to congregation of people and community.

It seems the seeds planted by Dr. Yan had grown to be the unusually tall, flourishing trees fronting his former home on Wukang Road, which are still benefiting and protecting people of this city.

Yesterday: Dr. Yan's residence   **Address:** Building 4, 40 Wukang Road
Tips: Two buildings in this "star-rated lane", No. 1 and No. 4 have housed influential figures in modern Chinese history. This is a yard worth wandering and pondering over.

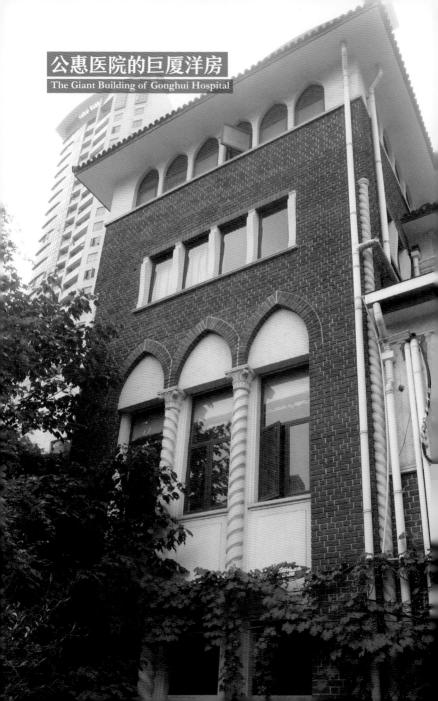

公惠医院的巨厦洋房

The Giant Building of Gonghui Hospital

上海南京西路地铁站附近的一条里弄深处，藏着一座设计精良、保存完好、但鲜为人知的历史建筑—斜桥弄巨厦，如今是公惠医院。

斜桥弄巨厦高达三层，建筑面积2000平方米，是一座体量很大的花园洋房。1931年，这座建筑由东欧建筑师邬达克（L. E. Hudec）为花旗银行买办吴培初（P. C. Woo）设计，1934年出版的《中国月刊》刊登了设计图。

《上海邬达克建筑地图》作者、同济大学华霞虹教授研究发现，斜桥弄巨厦在设计草图上是一座精致的折衷主义建筑，但真实的建筑比设计稿还要好。

"建筑外形以西班牙风格为主调，兼有其他风格的要素。典型的西班牙建筑特征包括：平缓的筒瓦屋面、螺旋形柱式、南向敞廊和阳台，窗、门廊乃至烟囱顶部均为尖券形。外墙除拉毛粉刷外，还辅以面砖、人造石、斩假石。室内公共部位的地面和柱式均采用大理石，门廊内的柱式和山花为巴洛克风格。堂屋暖气片的铸铁盖板被塑成各种中国传统吉祥图案，如'五福同祥''喜上眉梢'等。中式元素在邬达克的作品中非常少见。"华教授评价道。

邬达克毕业于布达佩斯的匈牙利皇家约瑟夫技术大学建筑系，1914年应征入伍参加一战后被俘。奥匈帝国在一战后解体，邬达克在遣返途中隐藏了战俘身份，几经辗转于1918年逃至上海，成为一位"国籍不明"的流亡者。

20世纪二三十年代的上海是远东最大的贸易、金融和工业中心，房地产和建筑业蓬勃发展，邬达克身无分文且有腿伤，但这个受过专业建筑教育的年轻人正是当时上海需要的人才。他先在美国建筑师罗兰·克利（Rowland Curry）的克利洋行找到绘图员的工作，后自立门户，至1947年离开上海时，他设计建成了包括远东第一高楼——国际饭店、远东第一影院——大光明大戏院、远东第一豪宅——吴同文住宅、远东最豪华医院——宏恩医院、中国知名学府交通大学的扩建规划及其工程馆、中国最大的啤酒厂——联合啤酒厂等54个项目，近百个单体建筑。

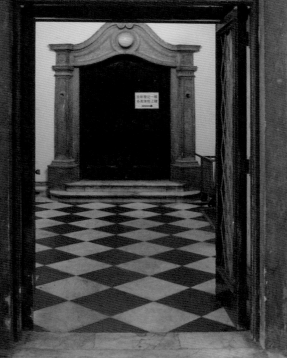

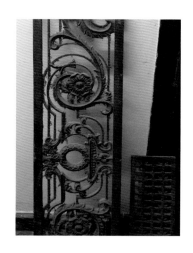

2008年匈牙利驻沪总领馆和上海市政府举办"邬达克年"活动后，一系列邬达克活动和话题持续激发着公众的兴趣。在上海市旅游局发布"上海99个经典符号"名单里，邬达克与他的两件名作——国际饭店和武康大楼被近百万参评者列为"喜欢上海的理由"。

与邬达克这些知名的作品相比，大隐隐于市的斜桥弄巨厦十分低调，知道的人不多。这里曾经由隶属上海市工会的公惠医院使用，为低收入患者提供医疗服务。

华教授推测，邬达克将斜桥弄巨厦设计为加入中国元素的西方古典主义风格，应该是根据客户的需求，因为当时他已开始设计大光明电影院这样的现代建筑了。

可能的确如此。斜桥弄巨厦主人（P. C. Woo）的神秘身份终于揭开了。他70多岁的孙子马丁（Martin）与夫人来到中国，跟华教授确认这座巨厦就是爷爷吴培初的家。

根据安徽师范大学李晓春的论文《近代中国外商银行买办群体分析》，吴培初于1932年到1941年担任花旗银行买办。他投资了不少产业，是余纶绸缎局的股东，担任中和商业储蓄银行和华安合群保险公司董事，还是裕发祥和大兴水金号店的店主。

买办，亦称"康白度"，原指欧洲人在印度雇佣的当地管家，后指旧中国替外国资本家服务的中国经理人。1902年，花旗银行在上海开设分行，这是美商在中国最早开设的分行，一开始就实行了买办制度。第一任买办是袁恒之(1902—1919年)，第二任是王俊臣(1919—1932年)，第三任是吴培初(1932—1941年)。

吴培初也曾撰写一篇《旧上海外商银行买办》回顾自己的人生

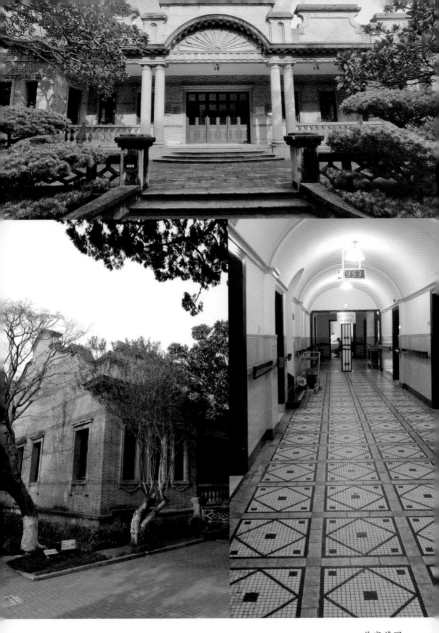

黄家花园

经历。

"我原籍苏州，1878年生于上海，父亲是布商人。我十二岁时到河南路天津路章东明酒店楼上向吴衡之学英文。1900年，十四岁，进上海电话公司做接线生。1903年，进俄国政订商约办事处任英文打字，该处主任是巴斯德纳也夫，后来在华俄道胜银行做事。约半年后，商约改好，这个机构结束，我进荷兰银行工作，同时利用晚上时间教上海地皮大王程霖生的兄弟、外甥和侄子三人读英文，并代办他家外文往来信件。"吴培初在这篇收录在《旧上海的外商与买办》（1987）一书里的文章中写道。

他回忆，离开荷兰银行后曾担任盘美花园（Boehmer Green House）会计工作，又任麦加利银行英文打字。麦加利银行买办王宪臣的弟弟王俊臣担任花旗银行买办后，给吴培初介绍了花旗银行副买办的职位。1932年，王俊臣辞去花旗银行买办职务后吴培初接替了这个职位，获得每月800两的高薪。

吴培初在文中透露，买办除了从事银行业务活动，还投资工商业，进行金融和其他投机活动。他本人就利用花旗银行职务，在标金和外汇方面进行投机，还投资美国物品和上海地产。

吴培初的地产投机起初很顺利。1929年，他花费五十万两贷款买入一块位于华安大楼旁的地皮，一年多后以110万两的价格售与邮政储金汇业局，获得巨额利润。这笔巨款也许是吴培初建造斜桥弄巨厦的资金来源之一。不过他坦言，这次投机成功也导致他后来过分热衷地产投机，盲目追求地价上涨。1932年后世界经济恐慌对中国带来很大影响，加上九·一八和一·二八两次事变，上海发生金融恐慌，吴培初手中持有的地产卖不出去，负债累累。

1934年，吴培初仍为上海交通大学助银五千元建造校门。交大建校初期的校门原为木质牌楼门，1935年由吴培初捐资改建的新校门式样为仿旧京城宫门式，朱门碧盖，颇为美观，沿用至今。

吴培初的孙子马丁回忆，吴氏夫妇与15位子女一起住在斜桥弄巨厦里。吴家的生活方式中西合壁，建筑的平面布局也兼顾中西。东面带有门廊、螺旋形大楼梯和车库，每个房间都设有壁炉，充满现代生活的气息。而西面设有客堂、餐厅、私塾、中式厨房和佣人房，风格更加传统。吴家有舞厅和弹子房，客堂间平日以字画装点，岁末会悬挂祖宗画像祭拜。

马学强、张秀莉在《出入于中西之间：近代上海买办社会生活》一书中提到，买办是与外国人交往最多的人，他们过着一种半西化的生活。作为近代上海新兴的富裕基层之一，买办有丰厚的收入，是近代中国口岸城市中最具消费能力的阶层之一。他们把财富用于消费，建造奢华的住宅，热衷于举行各种派对，赶时髦追时尚，享受着快乐的生活。

两位学者研究发现，普通职员、工人在上海大多是租用房屋，有能力购置者较少，而且购买的也只是面积较小的里弄房子。而对于腰缠万贯的买办来说，置地买房是轻而易举的事情。很多美轮美奂的建筑都是买办们苦心经营的杰作，如汇丰银行买办席鹿笙位于福熙路（Avenue Foch，今福煦路）191号的住宅、法商买办吴伟臣的大西路花园洋房，以及荣泰洋行买办、浙江定海人范珊琳在劳神父路（今合肥路）建造的独立花园住宅等。

值得一提的是，上海还有不少花园洋房后来用于医院功能，如青海路岳阳医院北楼（周湘云宅）、上海文艺医院（张叔驯宅）和上海健康医学院附属崇明医院（黄家花园）等。

1952年，吴家搬离斜桥弄巨厦，如今大多旅居美国和加拿大。1995年，几位吴家后代曾到公惠医院寻根。

"他们都是80多岁的年纪，从美国来看看小时候的家，回忆了在这座大房子里度过的童年时光，从螺旋型楼梯上滑下来玩得很开心。" 接待过吴家后代的公惠医院谢晓方回忆道。

如今，昔日的"巨厦"隐藏在公惠医院门诊大厅的后面。这座建筑虽然体量不小，却让人感觉尺度适宜。绿色常春藤浪漫地缠绕在红色砖墙上，造型别致的门窗背后，穿白大褂的医生与患者交谈。美好的花园十分安静。花园里有一排中医治疗室，弥漫着一股浓浓的草药味。

1953年建院的公惠医院原为公用事业职工医院，本着"医疗帮困，施惠于民"的理念，在面向全社会开放的同时，主要承担了对低收入困难群体实施医疗帮困的职能。斜桥弄巨厦现为医院三号楼，底层是检验科，二三层是综合病房。

走进大楼，华丽的螺旋形楼梯让人想起邬达克的一些其他作品。左琰、张飞武和马思雨在《从楼梯艺术看近代上海花园洋房装饰风格演变》一文中提到，20世纪二三十年代上海建造的花园洋房中，西班牙风格占据很大一部分。此风格当时在英美等国风靡，藉由来自英美或在英美等国受过教育的建筑师带入上海并迅速流行起来。西班牙洋房的楼梯样式相对比较自由。金属花饰栏杆和木扶手组合成为西班牙式花园洋房楼梯的流行风尚，20世纪30年代初期邬达克设计的孙科别墅和斜桥弄巨厦的楼梯均采用了这一装饰语言。前者采用了双跑梯段、木质踏步，而后者为水磨石踏步，其楼梯样式跟刘吉生住宅（今巨鹿路上海作家协会）楼梯样式相吻合。

作为国内最知名的邬达克建筑研究者，华霞虹对这位东欧建筑师的印象是"一位传统而专业的建筑师，始终为客户着想"。

"他不是那种非常前卫的人。邬达克虽然才华横溢、技术精湛，但他从不强迫客户接受自己的风格，并且始终注重施工的实用性。他不是那种想给世界带来惊喜并在建筑史上青史留名的人。这些年来很少有人关注斜桥弄巨厦，但是当我第一次见到它时，有一种找到宝贝的感觉。"华霞虹说。

还记得在一个夏日初次来到这座闹市中的洋房。七月炎热的阳光下，走过满是病人的诊所大厅，来到螺旋柱、常春藤和浓郁中草药气息包裹的花园中央时，不禁有同样的感觉。

昨天： 斜桥弄巨厦（吴培初住宅）　　**今天：** 公惠医院（改造中）　　**地址：** 石门一路 315 号
建筑风格： 西班牙风格　　**建筑师：** 邬达克
参观指南： 斜桥弄巨厦隐藏在车道内，很容易错过。医院周围的小巷也值得漫步。

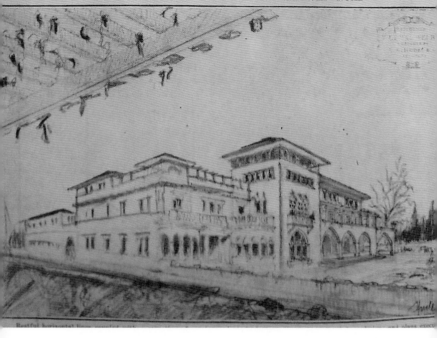

In the depth of a lane near the bustling Nanjing Road West, conceals a well-designed, well-preserved but rarely known edifice named "the Large Building in Hsiai Lane" designed by famous architect Laszlo Hudec. The building has been used by Gonghui Hospital for many years.

The 2000-square-meter building of three stories is a big-sized garden villa as its name indicates. It was designed by Hudec for P. C. Woo (or Wu Peichu), comprador of City Bank of New York, predecessor of Citibank.

Tongji University professor Hua Xiahong first discovered this historical building from blueprints published on an architectural journal of the 1930s.

"The blueprints display a delicate eclectic building but the real one looked even better than the design," Hua recalls her first visit.

"This beautiful building was designed in rich Spanish style but added with eclectic elements," says Hua, author of the book *Shanghai Hudec Architecture*.

"It was hidden inside and green ivies climbed all over the walls up to the third floor. The garden was nice and quiet. Among a rainbow of spiral columns and Spanish arches, I was surprised to find

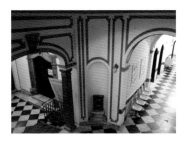 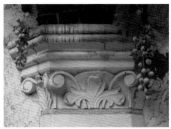

Chinese lucky patterns on the iron cover of the heating units, such as 'five bats' (meaning five lucky things in Chinese). Chinese elements were rare to find in Hudec's architectural works," she comments.

Laszlo Hudec was a legendary Slovakian-Hungarian architect who escaped to Shanghai in 1918 from a Siberian prison camp and designed around 100 buildings in Shanghai during 29 years. In recent years, Hudec was voted as one of the 99 Shanghai symbols by netizens.

Compared with his more famous masterpieces like the Park Hotel or the Grand Theater, this "large building" is quite unknown and has been used as Gonghui Hospital under the management of Shanghai Labor Union to serve low-income patients.

In 1931, this giant building was designed serve as private residence of the wealthy Chinese Family of P. C. Woo.

"In the early 1930s Hudec had already started to design contemporary buildings like the Grand Theater. I guess the classic style added with Chinese elements is according to the needs of his client," says Hua.

In recent years, Woo's grandson Martin confirmed with professor Hua of his grandfather's identity during a trip to Shanghai. P. C. Woo, the owner of the giant building, served as comprador of the American bank from 1932 to 1941. He also invested in silk and satin, banking, insurance and real estate.

In an article named "Compradors of Foreign Commercial Banks in Old Shanghai", Woo recalled his career development in old Shanghai.

"Originally from Suzhou, I was born in Shanghai in 1878. My father was a cloth merchant. When I was 12, I went to learn English from Wu Hengzhi on the upper floor of Zhangdongming Hotel on Henan and Tianjin Roads. In 1900, at the age of 14, I joined the Shanghai Telephone Company as an operator. In 1903, I entered the Russian Political and Commercial Contract Office as an English typewriter," he wrote in the article included in the 1987 book *Foreign Businessmen and Compradors in Old Shanghai.*

He later worked for ABN AMRO Bank, Boehmer Green House and the Chartered Bank of India, Australia and China. In 1932, he was appointed comprador of the City Bank of New York and received a high salary of 800 taels per month.

In the article, Woo released that old-Shanghai compradors invested extensively, conducting financial and other speculative activities. Woo himself also made use of his position in the bank to speculate on gold and foreign exchange, as well as investing in American goods and Shanghai real estate.

His real estate investment went smoothly at first. In 1929, Woo spent 500,000 taels to buy a piece of land next to the United Assurance Building, and sold it for 1.1 million taels more than a year later. The huge profits from the deal might be the source of funds for the construction of the giant building.

However, the success also led him to be overly enthusiastic about real estate investment. After 1932, he was unable to sell properties and heavily in debt as the world economic depression had a great impact on China and Shanghai.

According to his grandson Martin's narration, Woo and his wife lived with their 15 children in the giant home. The wealthy family's lifestyle was a combination of Eastern and Western styles, which was mirrored in the East-meet-West layout.

The east side had a porch, grand spiral staircase and garage, and every room had a fireplace, giving it an air of modern living. On the west side, there were living rooms, restaurants, private schools, Chinese kitchens and maid rooms, and the style was more traditional. The family had a dance hall and a billiard room. The living room was decorated with calligraphy and paintings. At the end of the year, portraits of ancestors would be hung up for worship.

In the co-authored book *Going Between China and the West: The Social Life of Compradors in Modern Shanghai*, scholars Ma Xueqiang and Zhang Xiuli note that most ordinary employees and workers rented houses in old Shanghai. Very few people could afford to buy a residence or they could only buy small lane houses. For wealthy compradors, buying a house was a breeze. Many beautiful villas in Shanghai were former villas of the compradors, such as the residence of HSBC comprador Xi Lusheng at No. 191 Avenue Foch (now Fuxu Road).

It is noteworthy that some old Shanghai garden villas were later used as hospitals, such as the North Building of Yueyang Hospital on Qinghai Road (tycoon Zhou Xiangyun's House), Shanghai Literature and Art Hospital on Tianping Road (famous collector Zhang Shuxun's House) and Chongming Hospital Affiliated to Shanghai University of Medicine and Health Sciences (Huang's Garden) etc.

In 1952, the Woo family moved out of the building. Most of the family members live in the United States and Canada today. Hospital employee Xie Xiaofang happened to meet several descendants of the Woo family in 1995.

"They were all in their 80s and came from the US to see their former home. They recalled their childhood days in this big house such as sliding through the spiral staircase for fun," Xie recalls.

Founded in 1953, the Gonghui Hospital provided medical services for low-income patients. The giant building is used as Building 3 of the hospital with clinical laboratory on the ground floor and wards on the above two floors.

The impeccable beauty of the building greatly touched me when I visited it in a hot July afternoon. Tucked away in a deep lane and hidden behind the clinic hall, the large building appeared to be colossal but not aggressive. Green ivies and even green grapes were swirling around the red-brick walls in a romantic way. Behind the doors and windows in interesting shapes, white-uniformed doctors were talking with patients. A strong Chinese herbal smell were lingering in the garden coming from a line of TCM treatment rooms.

According to book *Shanghai Hudec Architecture*, the facade was composed of typical Spanish architectural elements, such as Spanish roof tiles, open loggia, spiral columns and cast iron rails.

Inside the decoration was luxurious and east-meet-west. In the Western-style east part of the building, the centerpiece, the gorgeously curved staircase reminded of other Hudec works, such as

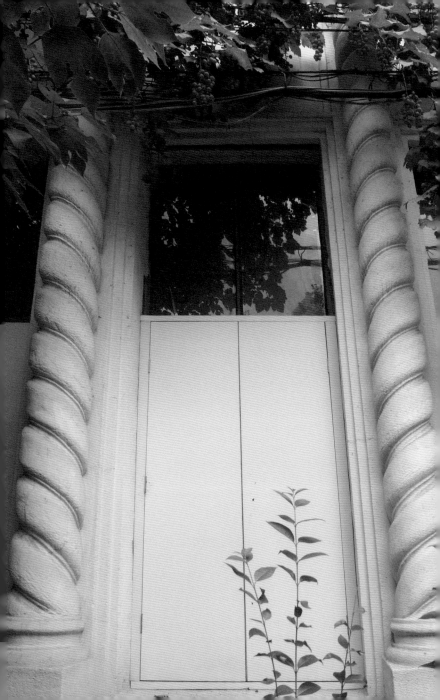

Ho Tung's Residence on Shaanxi Road. The three floors were paved with different colors and materials to offer an aesthetic variety, black-and-white marbles on the ground floor, yellow-and-black cements on the second and black-and-white mosaic tiles on the third.

The west part of the house contains several Chinese rooms decorated with stunningly exquisite Chinese wooden carvings all over the floors and walls.

"Hudec was a traditional and professional architect. He was not the avant-garde kind. Although he had great talents and techniques, he never forced his clients to accept his own styles and always paid attention to the practical side of construction," says professor Hua.

"He was not the kind of designer who wanted to surprise the world and become part of architectural history. Little attention had been paid on this building during the years. And that

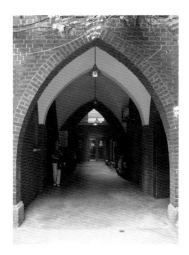

has made it uncharted and very unique. When I first visited it, I felt like finding a gem," says Hua.

And I had the same feeling when I walked through the hot sunlight of July, passed through an outpatient hall full of patients and finally stood in the middle of the garden surrounded by Spanish columns, green ivies and strong Chinese herbal smells.

Yesterday: The Large Building in Hsiai Lane
Today: the Gonghui Hospital (under renovation)   **Address:** 315 Shimenyi Rd.
Tips: The building is hidden inside the lane and quite easy to miss. The lanes around the hospital are also worth a walk if it's not too hot.

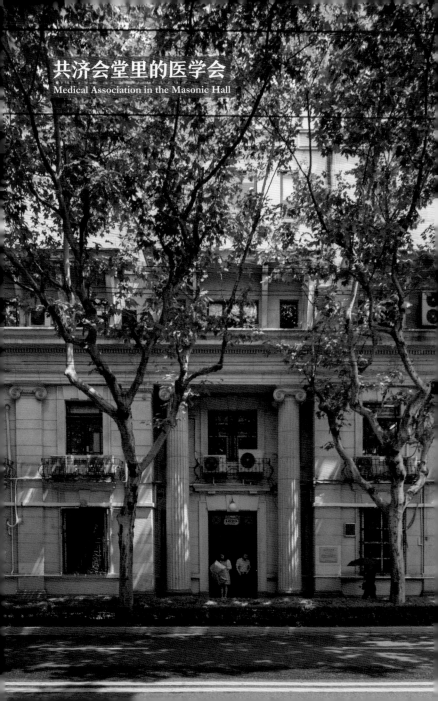

美国作家丹.布朗（Dan Brown）的畅销书《达·芬奇密码》（*The Da Vinci Code*）点燃了公众对神秘组织共济会的兴趣。在上海市中心，一座新古典主义风格的共济会堂至今犹存，半个多世纪以来一直由上海市医学会使用。

共济会堂原来在外滩，1931年迁到北京西路1623号现址，老会堂在被卖掉后遭拆除。

著名学者何新撰文提到，共济会在明清之际就进入中国，北京西路大楼是共济会在上海的一处遗迹。大楼正面的六芒大卫之星纹饰是共济会的重要标志之一，但关于这幢楼房的来历和资料，在目前已出版的介绍上海老建筑的书刊上都没有提到过，"好像这幢大楼从来不存在似的"。

圣约翰大学原校长卜舫济（F. L. Hawks Pott）在1928年出版的《上海简史》（*A Short History of Shanghai*）中提到，共济会在上海生活中扮演过重要角色。

"我们发现第一家分会——

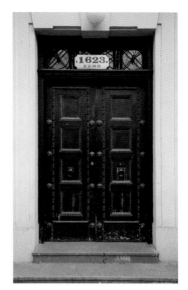

北华分会（Northern Lodge of China）——成立于1849年，紧随其后的是1863年的皇家苏塞克斯分会（Royal Sussex Lodge），最早设在花园弄（Park Lane，今南京路）。而外滩共济会堂（the Masonic Hall）的奠基石是1865年7月安放的，那是在外滩滨水区最早出现的吸引人的建筑之一。"卜舫济写道。

上海历史学家吴志伟研究发现，共济会起源于欧洲中世纪的石匠组织。

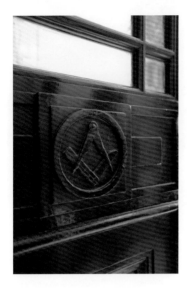

"1843年上海开埠后，共济会在这里成立了十几个分支机构，其中的北华分会、皇家苏赛克斯分会和塔司干分会（Tuscan Lodge）共同建造了外滩共济会堂。几个世纪以来，共济会的组织以神秘而闻名。作为世界上最大的秘密组织之一，其大部分的成员都是白人男性、自由思想者和社会精英。"吴志伟说。

外滩共济会堂的位置就在外滩29号东方汇理银行大楼和33号英国领事馆之间，原址如今是上海半岛酒店。共济会堂中文被译为"规矩会堂"，这是因为共济会的标志是圆规和矩尺，中世纪建造教堂的石匠们常用的两件工具。何新认为，会堂当年能在外滩这样的黄金地段占上一席之地，这从另一个方面也反映了共济会的实力。

共济会堂每两年举行一次慈善募款舞会，此时会堂就会对公众开放。舞会是上海最大型的宴会活动之一，非常受欢迎，共济的神秘特色也为活动增色不少。参加舞会的人数从1886年不到400人攀升到1910年的1200多人。原先宽敞的大厅变得拥挤，所以此时规矩会堂迎来一次改造。不幸的是，1918年一场大火部分损毁了这座美丽的大楼，后来共济会又把会堂卖给日本邮船株式会社（Japan Mail Shipping Line）。后者拆除了大楼，但却没有建造新楼。

1930年4月15日，英文《北华捷报》（the North-China Herald）刊登了一张新规矩会堂的设计图，与今日北京西路1623号的建筑十分相似。

"可能大家会记得外滩旧规

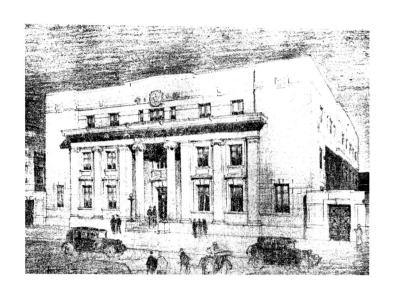

矩会堂在3年前卖给了日本邮船株式会社。今年初，共济会用这笔钱在爱文义路（今北京西路）和胶州路的东南角买到一块合适的基地。为了新会堂设计方案，共济会举行了一个小型设计竞赛，有6位建筑师参加。获胜的设计师J. E. March先生是英国皇家建筑师学会注册建筑师，来自新马海洋行（Messrs Spence, Robinson & Partners）。这张图显示设计方案面向爱文义路。建筑内部根据共济兄弟会的需求而规划，外观庄严美观。"报道写到。

报道还提到，大楼将由英国、苏格兰和爱尔兰的共济会员使用，而美国分会（the American lodges）两年前已在贝当路（Avenue Petain，今衡山路）建造了一座会堂。

根据静安区房地局资料，这座共济会堂是一座砖混结构建筑，呈现新古典主义风格，顶部有三角形大山花，立面装饰有两根巨大的爱奥尼石柱。

20世纪50年代后，这座美丽的会堂主要由上海医学会使用。上海市医学会缘起于1915年成立的中华医学会。

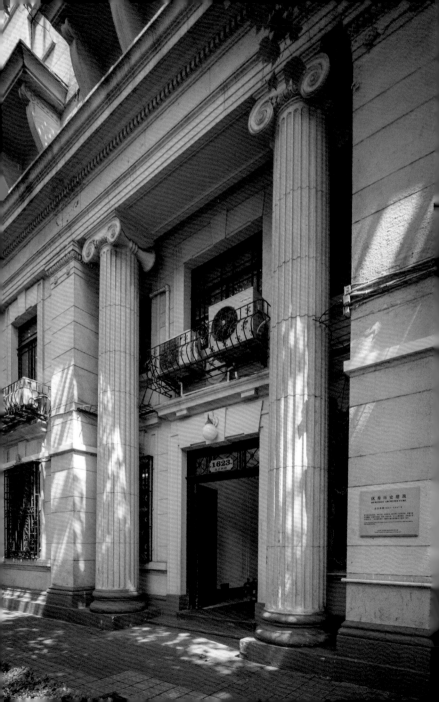

根据《中华医学会史概览》（1915—2010），在中国近代医学史上，最早的西医团体由在华的欧美教会医院发起的中国博医会（The China Missionary Medical Association，1925年改称The China Medical Association），于1886年在上海成立。中国博医会在相当长的时间内不允许中国医师加入，直到1910年2月才吸收留美归国的颜福庆博士成为该会的第一个正式会员，1911年辛亥革命后允许我国从国外学成回国的西医师参加，但人数依然很少。

1915年2月5日，当时已是中国博医会会员的伍连德、颜福庆、俞凤宾、刁信德、丁福保、石美玉等21位医师，趁出席博医会大会的机会，在上海一家饭店（Yi Lung Lao）开会宣布成立"中华医学会"（英文名为The National Medical Association of China），由颜福庆担任会长，伍连德为书记，暂借南京路34号俞凤宾医师诊所作为临时会所。

中华医学会在上海成立后受到全国广大医生的欢迎和支持，并于1932年合并了中国博医会，成为当时中国医学界的真正代表。在后来的动荡岁月里，中华医学会克服困难组织会员参与医疗救护工作，还举办学术活动、编译医学名词、出版医学书刊、推动卫生行政、促进现代医学教育、推广公共卫生及预防医学、普及医学卫生知识，为中国近代医学事业的发展做出重要贡献。到1949年时，中华医学会有4000余名会员，下设30多个支会和13个专科学会，出版《中华医学杂志》（中英文）等6种期刊和60余种书籍，为近代中国医学事业奠定了基础。

1917年1月，医学会第一个地方支会广东支会成立后，上海支会也于同年4月2成立，名医唐乃安当选为会长。如今，已有百年历史的上海市医学会凝聚了全市最优秀的医学科技工作者，开展学术交流、科普宣传、人才培养、科技奖励和医学期刊出版等活动，同时承接医学鉴定、医疗服务标准化、技术评估、临床重点专科建设等工作，促进了上海医药卫生事业的繁荣和市民健康

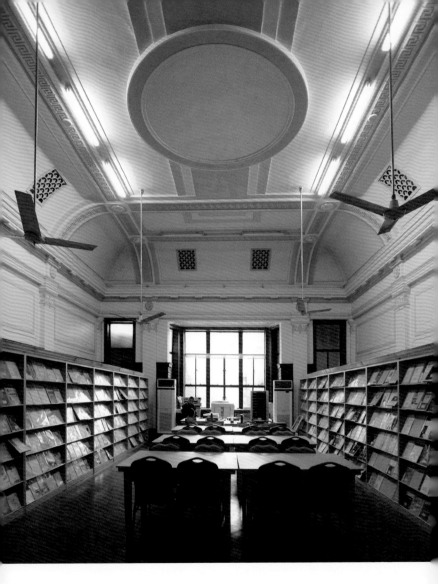

水平的提高。

　　上海市医学会办公的共济会堂在1985年加建了一层，2003年和2015年历经两次大修。医学会还使用与共济会堂毗邻的原基督教科学会堂（First Church of

Christs' Scientist）。

如今，共济会堂仍保留着原始的柚木地板、楼梯和礼堂。浅绿色调的礼堂设计简洁，装饰着神秘的图案与符号。礼堂的一扇门通往幽深的藏书室。藏书楼里有高达两层的巨大书架，有些神似电影《哈利波特》中魔法学校的图书馆。

上海市医学会图书馆副馆长张燮林介绍，这里藏有2000多本医学文献典籍，其中大多数都是中医书籍。医学会曾接待过来参观的海外共济会会员，他们辨认出了礼堂里的符号。这座大楼的红色木门仍装饰着共济会的标志--圆规和矩尺。

学者何新提到1949年以前，上海、威海、天津和厦门都有共济会的建筑遗迹。北京西路这座新共济会堂有一块石碑，上面刻有上海几位共济会成员的名字和大楼建造日期——1931年1月。

有趣的是，1931年在这块石碑上被写为"AL 5931"。"AL"是Anno Lucis的缩写，意思是"光年"。根据共济会的日历系统，公元1931是光历5931年，因此写成"AL 5931"。

"在维修大楼时，我们在这块石碑后面的墙壁里发现了一个铁盒，里面装着圣经和两支古董钢笔，还发现在一楼护墙板后的墙上刻有该建筑捐建者们的名字。"张馆长说。

2017年上海医学会创办百年纪念之际，这座鲜为人知的共济会堂被列入第五批上海市优秀历史建筑名录。医学会将绿色礼堂改造成一个面向医学专业人士和学者的"医学人文之家"，促进医学研究与交流。

昨天： 共济会堂　**今天：** 上海市医学会　**地址：** 北京西路 1623 号
建造年代： 1931 年　**建筑风格：** 新古典主义
设计师： 新马海洋行（Spence，Robinson & Partners）J. E. March
参观指南： 该建筑物不对公众开放，但可欣赏立面左下角奠基石上的原始铭文。

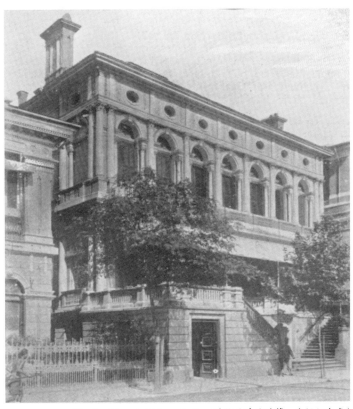

The first Masonic Hall on the Bund（位于外滩的第一代规矩会堂）

Dan Brown's best-selling novels *The Da Vinci Code* and *The Lost Symbol* aroused international interest in Freemasonry. And while people may read the books and view the resulting movies to satisfy their curiosity, it is rarely known that a former three-story Masonic Hall in neoclassical style still stands in downtown Shanghai. It's been used by Shanghai Medical Association for more than a half century.

The masonic hall moved to the current position after its structure on the Bund was sold and demolished in the 1930s.

"The building at 1623 Beijing Road W., now the office of the Shanghai Medical Association, is

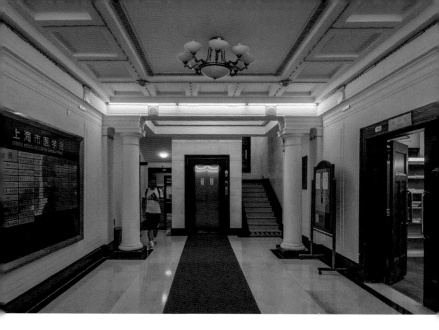

an important relic of Freemasonry in Shanghai," Chinese historian/economist He Xin wrote in his book *Who Rules the World*.

"However, the building is often missed out by publications on Shanghai historical architecture, Shanghai, Weihai, Tianjin and Xiamen all have relics of Freemasonry before 1949," he noted, who had studied and written about the secret society.

According to F. L. Hawks Pott's 1928 book *A Short History of Shanghai*, Masonry played an important part in Shanghai life.

"We find that the first Lodge — the Northern Lodge — was established in 1849," Pott wrote.

"This was followed by the Sussex Lodge in 1863. Its first home was in Park Lane (now Nanjing Road). The foundation stone of the new hall on The Bund was laid in July 1865, and was one of the first buildings of pleasing character to appear on the water front."

Shanghai historian Wu Zhiwei said the Freemasons have their origins in organizations for Medieval masons.

"Freemasonry founded over a dozen branches in Shanghai after the city opened as a port in 1843, among them were Northern Lodge of China, Royal Sussex Lodge and Tuscan Lodge that co-funded the construction of the Bund," Wu said.

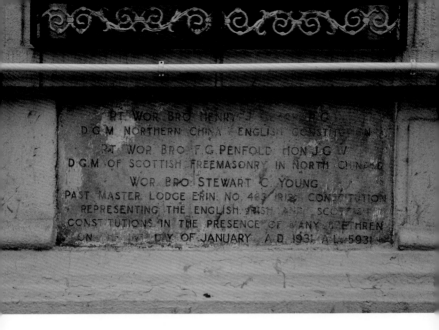

RT WOR BRO HENRY J [...]
D G M NORTHERN CHINA - ENGLISH CONSTITUTION [...]
RT WOR BRO F G PENFOLD HON J G W
D G M OF SCOTTISH FREEMASONRY IN NORTH CHINA
WOR BRO STEWART C YOUNG
PAST MASTER LODGE ERIN NO 463 IRISH CONSTITUTION
REPRESENTING THE ENGLISH IRISH AND SCOTTISH
CONSTITUTIONS IN THE PRESENCE OF MANY BRETHREN
ON THE [...] DAY OF JANUARY A D 1931 A L 5931

They also had a reputation for secrecy for centuries.

"As one of the world's largest secret societies nowadays, most of their members are white male Protestants, free thinkers and social elites," Wu added.

The site of the former Masonic Hall on the Bund is now occupied by the Peninsula Hotel.

The Chinese name "Kwei-Ken-Tang" meant "Compass and Square Hall" according to Masonic symbols "compass and square". two crafting tools used by masons who built stone churches.

The society's most revered room would be open to the public when hosting the famous biannual Masonic Ball for charity fund raising.

Symbolic mysteries added glamor to the ball, which was regarded as the city's largest feast and enjoyed great popularity.

The fewer than 400 participants in 1886 soared to 1,200 to 1,300 in 1910. The once spacious hall became crowded, which lead to a renovation in the 1910s. But unfortunately the building was partially damaged by a fire in 1918 and later sold to the Japan Mail Shipping Line (NYK), which demolished it and left the lot vacant.

On April 15, 1930, *the North-China Herald* published a drafting of the new Masonic Hall, which looks very like the one on today's Beijing Road W.

"As may be remembered the old Masonic Hall on the Bund was sold to the NYK nearly three years ago," the article states.

"With the proceeds a desirable site at the southeast corner of the Avenue Road and Kiaochow Road crossing was bought at the beginning of this year. For the design for the new building a limited competition was held, six architects taking part. The author of the winning design is Mr J. E. March, A.R.I.B.A., of Messrs Spence, Robinson & Partners. The picture shows Mr March's design as it will front on Avenue Road (today's Beijing Road W.). The interior of the building is as well planned for the needs of the Masonic fraternity as the exterior is handsome and imposing."

The report noted that the building would house English, Scottish and Irish Masons. The American lodges had built a hall adjoining Avenue Petain (today's Hengshan Road) two years ago.

According to archives from Jing'an District House and Land Management Bureau, the building is a brick-and-concrete structure in neoclassical style with a triangle gable over the top. The facade is adorned with two gigantic Ionic Orders.

In the 1950s it was assigned to six academic societies, including the Shanghai Medical Association, which originated from the Chinese Medical Association established in 1915.

According to the book *An Overall History of the Chinese Medical Association (1915—2010)*, the earliest Western medical group in the history of modern medicine in China was the China Missionary Medical Association initiated in 1886 in Shanghai by European and American missionary hospitals in China. It was renamed the China Medical Association in 1925.

For a long time, Chinese doctors were excluded from the association. It was not until February 1910 that Dr. Yan Fuqing, who had returned from studying medicine in the United States, became the first official Chinese member of the association. After the 1911 revolution, some Chinese doctors who had studied abroad were also allowed to join the association, but the number was still small.

On February 5, 1915, 21 Chinese physicians, including Wu Liande, Yan Fuqing, Yu Fengbin, Diao Xinde, Ding Fubao and Shi Meiyu, who were members of the Chinese Medical Association, took advantage of attending the association's meeting to gather in a Shanghai hotel and held a meet-

ing to announce the establishment of "The National Medical Association of China". Dr. Yan Fuqing was the president while Dr. Wu Liande was the secretary. Dr. Yu Fengbin's clinic at No. 34 Nanjing Road was used as the temporary office of the association.

After its establishment in Shanghai, the National Medical Association of China was welcomed and supported by doctors all over the country. In 1932, it merged with the Chinese Medical Association and became the genuine representative of the Chinese medical circle.

In the turbulent years that followed, the association overcame difficulties and organized members to participate in medical rescue work. It also organized academic activities, compiled and translated medical terms, published medical books and periodicals, spread medical knowledge, promoted modern medical education, public health and preventive medicine.

By 1949, the association had more than 4,000 members, established over 30 branches and 13 societies in different medical fields, and published six journals and more than 60 books. It had laid a solid foundation for medical work in China.

The Shanghai branch of the association was established on April 2, 1917. Famous doctor Tang Naian was elected as the president. Today, the century-old Shanghai Medical Association has gathered the best medical workers in town to carry out activities such as academic exchanges, training and publication of medical journals. It has contributed to the prosperity of Shanghai's medical and health services and the improvement of citizens' health.

The Freemasonry Hall of the Shanghai Medical Association was added an extra floor in 1985 and underwent two major restorations in 2003 and 2015. The medical association also uses the adjacent former First Church of Christs' Scientist building.

Currently housing a myriad of medical societies and organizations, the building is well preserved with the original teak wood flooring, staircase and most amazingly, a green-toned grand hall adorned with patterns and symbols.

A door in the hall leads to a dim-lighted old bibliotheca with a high ceiling and double-level book shelves, reminiscence of another era and a library in a "Harry Potter" movie.

Zhang Xielin, deputy director

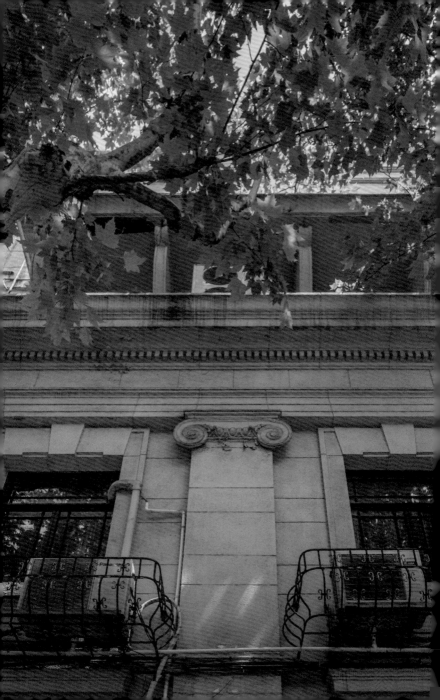

of the Shanghai Medical Association's bibliotheca, said it has more than 2,000 antique medical books, most of which are on traditional Chinese medicine.

Officer Hua Fei from the Shanghai Medical Society recalled receiving Freemason guests from overseas, who recognized symbols in the hall. Some red wooden doors of the building are still graced with the society's signature — "Compass and Square".

In his book, scholar He Xin specifically mentioned a stone tablet in the new Masonic Hall, which is inscribed with the names of several Freemasons in Shanghai as well as the construction date — January 1931.

The year "1931" was also written as "AL 5931" on the stone according to a calendar system within the Freemason fraternity. "AL" is an abbreviation for Anno Lucis, which means "Year of Light".

"We found an iron case hidden in the walls behind this stone tablet which contained a bible and two antique pens," Zhang with the medical association added.

"Another wall behind the dado is inscribed with names of expatriates who gave donations for the construction."

In 2017, the building was listed in the fifth batch of Shanghai Historical Buildings upon 100 years' anniversary of Shanghai Medical Association. And the green bibliotheca hall has been converted to "a family for medical professionals and scholars" for better research of medical work.

Yesterday: Masonic Hall   **Today:** The Shanghai Medical Association

Address: 1623 Beijing Road W.   **Built in:** 1931   **Architectural Style:** Neoclassic

Architect: J. E. March, A.R.I.B.A., of Messrs Spence, Robinson & Partners.

Tips: The building is not open to the public but you can admire the original inscription at the left bottom base stone.

毗邻共济会堂的第一基督科学会堂（上海医学会使用）

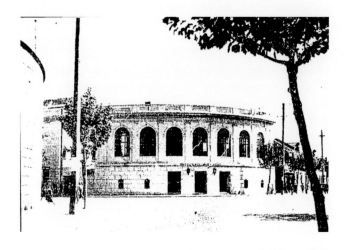

　　1934年11月4日（星期日），上海第一基督教科学教会在这幢新的教堂大楼内举行了仪式。新教堂位于爱文义路和胶州路转角处。这是在中国建造的第一座基督教科学教堂，开幕式将是奉献典礼之一，教堂完工准备投入使用，没有任何债务。1934年3月22日奠基的教堂结构已接近完成。这座建筑是一些人寄予目标和希望的物质体现。在过去的20年里。他们因为基督科学教而相识。教堂根据哈沙德洋行（the firm of Elliott Hazzard Architects）的设计建造，弧形立面所遵循的风格源自经典罗马风。教堂用灰泥覆盖的砖建造，其外观与浅黄色石灰石相似。入口门的上方用铜字写着"First Church of Christs' Scientist"（第一基督科学会堂），两侧是艺术设计的铸铁灯笼。

　　根据该建筑基地的形状，半圆形或扇形平面似乎是唯一可能的解决方案。但这被证明是一个理想的机会，因为随之而来的安排特别适合于基督科学教的仪式，从而允许面向读经师的桌子进行方便的座位安排。〔注：基督教科学派或称科学教派，The Church of Christ, Scientist，是基督教新教的一个边缘教派，由Mary Baker Eddy于1879

年创立，礼仪简朴严格，由读经师主持）

整个建筑的内部装饰在各方面都保持现代和艺术性，同时又简约而节制，其设计想法是保持一种安静庄严的氛围。必须承认，整个建筑无论内部外部，都是装饰性的经典设计方面一项令人称赞的成就，再加上最富有吸引力又很柔和的家具，为快速发展的上海精美建筑又添加了显著的一笔。1914年，第一个基督科学教派的阅览室开幕，自那时以来，阅览室一直运营，现在的阅览室位于南京路49号中央拱廊8b室。1915年，基督教科学派举行了第一次免费公共讲座。1928年，该组织获得了足够的会员资格，成为上海基督科学派第一教会，就是今天的名字。

教会仪式一直在外滩共济会堂举行。该建筑被拆除后，又在皇家亚洲学会位于博物馆路（今虎丘路）的建筑中进行。当美国共济会堂在杜福路（今乌鲁木齐南路）上建成时，他们就在那里举行活动，直到现在。

1934年12月2日晚9点15分，一个星期天的晚上，来自马萨诸塞州波士顿市的曾长期居住在科学教派创始人玛丽·贝克·埃迪（Mary Baker Eddy）家中的第一科学教派会员，将在这座新教堂发表演讲。

摘自 1934 年 11 月 7 日《北华捷报》

the First Church of Christ, Scientist

On Sunday, November 4, 1934, the First Church of Christ, Scientist, Shanghai held services in this new church building, located at the corner of Avenue and Kiaochow roads.

This is the first Christian Science church to be erected in China, and the opening service will be one of dedication, the edifice being finished and ready for occupancy, free from all debt.

The cornerstone for this building was laid on March 22, 1934, and this structure, now almost completed, is the material embodiment of the aims and hopes of a small group of people who, for the past twenty years, have met for the holding of Christian Science services.

It is built according to the designs of the firm of Elliott Hazzard, Architects, and the style adhered to in the curved facade is derived from the classic Roman.

Brick, covered with plaster, was used in its construction, and the exterior is similar in appearance to buff limestone. Above the entrance doorway, in bronze letters, are the words "First Church of Christs' Scientist" and wrought-iron lanterns of artistic design flank the central doorway.

In conforming to the shape of this building site, the semi-circular or fan-shaped plan seemed the only possible solution.

This necessity, however, proved a desirable opportunity, as the arrangement ensuing is especially well adapted to Christian Science services, permitting a convenient seating arrangement with respect to the Readers' desk.

The interior finish throughout of this building, while modern and artistic in every respect, has been kept simple and restrained, with the idea of preserving an atmosphere of quiet repose and dignity. It must be conceded that the entire edifice, within and without, is an admirable achievement in decorative and classic design, combined with most attractive though subdued furnishings, a notable and outstanding addition to the fast-growing collection of Shanghai's fine buildings.

In 1914, the first public Christian Science Reading Room was opened and since that time a Reading Room has been constantly maintained, the present one being located at Room 8b, Central Arcade, 49 Nanking Road. The first free public lecture on Christian Science was given in 1915.

In the year 1928 this Society had attained a membership sufficient to become organized as First Church of Christ, Scientist, Shanghai, and thus it is known today.

Services were held in the Masonic Hall on the Bund until that building was demolished, when they were held at the Royal Asiatic Society's building on Museum Road (today's Huqiu Road). When the American Masonic Temple was built on Route Dufour (today's Urumqi Road S.), they arranged to hold their services there, and have been in that location ever since.

The First Church of Christ, Scientist of Boston, Mass, and for many years resident in the home of Mary Baker Eddy, the founder of Christian Science, will lecture in Shanghai, in this new church edifice, on Sunday evening, December 2, 1934, at 9:15pm.

Excerpt from *the North−China Herald* on November 7, 1934

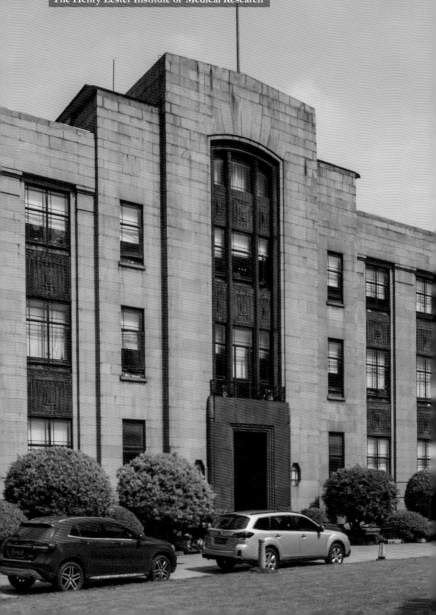

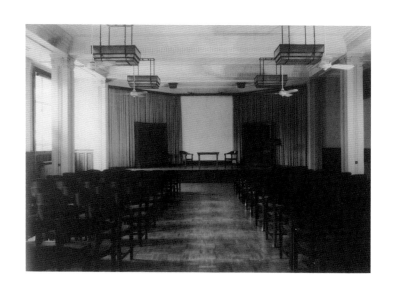

1932年9月，雷士德医学研究院（Henry Lester Institute of Medical Research）即将在爱文义路（今北京西路）落成。简洁现代的大楼高达三层，阳光充足，设有演讲厅、医学图书馆、会议室和实验室等，英文《大陆报》称这是"远东地区最大、设备最好的研究型医院，可与国际上任何同类机构媲美"。

这所医学研究院根据英国富商、慈善家雷士德（Henry Lester）的遗愿建造，建筑今日犹存，位于北京西路1320号。

这是一家专注于公共卫生研究的机构，由临床部，生理部和病理部组成，有近百名员工。1932年开办的研究院抗战时暂停工作，虽然时间不长，却汇聚一批优秀的化学家、生理学家、病理学家、昆虫学家、内科外科医生。他们在此潜心研究，发表了很多研究成果，也为中国培养了一批医学专业人才。

研究院的主楼由雷士德开办的德和洋行设计，高达三层，大门摩登现代，很多知名医学专家曾在大门前合影留念。

"正门大厅的门廊一侧是门房间和电话室，另一侧面向电

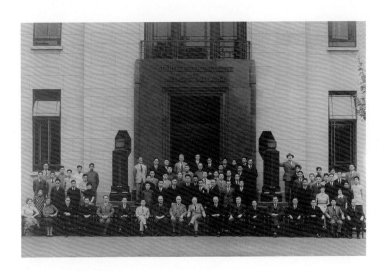

梯。长长的走廊向两侧延伸开来，在这些走廊上分布着办公室。"1932年的英文报纸写到。

走廊的西端是主演讲厅（main lecture hall）和小演讲厅（small lecture hall）。主演讲厅设计有宛若小舞台的讲台，配有准备间（preparation rooms）。在1930年代的上海，这里每周举办专业讲座。著名病毒学家汤非凡（Dr. F. F. Tang）从美国哈佛大学留学归来后曾担任雷士德医学院的细菌学系主任，他在这里做过病毒主题的讲座。而雷士德医学院的生理科学组主任、英国生理学家伊

博恩（Bernard Read）则在此分享了他关于上海食物营养分析的研究。伊博恩重视对中国药物、药用植物和当地食品的研究，他对促进中药材科学研究方面的贡献尤其重大，出版了多部专著，还将李时珍的《本草纲目》和朱元璋之子、植物学家朱橚所著的《救荒本草》翻译成英文。

走廊的东端是雷士德医学院著名的图书馆（Library）以及期刊室(Journal Room)。因为馆藏大量原版医学专业书籍，当时很多学者都申请到这个图书馆查资料。除了书籍，雷士德研究院还收藏了很多名贵的动植物标

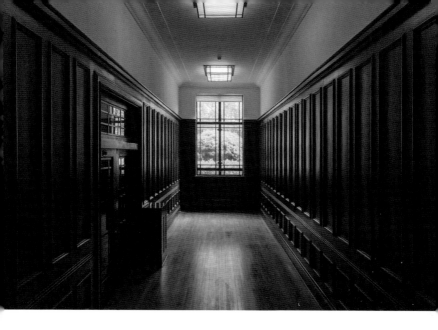

本，包括骨化石和中国草药标本。

主楼的二楼和三楼分别是病理学组和生理学组的实验室和办公室。这些实验室由一个个"单元"组成，可以拼接或分隔。由于分隔这些单元的隔板由不承重的轻质混凝土制成，可以根据研究工作的需求灵活地变化调整。主楼还有地下室，设有焚化间和储藏室。

大楼是平屋顶，阳光充足，空间开放而且充足。建筑挑高4米左右，窗户大，采光好，冬暖夏凉。室内地板、门墙都为柚木，质量优良经久不变。

除了主楼，雷士德研究院还有员工宿舍、所长住宅等配套建筑。最有特色的是一座专门饲养实验动物的小楼，房间围绕着一个中央庭院而建造。

抗战爆发后的动荡岁月里，研究院的工作大受影响。这座为了实现科学理想而建造的建筑在战争中作为公济医院的应急医院使用，大部分外国工作人员被送回英国，研究工作停滞不前。1941年，研究院又被日军占领。

美国埃默里大学助理教授傅家倩研究发现，雷士德研究院是

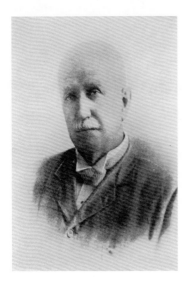

"一家主动尝试根植于中国土壤的西方机构"。

"根据1932年至1940年担任研究院院长的厄尔（H. G. Earle）的说法，雷士德医学研究院能够发挥重要作用，正是因为它是一个有组织的研究机构，而不是一所大学或医学院。有组织的研究机构是必要的，以便研究的主体可以一直向前推进，并且可以积累大量准确的知识，预备着留给天才的头脑对其进行阐释。在中国这样的国家，'西方医学的历史不长，发展欠缺，雷士德医学研究院确保基础性研究

的开展既有场所，也有必要的物质资料。'"傅家倩(Jia-Chen Fu)在论文《实验之屋：为民国科学创造空间》（*Houses of Experiment: Making Space for Science in Republican China*）中写道。

多年以来由于围墙很高，从外面只能看到建筑顶部和绿树，研究院的大楼一直披着神秘的面纱。1949年后，这里先后挂牌"华东工业部上海工业试验所""轻工业部上海工业试验所""食品工业部上海科学研究所"，直至1957年，这里成为"化工部上海医药工业研究所"，1960年改名为"上海医药工业研究院"，如今大楼空置。

雷士德医学研究院是根据雷士德的遗嘱而建立的三个主要慈善项目之一，另外两个项目是雷士德医院（今仁济医院）和雷士德工学院（曾用作海员医院）。这三个历史建筑今日犹存，都是雷士德留给上海这座城市的遗产。

1840年2月26日，雷士德（Henry Lester）出生于英国南

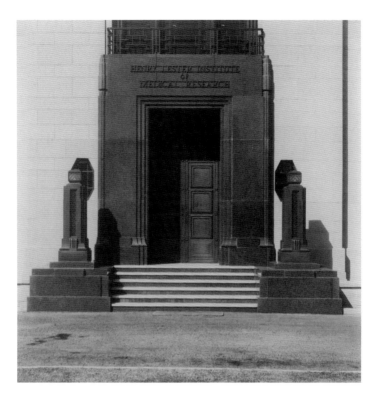

部港口城市南安普敦市。他曾在伦敦接受建筑师和土地勘测师的训练，1863年到上海后受雇于工部局负责公共租界土地测量的工作，后来也为法租界测量土地。这些工作都完成后，雷士德回归建筑师的角色。他先与一名建筑师合作，但很快独立创业，沿着黄浦江岸设计建造了许多著名的洋行、码头和仓库。

1913年，雷士德又与强生(George A. Johnson)和马立斯（Gordan Morriss）联合创办德和洋行（Lester, Johnson & Morriss），专营建筑设计、土木工程、测绘检验、房地产抵押放款等业务。德和洋行发展成为近代上海实力最强的设计事务所之一，承接的项目包括外滩5号日清大楼、外滩17号字林西报大楼和南京路先施公司大楼等。

1926年5月14日，雷士德在上海公济医院（General Hospital，今上海第一人民医院）病逝，安葬于静安寺公墓（今静安公园）。《北华捷报》和《大陆报》等英文报纸纷纷撰文回顾雷士德的一生，评价他是一个有远见的人，很早发现了上海的潜力，大量投资不动产。而他在上海的运气特别好，从一开始就很成功，无论做什么都能"点石成金"，做成了上海历史上最大的几笔土地交易。雷士德在去世前已成为上海最大的土地拥有者之一。

报道估算，雷士德拥有价值约300万英镑的财富，也有传闻称他的财产达500万英镑之多。英国学者Peter Hibbard曾在《上海外滩》中评价，雷士德的洋行既做建筑设计与建造项目，又做土地和地产交易，开创了先河，堪称在上海投资最成功的英国建筑师。

不过虽然投资如此成功，雷士德的个人生活却与住华丽别墅的上海富豪们形成强烈反差。终身未婚的他生活非常简朴，穿别人的旧衣，交友不多，喜欢步行和乘公交汽车，被认为是上海英侨社区最吝啬的人。

雷士德在外滩共济会堂和上海总会居住多年，被认为是总会"最早、最奇怪的会员"。"点石成金"的雷士德却很少去总会著名的长吧（long bar）消费，除了为会员提供免费葡萄酒和蛋糕的平安夜。

富豪雷士德简朴生活的谜团在他去世后揭开。雷士德去世时除了一名在军中服役的侄子没有亲属，他留下一份惊人的遗嘱，除了少量遗产赠予个人，将几乎所有遗产留在上海用以成立"雷士德基金会"，发展医疗、教育和慈善事业。

他生前指定用遗产资助建造任济医院新大楼、雷士德医学研究院和雷士德工程研究院和学校。此外，上海聋哑学校、虹口华德路圣路加医院、虹口黄包车夫会等慈善组织也得到捐助，遗嘱还为在上海就学的所有国籍、任何宗教信仰的14岁以下的男女学生设立雷士德奖学金。从这份遗嘱可以看出，雷士德十分关心城市弱势群体，同时重视医学和教育事业，富有长远发展的眼光。

1927年，雷士德基金会即按照这份遗嘱开展筹建工作，由雷士德创办的德和洋行三大项目的负责设计。这三大项目在20世纪30年代陆续建成使用。

1931年，仁济医院位于山东路的新大楼首先落成，展开作为现代化医院的新一页。仁济医院新大楼原计划盖5层，因为后来决定让雷士德医学研究院使用其中一层，加建为6层。

1932年，选址在爱文义路的雷士德医学研究院是第二个落成的遗产项目。有意思的是，雷士德捐建的两家医学机构——仁济医院与雷士德医学研究院，不仅曾在一起办公——研究院一度设在医院新楼五楼，还开展良好的密切合作。研究院接办了医院的化验部，帮助其开展细菌学、血清学、临床化学、病理学、临床造影等方面的研究应用。研究院的医学专家对医院提供了给力的帮助，而供研究院使用的五楼保留了一些病房，以供专家研究临床疾病。合作有机结合了基础研究与临床治疗，而两家医学机构都为近代中国培养了很多医疗技术人才，也为今天上海的医疗卫生事业奠定了一定的基础。

1934年，根据遗嘱兴建的第三个项目——雷士德工学院及学校在东熙华德路（今东长治路）完工。占地达10000平方米的工学院是一座引人瞩目的装饰艺术风格建筑，提供科学技术方面的培训教育。

如今距雷士德逝世已近百年，但他留下的遗产保存至今。仁济医院已发展为一所集医疗、教学、科研于一体的综合性三级甲等医院。雷士德工学院及学校培养了数百名杰出的"雷士德男孩"，工学院大楼也保存至今，由海员医院使用多年。

1957年，雷士德医学研究院这座伟岸的建筑成为化工部上海医药工业研究院，延续了昔日功能。这里荟萃了一大批来自各大药厂的知名专家和科研人员，如雷兴翰、童村等，声名远播，成为中国医药工业系统中科研实力

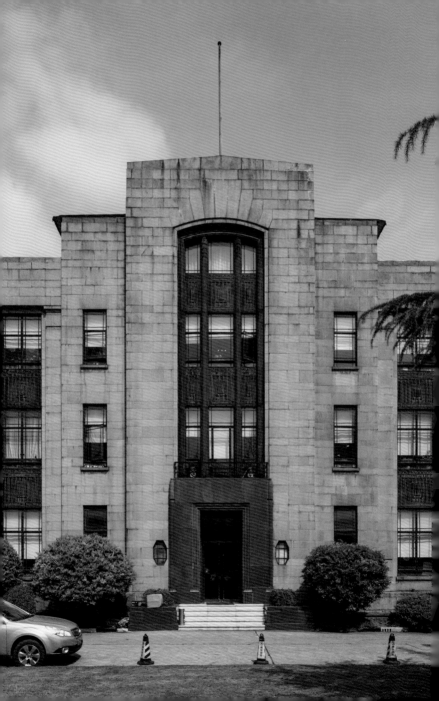

最强的研发机构之一。医工院迁往张江后，这里由和睦家医疗使用。

在为《遗产与记忆—雷士德、雷士德工学院和她的学生们》一书撰写的前言里，熊月之写道："在数以万计的近代寓沪外侨中，来自英国的雷士德特立独行，品德高尚，闪射出夺目的光彩……雷士德以其毕生的辛劳，全部的积蓄，书写了一个大写的'善'字，也是一个大写的'爱'字，对弱势群体的善与爱，对儿童的善与爱，对上海的善与爱。"

在上海这座城市，孤身一人的雷士德深居简出，度过了63年漫漫人生岁月。在那份写满"善"与"爱"的遗嘱中，他还写下一段话："在将近60年中，我主要和永久的家一直在中国的上海，现在如此，以后也将如此。自从很久以前我选择中国作为定居地以来，这里就是我的家了。"

如今，雷士德设立于1926年的信托基金仍在运作，为赴英深造的中国学者提供奖学金资助。基金会英文网站的首页写着两个中文字——"上海"。

上海曾经给雷士德带来巨大的机遇和财富，他又将获得的财富回馈给这座城市，仿佛形成了一个爱与能量的完美闭环。而雷士德医学研究所这座大楼幸运地保留至今，在上海的城市中心，闪耀着科学与爱的光芒。

昨天： 雷士德医学研究院　**今天：** 和睦家医疗
地址： 北京西路 1320 号　**建造年代：** 1934 年
建筑师： 德和洋行（Lester Johnson & Morris）
参观指南： 大楼不对外开放，但可以从北京西路欣赏建筑的立面。雷士德工学院旧址位于东长治路 505 号，现在是上海创新创意设计研究院。

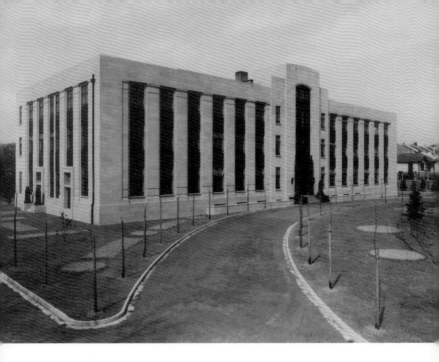

When the building at 1320 Beijing Road was near completion in September 1932, *The China Press* said it would be "the largest and most finely equipped research hospital of its kind in the Far East and is equal to most anywhere in the world".

This institution focused on public health research, consisting of clinical, physiology and pathology departments, with nearly 100 employees. The research institute opened in 1932 and its work was suspended after World War II broke out in 1937. Although it did not operate for long, the institute brought together a galaxy of outstanding chemists, physiologists, pathologists, entomologists, and medical surgeons. They had devoted themselves to research, published a number of research findings and trained modern medical professionals for China.

The establishment of the Henry Lester Institute of Medical Research realized the Last Will and Testament of Henry Lester, a British millionaire landowner and philanthropist whose name is intimately associated with early Shanghai history.

"Among the tens of thousands of expatriates living in modern Shanghai, Henry Lester with his unique character and noble virtue glittered brilliantly," famous Shanghai historian Xiong Yuezhi wrote in the preface for the book *Bequest and Memory* by Fang Yunfang.

The medical research institute had been built entirely for research purposes where a staff of physicians and scientists had some headquarters. Sitting well back from the street, the institute was surrounded by a brick wall; the entrances were guarded by heavy bronze grills. There was a three-story building and on either end of the ground floor were large rooms, one of which had been used as a lecture room and the other as a medical library.

According to *The China Press* on September 15, 1932, the lecture room contained a stage and preparation rooms behind it. In the 1930s, lectures in a variety of medical topics were held here every week.

Famous virologist Dr. F. F. Tang (Tang Feifan), who had studied in the Harvard University in the US and served as director of Department of Bacteriology, gave a lecture on filtrable virus. British physiologist Bernard Read, who headed physiology team of the institute, shared his study on the nutrition of Shanghai food.

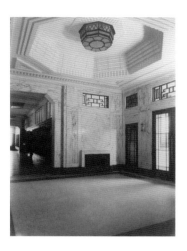

Read attached great importance to the research on Chinese medicine, medicinal plants and local food. He had made a great contribution to the promotion of scientific research on Chinese medicinal materials, having translated Ming (1368—1644) dynasty prince Zhu Su's *Famine Rescue Materia Medica* into English.

With a journal room in connection with it, the library boasted of a rich collection of imported medical books. Medical experts of the times would apply to research in this famous library. The remainder of the ground floor was used for conference rooms and offices.

"On entering the main entrance hall, flanked on either side by the porter's office and telephone office, one faces the elevator. Long

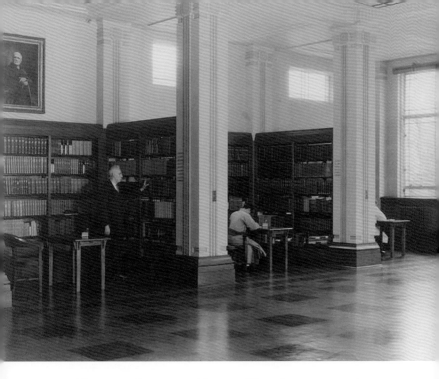

corridors extend away on either side, on to which open the offices. Ascending to the first floor, which will house laboratories, one finds a similar arrangement of space. Each room will be devoted to a special use. The third floor, beside housing other laboratories and offices, will contain a large museum of medical research. The roof is flat and is open and sunlit, containing much space," *The China Press* said.

The medical research institute was one of the two major philanthropic projects constructed to realize Lester's will.

The other one was a three-story structure in Art Deco style for a combined Lester school — the Henry Lester Institute of Technical Education, which is located on today's Dongchangzhi Road in Hongkou District.

The object of the school was to provide sound fundamental training in the sciences and technology for boys preparing to enter the building and allied trades. In the technical institute more advanced and more theoretical training would be given.

Both the medical research institute and the institute of tech-

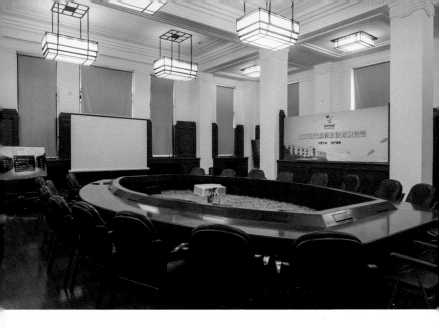

nical education were designed by the architects of Lester Johnson and Morriss, a firm co-founded by Henry Lester.

Born in 1840 in Southampton, Lester, who had received his training in London as an architect and land surveyor, came to Shanghai in 1863—1864 to survey the settlement for the Shanghai Municipal Council. He also served in the Public Works Department of the French Council. It is said he followed a doctor's advice and embarked on a journey to Shanghai after an unknown disease took the lives of all three of his brothers.

It seemed he made the right choice and Shanghai became his lucky city. After his service in the municipal council was completed, he started his own business.

His company, Lester Johnson & Morris, became one of the most well-known architectural firms in town. A man of great foresight, he saw the potential of Shanghai and made large investments in property. Prior to his death, he was one of the largest landowners in Shanghai. Most of his property was used for the purpose of Chinese buildings.

With so much money and land in hand, Lester was unlike most tycoons in modern Shanghai who often lived an extravagant life by building gorgeous mansions and hosting parties night after night.

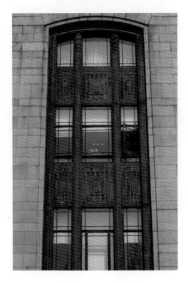

He never married, lived in the dormitory of Shanghai Club on the Bund, had no cars and often took buses. He seldom bought new clothes and many of his clothes were gifts from friends.

Before he died in May 1926, Lester bequeathed most of his assets to philanthropy, including the St Luke's Hospital, the Institution for the Chinese Blind, the Children's Refugee, The Little Sisters of the Poor, The Shanghai Mission for Ricsha Men and St Joseph's Asylum for the Poor.

He also left the bulk of his fortune for the re-establishment of the Cathedral School, for the building of the Lester Chinese Hospital and a Henry Lester School and Institute of Technical Education.

In carrying out the latter provisions, the Trustees and their advisors decided to establish two institutes, one for medical research and the other for technical education. The Lester school was to be closely associated with the technical institute.

"I declare that for about 60 years my principal and permanent home has always been and that it still is and will be in Shanghai in China and that long since I chose China as my domicile and such is my domicile now," Lester stated in his will.

Time flies but Lester's legacy is well preserved in the city he loved.

The Lester Chinese Hospital turned to be today's Shanghai Renji Hospital on Shandong Road. The Lester school lasted only for less than 10 years due to World War II but nurtured hundreds of outstanding "Lester Boys" who grew up to be Chinese professionals in all aspects of life.

The medical research institute was fortunate to always be tied with medical or scientific research after the Shanghai Institute of Pharmaceutical Industry was founded here in 1957.

"The walls of the building at 1320 Beijing Road W. were tall and people could only see the top of a grand building and lush green trees. They had to admire the grandeur of the building only when the gate opened occasionally. Our institute has always been shrouded with a mysterious veil until the solid surrounding walls were replaced by railings during a renovation in the 1990s. Our institute had congregated a large amount of renowned experts and excellent technicians from large medical factories, such as Lei Xinghan and Tong Cun. It was reputed as the best comprehensive medical and pharmaceutical research institute in China," Hu Guoliang, the late office director of the institute, wrote in an article about the building.

After Shanghai Institute of Pharmaceutical Industry moved to Zhangjiang, the building is now used by United Family Healthcare.

After Lester died in 1926, he was buried 10 minutes' walk from this institute built according to his will. He rested in peace in the now Jing'an Park, which had been Bubbling Well Cemetery for local expatriates since 1898.

"Many American and European expatriates who first came to Shanghai boasted cultural privilege and despised Chinese culture. But with extensive contact with and a deeper understanding of Chinese people, some of them gradually paid more attention to or even loved Chinese culture. They became more friendly to the country. Lester was a typical example of its kind," Xiong said during a recent lecture.

Today, the Lester Trust still supports Chinese students and scholars to study or research in the United Kingdom. In the conditions for applications, "the grant will give a Chinese citizen, whose knowledge and skill obtained, will be for the benefit of the people of China." The official English website for the Lester Foundation contained two big Chinese characters which are "Shanghai".

And in the city center of Shanghai, the Henry Lester of Medical Research building survives and glistens with light of science and love.

Yesterday: Henry Lester Institute of Medical Research
Today: United Family Healthcare   **Address:** 1320 Beijing Road W.
Built in: 1934   **Architect:** Lester Johnson & Morris
Tips: The building is not open to the public but you can see the façade on Beijing Road. You can also visit the Henry Lester Institute of Technical Education at 505 Dongchangzhi Road.

研究古代中医药

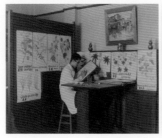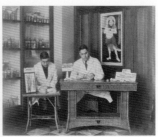

雷士德医学研究院发现古老的疗法有许多治疗作用。

很多人认为，驴皮、羊眼、鹿角、狗脑、奇怪草药等的疗愈用途，在民间传说和妖魔论中交织在一起，实在是空洞的中国迷信。

不过，生理科学部负责人伊博恩博士（Dr. Bernard Read）和雷士德医学研究院的同事们正在进行广泛的调查，这可能会大大减少人们对中医药的怀疑态度。

雷士德医学研究院的态度是，在可以将当今西方世界的医学科学强加给中国人民之前，必须对传统中医实践的基础进行实验性观察。

有理由相信，当某些治疗方法不仅在中国、印度已经持续使用了多个世纪，而且有历史文献表明，尽管没有直接的联系，这些疗法在更古老的文明也有使用，那么基本可以认为这些疗法是有疗效的。

在中国被称为"阿胶"的熬煮驴皮被广泛用作血液再生剂和体内止血药，并且是体弱人士、尤其是那些患有肺结核的人们的普遍营养品。这种现象引发人们对其特性的化学和生理研究。T. G. Ni博士发现阿胶中含有大量的甘氨酸、胱氨酸、赖氨酸、精氨酸和组氨酸，口服后可提高钙氮的吸收并提高血液中的钙含量，而静脉注射阿胶可有效恢复出血和休克后的循环低下。进一步关于阿胶在肌肉萎缩中的有益作用正在进行中。去年在杭州，仅一家商店就交易了25万元的驴皮。

伊博恩在关于"新型药理和古代医学"的报告中说："值得注意

的是，1909年英国药典的现代医学仅包含9种动物来源的物质，而几乎所有这些物质，都是像猪油和蜂蜡一样无害的东西。当现代科学转向肝脏、胃、来自眼睛的维生素A、肾上腺素等时，在古代医学中发现了这么多动物组织的应用是令人惊奇的。

在上述最新发表的报告中，伊博恩博士用一张表格列出了传统中医使用的6种家畜的26个部位，这些动物包括牛、马、猪、鸡、绵羊和狗。

梅花鹿等物种的天鹅绒质地的角制成的粉末状药物，受到中国人的高度认可。俄罗斯科学家最近的研究表明鹿角含有雄性荷尔蒙激素。

羊眼的虹膜和晶状体用来治疗视力模糊和结膜炎。鹰、鹦鹉和鲭鱼的眼睛用于治疗夜盲症。最近，瓦尔德（Wald）从绵羊、猪、牛和青蛙的虹膜中分离出维生素A。

在传统中医里，建议猪肝治疗夜盲症、脚气病等，最近人们发现猪肝富含维生素A、B、C、D、E。有很多这样的例子，比如荠菜。因为草药明显缺乏强大的原理，因此被抛在一边，现在已被证明荠菜适度地富含三种维生素，这也很好地证明了中国古人使用荠菜来治疗很多疾病的科学依据。

在中国，人们保存有30到50个世纪的非常准确的医学经验记录。这些记录并非神圣机构的积累，而是迄今为止的经验发现，只是在20世纪科学的相当粗糙的筛子中才被筛选出来。

摘自 1935 年 7 月 24 日《北华捷报》

Ancient Chinese Medicine Studied

Lester Institute of Medical Research Finds Many Healing Properties in Old Remedies.

It may seem to many that the healing use made of donkey skin, sheeps' eyes, deer's horn, dog's brain, odd herbs, etc. All interwoven as they are in folk-lore and demonology, is just so much empty Chinese superstition, and that it is unfortunate that such great faith is placed in such absurd remedies.

However, an extensive survey now being undertaken by Dr. Bernard Read, head of the Division of Physiological Sciences and his associates at the Henry Lester Institute of Medical Research may greatly diminish popular skepticism.

It is the attitude of the Lester Institute that before today's medical science of the western world can be imposed on the Chinese people, due regard must be given to the empirical observations which form the basis of the old Chinese medical practice.

Reason has suggested that when certain therapeutic practices have been in constant use for a great many centuries not only in China but in India and with no apparent relationship in the still more ancient civilizations, as revealed in old manuscripts, it is at least likely that some real benefit is derived.

The phenomenally widespread use in China of boiled down donkey skin, called "Ah-Chiao", as a blood regenerator, and internal styptic, and a general nutritive for weak people, especially those suffering from tuberculosis, has led to an investigation into its particular character both chemical and physiological. Dr. T. G. Ni finds that it contains a large amount of glycine, cystine, lysine, arginine and histidine. Administered orally it improves the calcium nitrogen absorption and raises the calcium level of the blood. This Ah-Chiao used intravenously was found to be effective in restoring a depressed circulation after hemorrhage and shock. Further work is proceeding on its beneficial effects in muscular atrophy. In Hangchow last year there was a quarter-million dollars trade of the donkey skin in one store alone.

"It is of interest to note," states Dr. Bernard Read in his report on "The Newer Pharmacology and Ancient Medicine", "that the modern medicine of the 1909 British Pharmacopoeia only included nine substances of animal origin, and those nearly all, quite innocuous things like lard and wax. While modern science is turning to liver, stomach, vitamin A from the eye, adrenalin, etc., it is remarkable to find the use of so many animal tissues in ancient medicine."

In his recently published report mentioned above, Dr. Read presents a table showing twenty-six parts of six domestic animals used in old Chinese medicine. These animals include the cow, horse, pig, chicken, sheep and dog.

The velvet horn of the Skia deer and other species is taken as a drug in powder form and is very highly regarded by the Chinese. Recent studies by Russian scientists show that the male sex hormone is present.

The iris and lens of the sheep's eyes were given for dimness of vision and conjunctivitis. The eyes of the hawk, parrot and mackerel, were administered for night blindness. Recently Wald has isolated vitamin A from the iris of sheep's, pig's, cattle and frogs.

In old Chinese medicine, pig's liver was recommended for night blindness, beri-beri, emancipation etc. And has fairly recently found to be rich in vitamins A, B, C, D and E. A great many instances of this sort are cited. Shephard's purse is given as an excellent example of a medicinal herb cast aside for its apparent lack of potent principles which has been shown to be moderately rich in three of the vitamins and well justifies the old Chinese use of it for a number of maladies.

In China there has been preserved for something between 30 and 50 centuries remarkably accurate records of human experience in the field of medicine. These records are not accumulations of divine institutions but empirical findings which up to the present have only been sifted with the very coarse sieve of last century science.

Excerpt from *the North-China Herald* on July 24, 1935

汤教授的病毒专题讲座

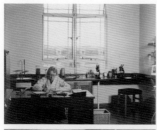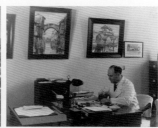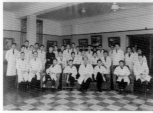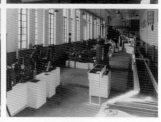

昨晚在雷士德医学研究院举办的讲座中，汤飞凡教授指出，过去几年的研究表明，不可滤病毒是包括流感与黄热病在内的众多具有高度传染性的疾病的致病原。

汤教授说，过去几年，不可滤病毒的相关研究已经取得重大进展。

由于不可滤病毒形态更小，无法用肉眼观察到，科学家们对于这些生物体在诸多方面的特性都尚未完全了解。

但学界确信，这类微生物就是引发黄热病、流感、麻疹、普通感冒、沙眼、脑膜炎以及其他诸多疾病的致病原，而这些疾病几乎都具有相当的传染性。同时，这些疾病大多也被认为能够赋予人体免疫力。

尽管巴斯德对于比微生物更小的生物体的存在表示出怀疑，有关方面的研究却成果甚微，直到过去几年，各类新型研究手段的发展才改变了这一状况。

根据汤教授的讲述内容得知，当前，有三种新型研究手段得到发展，分别是超过滤法、超离心法和超微缩法。

超过滤法中，采用了一种经由复杂化学工序制成的薄膜。这种薄膜的厚度薄到只能以微米（毫米的千分之一）为单位来测量。目前雷士德医学研究院已经预订了这类制品。

新型离心机的离心速度已经可以超过每分钟15000转，能够对这类病毒进行处理。此外，据汤教授称，一种真空新型离心机已经在过去数月间被研制出来。

拥有了这些新的研究工具，科学家们将更好地对这些微小生物体进行研究，从而进一步开展医学实践，朝着消除这类疾病的目标前进，造福全世界。

汤教授称，不可滤病毒具有众多已经明确的特性。小型的不可滤病毒虽然肉眼不可见，但均有固定的大小。它们是严格意义上的胞内寄生体，无法人工培育。

这些生物体会引致细胞质内封入体的形成。它们对于环境变化表现出极强的适应力，在严寒、干燥与50％丙三醇溶液作用下均能生存。

这一系列的下一场讲座主题为"与维生素A相关的天然色素"，时间为周三下午5点30分，地点是雷士德医学研究院主演讲厅，主讲人为马尔博士（Dr. P. G. Mar）。

摘自 1937 年 1 月 14 日《大陆报》

Invisible Organisms Discussed At Henry Lester Institute

Research during the past several years indicates that filtrable viruses are the cause of numerous highly infectious diseases, including influenza and yellow fever, declared Dr. F. F. Tang in a lecture yesterday evening at the Henry Lester Institute of Medical Research.

Much progress has been made during the past several years in the study of these filtrable viruses, he said.

Because the smaller filtrable viruses are invisible, scientists are still not entirely certain about many aspects of these organisms.

It is believed, however, that they are the cause of yellow fever, influenza, measles, common cold, trachoma, meningitis and a number of other diseases, nearly all of which are highly infectious. Most of them are also characterized as conferring immunity.

Suspected by Pasteur

Although the presence of organisms smaller than micro-organisms were suspected by Pasteur, little advance was accomplished until during the past several years when new methods of research were developed.

Three new methods have now been developed, according to Dr. Tang. They are ultra-filtration, ultra-centrifugation and ultra-microscopic work.

In ultra-filtration, a membrane developed through a complex chemical process is used. This membrane is so thin that it can only be measured by a micrometer which measures one-thousandth of a millimeter. Such an instrument has now been ordered by the Lester Institute.

New centrifuges that can concentrate these viruses have now been developed which have a speed of more than 15000 revolutions per minute. A new vacuum centrifuge has recently been developed during the past several months, he said.

With these new methods, scientists will be able to better study these tiny organisms and thus do further practical work toward ridding the world of these various diseases.

Definite Characteristics

Filtrable viruses have a number of definite characteristics, he said. The small ones are invisible, but all possess a definite size. They are strictly intra-cellular parasites and resist artificial cultivation.

The organisms induce the formation of cell-inclusion bodies. They show great adaptability to environmental changes. They are resistant to freezing, drying and the action of 50 percent glycerin.

The next lecture of the series will be given by Dr. P. G. Mar on Natural Pigments Related To Vitamin A on Wednesday at 5:30 p.m. in the main lecture hall of the Lester Institute.

Excerpt from The China Press on Jan 14, 1937

雷士德工学院（曾用作海员医院）

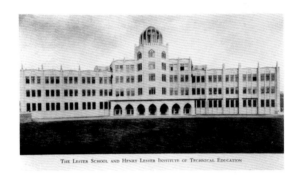

THE LESTER SCHOOL AND HENRY LESTER INSTITUTE OF TECHNICAL EDUCATION

　　雷士德工学院（Henry Lester Institute of Technology）占地10,000平方米，是一座气势宏伟的建筑。创办于1955年的上海海员医院曾经使用这座建筑多年。大楼的中央是四层高的塔楼，两翼为三层高建筑。

　　雷士德工学院的学校是为准备进入建筑和相关行业的男孩提供科学技术方面的基础培训，而工学院则提供更高级和理论方面的培训。

　　大楼建于1934年，由德和洋行设计。建筑体量很大，融合了哥特式和装饰艺术等多种建筑风格。

　　走进院落，参观者首先被一楼美丽的哥特式拱门所吸引，向上看又会发现一个巨大的圆顶。这座建筑看起来像是一艘远航的大船，从高处鸟瞰又觉得它像一架飞行的飞机。

大楼的墙面上装饰着小巧的方形黄油色瓷砖，楼梯上铺着水磨石地砖，没有过多的室内装饰。

由于战争等原因，雷士德工学院的历史不长，但在短短十年间培养了数百名"雷士德男孩"（Lester Boys）。他们成长为各领域的专业人士，其中包括著名的城市规划师、建筑师陈占祥。

1935年入学的陈占祥在传记中回忆了这所对他一生影响巨大的学校。他提到，雷士德学校几乎所有用品都来自英国，从粉笔到所有教师。学校只招收科技专业的男生，还为来自贫困家庭的有才华的学生提供奖学金。

他特别提到自己的老师米勒（H. Miller）是利物浦大学毕业的一名建筑师，"他教会了我建筑师的责任和终极力量……建筑师所做的不只是绘图和建造。"他写道。

1938年，在米勒的鼓励下，陈占祥前往利物浦大学建筑学院继续深造，开启了他传奇而曲折的建筑人生。

创建于1955年的上海海员医院曾使用雷士德工学院建筑多年。医院隶属于上海海运(集团)公司，日本外航船员医疗事业团在中国的特约医院，承担移民加拿大、澳大利亚、新西兰等国家的体检和上海市涉外婚检，是一所集医疗、教学、科研、预防、防疫、保健为一体的综合性职工医院。雷士德工学院大楼历经修缮更新，正改造为上海创新创意设计研究院。

Henry Lester Institute's legacy to architecture

Covering an area of 10,000 square meters, the Henry Lester Institute of Technical Education, also known as the Lester school at 505 Dongchangzhi Road in Hongkou, is an imposing three-story structure aligned on both sides of a four-story central unit and tower.

The object of the school is to provide a sound fundamental training in the sciences and technology for boys preparing to enter the building and allied trades. In the technical institute, more advanced and more theoretical training will be given.

Built in 1934 and designed by the Lester Johnson & Morriss Co, this was an unusually large building combining different architectural styles on one body.

Visitors are first struck by a beautiful array of Gothic arches on the ground floor. As you look up, a gigantic dome emerges. The building looks like a sailing ship from afar and in a bird's-eye view it resembles a flying plane. It's a mixture of Gothic and Art Deco styles.

The walls are delicately adorned with small square-shaped, butter-colored tiles. The staircase is paved with terrazzo tiles. No excessive interior decorations are seen for this former famous institute.

The Lester school during a decade of operation in Shanghai had trained hundreds of "Lester Boys" who grew up to be Chinese professionals in all aspects of fields, including Charlie Cheng, a renowned urban planner and architect who enrolled in the school in 1935.

According to his biography, the school used everything from the United Kingdom, from chalks to all the teaching faculties. The institute recruited only male students majoring in science and technology. It also provided scholarships for talented students from poor families.

"My teacher H. Miller, an architect who graduated from the Liverpool University, had taught me the responsibilities and the ultimate power of an architect ... An architect does more than just drawing and building," Cheng wrote.

In 1938 Cheng went to further his study in the School of Architecture, University of Liverpool, with the encouragement of Miller.

The building was used by Shanghai Seaman's Hospital since 1955. It's been renovated and converted to be the Design Innovation Institute Shanghai.

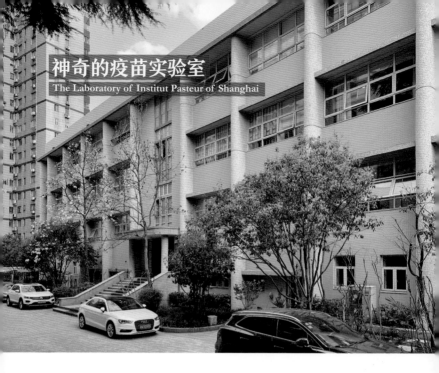

神奇的疫苗实验室

The Laboratory of Institut Pasteur of Shanghai

中科院上海巴斯德研究所因为在抗疫工作中做出的贡献，曾获得上海市政府表彰。在20世纪30年代的上海，上海巴斯德所的前身也为研制疫苗、防治流行病做了大量杰出工作，其简洁现代的大楼至今犹存。

这座米色建筑毗邻瑞金医院，位于瑞金二路207号的一个安静院落中，设计风格现代，有着十分特别的弧形转角。大楼目前由中国寄生虫病研究所使用。

1936年，米色大楼作为上海旧法租界公共卫生医学化验室隆重开幕，后来由上海巴斯德研究院负责运营，是中国最早研制疫苗的医学实验室之一。

《赉安传》作者吴飞鹏介绍，1933年初，旧法租界公董局委托法国建筑师赉安（Alexandra Leonard）设计一座由公益慈善基金资助建造的医学化验室。赉安与合伙人克鲁泽（A. Cruze）将这个项目设计为一座创新的现代公共建筑。

1935年7月27日，英文《大

陆报》（*The China Press*）刊登了一张医学化验室大楼的照片，立面简洁利落。

"法租界最新的医学化验室将成为远东地区最现代、最完备的医学化验室。外立面照片展示了注重功能性的现代建筑风格。" 照片的说明文字评价。

根据时任上海巴斯德研究院副院长刘永纯1941年撰写的文章，该院成立虽在晚近，然回溯来源则已久远。

"上海第二特区当局于巴斯德百年纪念之年（一九二二年）在广慈医院基地内设立抗疫诊疗所，即以'巴斯德诊疗所'名之，但成立之后，困难叠生；未及三年即改组为医学化验室，至今室址犹存，但已作他用；而化验室者，已迁入平民病舍之中，工作范围亦经缩小矣。在此变迁之中，第二特区居民日增，卫生机构逐渐发展；附设于卫生局之化验室不敷应用，于是筹建大规模卫生试验所一所，此所于一九三四年兴筑，一九三六年竣工，是年七月开幕。当其成立之前多年，沪地法籍士绅有在沪创立巴斯德研究院之议，曾与越南巴斯德研究院非正式交换意见数次；越南拟派专家来沪磋商，迄未实行，而试验所之建，又迫不及待。此所成立后，关于卫生及医学方面凡切于实用之技术，无不具备。工作二年，差强人意，然试验所直隶卫生局，其工作范围不能超出实用；其预算有规定，不容于实用工作之外再求进展，第二特区最高行政机关鉴于研究工作之重要，在沪熟商之后，遂与巴黎巴斯德研究员磋议，将试验所改组，于是上海巴斯德研究分院于一九三八年元旦正式成立。" 刘永纯在为震旦医学院第二十二届毕业纪念册撰写的报告中提到。

1936年7月1日，位于金神父路207号（今瑞金二路207号）的新医学化验室大楼隆重开幕，门前的台阶上站满了中外来宾。出席开幕典礼的来宾来自法方的政府代表和卫生官员，还有"在法租界执业的几乎所有医生"。他们"向上海的医学进步致敬，随后进入大楼参观闪耀的门厅"。

医学化验室由法国驻华大

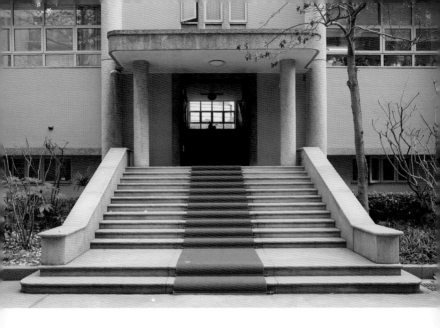

使纳吉亚（P. E. Naggiar）揭幕，在《马赛曲》的乐声中，法国驻华大使、驻沪总领事、公董局公共卫生处负责人贾斯帕（M. Jaspar）纷纷致辞。

"贾斯帕说医学化验室的建立是为了协助医生从事日常工作，充分发挥他们的技能与知识。通过研究危险疾病向当局提供帮助，生产疫苗，并与卫生局合作，对饮用水和食物进行有效监督。他赞扬了医学化验室主任雷纳尔医生（Dr. Reynall），并谈到了他在巴黎巴斯德研究所任职期间的研究工作经验。"

1936年7月8日的英文《北华捷报》（the North-China Herald）报道。

医学化验室为当时上海法租界居民提供的大部分服务是免费的。一些大型医院，如俄国医院、隔离医院和广慈医院也得到免费化验服务，只有私营机构和私人医生会被收取费用。

1936年的报道透露，这座以法国国旗装饰的新建筑外观很漂亮，内部装有当时最现代化的用于研究的设备。

"大楼通过一个宽敞的大厅进入，精美的楼梯通往大部分行政办公室所在的二楼。医学化验室设有一个装修豪华的图书馆，家具是超现代的管状风格的，而研究部门则装备精良。大楼里有一部分专门用于研究狂犬病，有一间装有铁丝笼的房间。这将是医学化验室的主要工作。有关伤寒、霍乱和其他本地流行疾病的研究工作将在这里展开。"1936年的报道说。

参加开幕仪式的来宾对走廊、房间和图书馆的优美装饰留下深刻印象。设计师努力使建筑结构尽可能地简单实用。

"光线、通风和完美的工作环境在很大程度上决定了外观设计的特征。据说该建筑是现代建筑设计中功能性的绝佳典范。"报道评价道。

负责大楼设计建造的赉安洋行（Leonard, Vesseyre & Kruze）是一家高产的设计事务所，由法国建筑师赉安（Alexandra Leonard）、韦西埃（Paul Veyssyre）和克鲁泽（Arthur Kruze）合伙经营。洋行的建筑作品大多风格现代，类型多样，有60多个建筑至今犹存。

"医学化验室大楼位于著名的圣玛利亚医院的西南角，是一座既浑厚稳重又现代感十足的5层建筑。赉安第一次大胆地将建筑的立柱全部置于建筑的外部，直上直下的立柱毫无装饰，还是一贯的抹圆。从远处看，竖向结构的半圆立柱间隔着整齐划一的排窗，做足了现代派建筑的气势。"吴飞鹏评价。

他提到，赉安认为建筑必须有合理的空间布局与舒适的居住或工作环境，外观只是这些合理性与舒适度的陪衬。由于资金有限，赉安在设计时充分考虑了建筑材料的成本，以及一座公共建筑应有的美观与稳重。

1938年，经过与巴斯德研究所巴黎总部的协商，公董局医学化验室被改组为上海巴斯德研究分院。巴斯德研究所是世界知名的生物医学研究中心，由法国科学家路易斯·巴斯德（Louis Pasteur）于1888年创立，在世界各地设有分支机构。

根据1938年8月10日的《北华捷报》报道，当年早些时候上

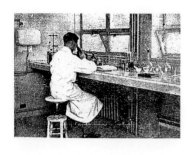

海巴斯德研究分院已在金神父路医学化验室大楼揭幕。雷纳尔医生专程从越南来到上海，负责管理这家新研究院。

刘永纯文章提到，上海巴斯德研究院直接为巴黎巴斯德研究所管辖，置院长一人，综理全院院务。院长之下分设四部，每部有主任一人，职工若干人，院长及主任人选，皆由巴黎委派。四部分工如下：

研究部：各项研究及病理学属之（此部主任暂由院长兼顾）。

微生物、血清检验部：凡系细菌，寄生物及血清检验皆属之。

疫苗部：凡制造普通菌苗（霍乱，伤寒等）卡介苗（B.C.G.）防疫苗等皆属之，防疫诊所附属于此部。

化学部：凡实业，食物，饮料，医学，毒物之检验皆属之。

其中，刘永纯负责疫苗部门。他出生于1897年，从上海震旦大学毕业后赴法留学，获医学博士，在巴斯德研究所巴黎总部以及法国斯特拉斯堡和越南西贡的分所从事过疫苗相关工作，曾负责管理西贡巴斯德分所。中华人民共和国成立后，他成为我国卡介苗防痨的创始人之一，对于狂犬病的防治也做出很大的成绩。

刘永纯在1941年的文章中透露，巴斯德研究院的唯一宗旨为服务于所在地方，使社会蒙其福利。

"上海巴斯德研究院于成立以来，根据上述宗旨，竭力进行。对于实用方面，因地方上之需要，已有相当发展。但对于研究及教育方面，因经济困难，尚未完全履行原定计划。"他写道。

1950年，上海巴斯德研究院由上海市人民政府接管，1951年中国人民解放军军事医学科学院在上海成立，巴斯德研究院并入该院，1958年前往北京。

此后，这座大楼由中国疾控中心寄生虫病预防控制所使用，2011年历经一次保护性修缮。

马克·吐温说过，历史不会重演，但有相似的韵脚。"非典"流行后的2004年10月11日，中科院与法国巴斯德研究所合办的上海巴斯德研究所举行揭牌仪式，法国总理希拉克（Jacques Chirac）、中科院副院长陈竺、上海市副市长唐登杰共同在上海合肥路411号为研究所揭牌。这家新的研究机构汇聚中法专家，聚焦病原微生物、重大传染性疾病研究，推动病原学、免疫学和疫苗学知识创新与学科发展。

巧的是合肥路411号恰好是赉安洋行设计的另一座现代风格建筑—震旦博物院（Musee Heude）。新诞生的中科院上海巴斯德研究所开始在这座历史建筑里工作，后因需要更多实验空

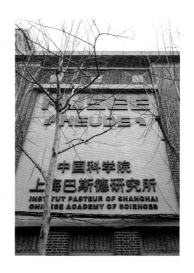

间，迁到岳阳路中科院。

更巧的是，中科院上海巴斯德研究所与使用巴斯德老楼的寄生虫病研究所都在抗击新冠疫情中做出贡献，巴斯德所参与病毒溯源、疫苗等工作，寄生虫所则派遣流行病专家支援。

如今，米色大楼仍完好保留着弧形转角、立柱、大理石门套与富有设计感的楼梯。这座现代建筑实用而美观，映射了人们为公共卫生健康付出的不懈努力。

昨天： 法国公董局医学化验室（1936年）、上海巴斯德研究院（1938年后）

今天： 中国疾病预防控制中心寄生虫病研究所　　**地址：** 瑞金二路207号　　**建于：** 1936年

建筑师： 赉安洋行　　**参观指南：** 在瑞金二路上可以欣赏到建筑物的外观。

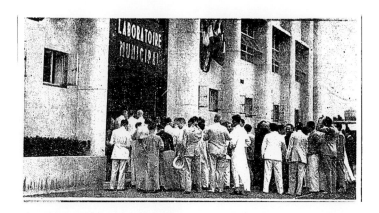

Mark Twain once said, "History never repeats itself but it rhymes". And the American writer's epigram is never more fitting when applied to the historic medical center situated at 207 Ruijin No. 2 Road.

The Institut Pasteur of Shanghai Chinese Academy of Sciences received a municipal prize for its work during the COVIC-19 pandemic in September last year, while ironically, in the 1930s, the medical center's predecessor also battled an epidemic.

Tucked away in a yard beside the Ruijin Hospital, the beige-hued building at 207 Ruijin No. 2 Road is a modern architecture with curved corners. It was built in 1934 to serve as the laboratory of the former French Concession and later operated as the Shanghai Pasteur Institute.

"In early 1933, the French municipal council commissioned French architect Alexandre Leonard to design and build a lab with public funding. Leonard and his partner Arthur Cruze made innovations on the modern design," said Wu Feipeng, author of an autobiography on the architect Alexandre Leonard.

A picture of the building's simply-cut façade was published in *The China Press* on July 27, 1935.

"The new Frenchtown laboratory will be one of the most modern and complete in all the Far East. The exterior photograph well displays the functional modern architecture used," the caption reads.

A 1941 article by Liu Yongchun, the then deputy director of the institution, revealed the history of the Shanghai Pasteur Institute traced back to 1922, when the local government established a clinic for epidemic prevention and control in the Ste. Marie's Hospital (today's Ruijin Hospital). The project also celebrated the 100th anniversary of the birth of French chemist/microbiologist Louis Pasteur (1822—1895). Pasteur was one of the most important founders of medical microbiology. And as a consequence, the clinic later became a medical laboratory.

As the population grew rapidly, a large-scale medical lab was constructed. On July 1, 1936, a large crowd gathering at the portals of the new French Municipal Laboratory on Route Pere Robert (now 207 Ruijin Road 2) "paid tribute to medical progress in Shanghai and later proceeded to inspect the glistening hallways within".

The building was opened by Ambassador P. E. Naggiar in the presence of French civic and governmental officials, health authorities and medical workers. After the playing of the "Marseillaise", addresses were given by the ambassador, the Consul-General and M. Jaspar, director of Public Works for the French Municipal Council.

"Jaspar stated the laboratory had been erected to assist medical practitioners in their daily duty, research into dangerous diseases, manufacture vaccines and cooperate with the Health Bureau in the effective supervision of drinking water and food. He paid tribute to the director of the laboratory, Dr. Reynall and spoke of his previous experience in research work while attached to the Pasteur Institute in Paris," *the North-China Herald* reports on July 8, 1936.

The laboratory offered most services free of charge to inhabitants of the former French Concession. A number of large hospitals, such as the Russian Hospital, the Isolation Hospital and Ste. Marie's Hospital, also received free services. Only private institutions and physicians were charged.

The report revealed the new building, which was bedecked with French national flags, presented a fine appearance from the outside. Inside, it was fitted with the most modern appliances of its times for the carrying on of research work.

"The building is entered through a spacious hall and a fine staircase leads up to the first floor, where most of the administration offices are situated. The laboratory contains a luxuriously fitted library, the furniture being of the ultra-modern tubular style, while the research department is ex-

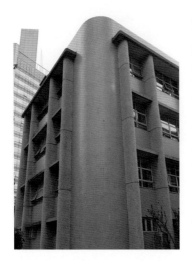

acter of the exterior design. The building was said to be an excellent example of the functional in modern building design," a preview report in *The China Press* noted on July 27, 1935.

The building cost over US$300,000. Leonard, Vesseyre and Kruze were the architects in charge of the design and construction. It was a prolific design firm managed by three French architects, Alexandre Leonard, Paul Veyssyre and Arthur Kruze.

"The laboratory building located at the southeast end of the renowned Ste Marie's Hospital is a solid, modern architecture of five floors. Alexandre Leonard adapted his signature curved corners. In addition, he made an experiment to place pillars on the external walls. Viewing from afar, the semicircular pillars divide identical windows and present a modern feel," researcher Wu said.

He adds that Leonard insisted proper space arrangement and a comfortable environment for living or working in his design. The appearance of a building was only a setting for its proper function and comforts. Owing to a limited budget, the architect had also taken building cost, as well as the beauty and steadiness of a public building into consideration.

tremely well fitted. In the section of the building set aside for research into hydrophobia, which will form a large part of the work undertaken by the laboratory, there is a room fitted with wire cages. Research work also will be carried on in connection with typhoid, cholera and other diseases prevalent here," the 1936 report said.

Visitors attending the ceremony were impressed by the beautiful finish of the corridors, the rooms and the fine library.

"Every effort had been made to make the structure as simple and practical as possible. Light and airy and perfect working conditions largely determined the char-

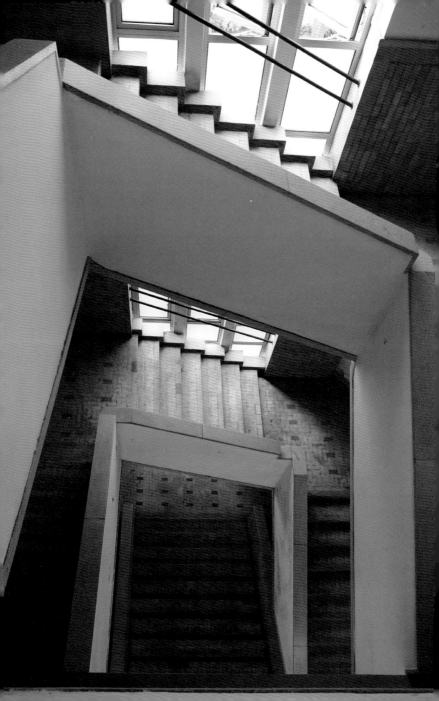

In 1938, the French municipal laboratory was reorganized into the Shanghai Pasteur Institute after a discussion with its Paris home center. Founded by Louis Pasteur in 1888, the Institut Pasteur is an internationally renowned center for biomedical research with branches all around the world today.

The North-China Herald on August 10, 1938, revealed the local branch of the Pasteur Institute was inaugurated earlier that year in the premises of the laboratory building on Rue Pere Robert. Dr. J. Raynal arrived from Indo-China to take charge of the new institute.

The Shanghai branch had four main departments-Pathological Anatomy, Microbiology and Serology, Vaccines, Organic and Industrial Chemistry.

Dr. Lieou (Liu Yongchun) who wrote the 1941 article directed the department of Vaccines. He had worked at the Paris Center of the Institute, in Strassbourg and Saigon, where he directed the branch of the Saigon Pasteur Institute.

Liu noted that the Shanghai branch of the Pasteur Institute had done much practical work during the three years. However due to financial difficulties, the institute did not carry on the

research and education work as scheduled.

The institute was taken over by the Shanghai government in 1950 and merged into the newly founded PLA Academy of Military Sciences in 1951 and moved to Beijing in 1958.

Since then, the building has been used by the National Institute of Parasitic Diseases, Chinese Center for Disease Control and Prevention.

In 2004, French President Jacques Chirac attended the inauguration of the Institut Pasteur of Shanghai co-founded by its Paris center and the Chinese Academy of Sciences. It was established to promote cooperation between France and China in the field of preventing and treating new infectious diseases. The new institute was opened in the former Aurora Museum at 411 Hefei Road, another modern-style building designed by Leonard and his firm in the 1930s.

Moreover, both Institut Pasteur Institute of Shanghai and the parasitic diseases institute using the former Pasteur building did great job during the COVIC-19 pandemic. The Pasteur institute organized a team to work on virus traceability, vaccine and antibody research while the parasitic diseas-

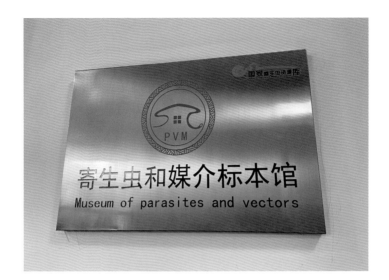

es institute sent epidemic experts to Wuhan and Italy.

Today, the beige-hued building is well preserved with the original curved corners and pillars on the facade, the stylish staircase and marble door pockets. These modern, functional details are living proof of the endless efforts for public health.

Yesterday: French Municipal Laboratory (in 1936) and Shanghai Pasteur Institute (after 1938)

Today: The National Institute of Parasitic Diseases, Chinese Center for Disease Control and Prevention

Address: 207 Ruijin No. 2 Road

Built in: 1936

Architects: Leonard, Veyssyre and Kruze

Tips: The façade of the building can be admired from Ruijin No. 2 Road.

巴斯德研究所巴黎总部的伯纳德教授访沪

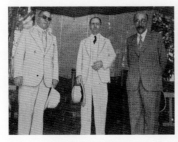
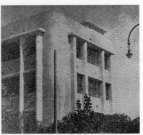

巴黎巴斯德研究所科学委员会的伯纳德教授（Prof. Noel-Bernard），同时也是巴斯德所远东事务部顾问和远东检查专员，昨日抵达上海视察巴斯德分院。他代表巴黎总部的巴斯德所所长向在上海工作的科学家们转达了问候，并对他们的工作表示鼓励。昨天早晨，他抵沪后旋即访问了位于金神父路207号的上海巴斯德研究院，院长雷纳尔博士（Dr. J. Raynal）带他实地参观研究院工作。视察结束时，伯纳德教授对《字林西报》（North-China Daily News）记者说，他很高兴地发现，上海巴斯德研究分院装备精良、组织得当、管理有序。

"由于得到了财政支持，该研究院拥有对本地疾病进行研究所需的一切条件，有各种类型的分析、疫苗的生产以及实际上服务当地卫生要求的一切必需。这些都超出了普通医学化验室的范畴。"

这位来访的科学家特别高兴地发现上海分院为分析各种类型的水做好了充分准备。"水质控制是在远东抗击流行病的一个非常重要的因素。令我感到极其高兴的是，上海分院具备条件处理此类水质分析，同时具有其他细菌学分析的能力。"

目前与霍乱的斗争需要大量疫苗，该研究院现在每月可生产近100万立方厘米霍乱疫苗。而抗伤寒和副伤寒疫苗库存始终保持足够的库存，以满足当地需求，这里同时也生产狂犬病疫苗。除此之外，该研究院还生产抗结核的卡介苗（B. C. G.）。该疫苗每周使用约300

剂，在父母的同意下，在广慈医院（今瑞金医院）为刚出生的婴儿接种卡介苗。疫苗接种已产生令人鼓舞的结果，目前正在进一步研究疫苗更广泛使用的可能性。

摘自 1938 年 8 月 10 日《北华捷报》

French Savant in Far East Tour

Prof. P. Noel-Bernard of the Scientific Committee of the Paris Pasteur Institute, Counsellor of the Institute's Department on Far Eastern questions, and their Inspector for the Far East, arrived yesterday to inspect the local branch of the Institute, on behalf of the Director-General and convey to local scientists greetings and encouragement in their work from the Home Center. Yesterday morning, immediately after his arrival, he visited the local Pasteur Institute at 207 Rue Pere Robert, where he was shown over the premises by Dr. J. Raynal, Director of the local branch. At the end of the inspection, Prof. Noel-Bernard stated to a "North-China Daily News" reporter, that he was very pleased to find, the local branch of the Institute excellently equipped, organized and administered.

"The institute, now, thanks to this financial support, possesses everything necessary for the study and research in local diseases, various types of analysis, production of vaccines, and in fact everything necessary to minister to local sanitary needs, which are beyond the scope of ordinary laboratory," he said.

The visiting scientist was particularly pleased to find the branch exceptionally well prepared to handle various types of water analysis.

"Water control is a very important factor in the struggle against epidemics in the Far East, and it gives me great pleasure to note that the

Shanghai branch of the Institute is well equipped to handle these types of analysis, as well as other types of bacteriological research," he said.

The present fight against cholera requires much vaccine and the institute's present monthly output of these vaccines reaches 1,000,000 c.c. A stock anti-typhoid and anti-paratyphoid vaccine is always kept in quantity sufficient to meet the local demand, while anti-rabic vaccine is also made. Besides these, the institute produces B. C. G. (Calmettes Guerin) anti-tuberculosis vaccine. This vaccine was used at the rate of some 300 doses per week, vaccinating, with the assent of the parents, newly born babies, at the Ste. Marie's Hospital. The vaccinations have given encouraging results and the possibilities of more extensive use of the vaccine, are at present further studied.

Excerpt from *the North−China Herald* on August 10, 1938

后 记

2022 年春夏之交,我因为上海疫情被封在武康路月亮书房。这是一段艰难又安静的时光,正好重读史料,写作此书。百年前的上海,人们也在做同样的事情,研究高度传染性的病毒、研制疫苗、建造类似方舱的隔离医院、普及传染病预防知识……

本书的缘起是 2020 年初爆发的新冠疫情。当时计划写一个"外滩第二立面建筑"专栏,但疫情后外滩建筑纷纷关上大门,抗疫工作让我的目光转向上海医院。

我曾写过邬达克设计的宏恩医院(华东医院)和同济医院(长征医院)。初步调研后,我发现上海各大医院里深藏着不少历史建筑,它们建造于不同年代,来自背景各异的医院,呈现丰富多样的建筑风格。这些映射了近代上海医学史的老建筑,默默诉说着百年前医疗工作的艰辛与不易。

我对上海医院建筑的选题兴趣浓厚。我的奶奶、外婆、母亲、姑母和姨母都是医生,她们有中医也有西医,注重卫生保健知识,让我从小耳濡目染。儿时我常跟随母亲到医院值班,在白色病房大楼里度过不少童年时光。

我还从奶奶于玲的传记中读到一段上海医院故事,她和爷爷乔信明都是新四军老战士。1942 年 10 月,年仅 25 岁的奶奶搭乘一条陈毅军长介绍的运咸肉的船,陪爷爷到上海看病。爷爷曾与方志敏一起在怀玉山被捕,因为坐水牢落下严重腿伤。他们一路艰险，掩盖身份辗转红十字会第一医院（华山医院）、红十字会第三医院和广慈医院（瑞金医院）等上海医院求医问药。1949 年后，他们又到上海，在中美医院（长征医院）得到著名骨科专家屠开元的手术治疗。爷爷从此可以拄拐杖走路，提高了生活质量，并重返工作岗位。

虽然我对上海医院建筑的选题很有兴趣，但深入调研却发现资料不多，属于上海建筑史书中的"冷门内容"。医院建筑以功能性为主，不如外滩的银行、南京路的商厦、武康路的洋房华丽精致。除了一些特别精美的作品，散落在上海各大医院里的历史建筑缺乏系统性研究。

幸运的是，我在老上海英文报纸等文献中查找到很多一手档案资料。在上海市医学会的帮助下，我还认识了原上海市第四人民医院图书馆陆明馆长。潜心研究医学史的他不仅提供了大量历史资料，还帮忙联系多家医院。复旦大学历史系高晞教授、同济大学建筑与城市规划学院华霞虹教授、张晓春教授及黄钰婷博士也对本书的研究写作提供了指点与帮助。

2020 年 3 月疫情还很严重时，我开始"逆行"采访一座座上海医院建筑，重访半个多世纪前爷爷奶奶去过的医院。在医院建筑探索之旅中，得到上海多家医院的支持帮助，有很多难忘的经历。

我采访第一人民医院时正好参加了该院的院志编纂会议，提供了一份 1914 年英文报纸关于医院建筑的报道作为参考。在写孙克基产妇医院（长宁区妇幼保健院）时，我发现 1936 年孙博士亲手接生过一个名叫彼得·雷文（Peter Raven）的美国男婴。在中科院朋友的帮助下，我联系到远在美国的雷文。他是世界知名的植物学家、美国科学院院士和中科院首批外籍院士，还是老上海金融地产大王弗兰克·雷文（Frank Raven）的后人。雷文院士一生热爱上海，家族相册中珍藏着孙博士抱着还是新生儿的他的照片。

2020 年 4 月，我的英文

上海医院建筑专栏"Shanghai Hospitals"在上海日报(*Shanghai Daily*）开始连载。

专栏从上海第一家西医院开始，先写西人创办的不同背景的医院：英国传教医生开设的仁济医院、日本医生开办的福民医院（第四人民医院）、法国天主教会创办的公济医院（第一人民医院）和广慈医院（瑞金医院）、英国富商捐赠的宏恩医院、德国医生为华人开设的同济医院等。

写着写着，中国人自己创办的医院：中国红十字会总院（华山医院）、中山医院、普慈疗养院（上海精神卫生中心闵行分院）、圣心医院（第一康复医院）、虹桥疗养院（徐汇区中心医院）、孙克基产妇医院（长宁区妇幼保健院）等登上历史舞台。

我曾写过多个上海建筑系列，"上海医院建筑"是调研难度最大的，也是收获最大、感受最深的专题。

1926年，英国富商查尔斯·雷纳（Charles Rayer）匿名捐建宏恩医院后，在英文《大陆报》（*The China Press*）上吐露心声。他说这是一家"没有国籍、种族或宗教歧视"的医院，因为"所有人都可能受到健康不良的折磨"。他希望这座医院能让人们怀有一种"开朗的善意精神"，对任何人都不恶意相加，由此团结居住在这座城市的人们。这种超越国籍种族的大爱与开朗的善意，正是疫情和危机四伏的今日世界最需要的。近年来，我国也在世界卫生大会呼吁共同建设人类卫生健康共同体。

历史最吸引人之处，就是一个个感人的故事，这些大上海医院的建筑故事让我深深着迷。上海医学建筑历史是一座宝库，内容丰厚，还有很多尘封的海内外档案在静静地等待有心人。本书分享的是阶段性的研究成果，由于篇幅等原因，还有一些医院历史建筑未及专门介绍，如上海健康医学院附属崇明医院（黄家花园）、上海市口腔医院（原中央储蓄会）、上海市儿童医院（原基督教中国内地会总办事处及医院，曾租给红十字会第三医院）、上海市第十人民医院（原上海铁路医院）、解放军455医院（中央银行俱乐部）、解放军 455 医院分院（基督教临安息日会上海卫生疗养院）等。期待未来有更多的发现。

这本书落笔之日，恰逢"大上海保卫战"进入新的阶段，武康路开始重现生机。这座城市迎来新的开始，也将需要一段时间来疗愈，恢复元气和光彩。通过一座座大上海医院建筑回望近代上海医学史，阅读这些匠心仁心的故事，可以带来不少信心和力量。

乔争月

2022 年 6 月 1 日

于上海武康路月亮书房

Epilogue

In Shanghai's epidemic lockdown caused by the Omicron virus from April to May of 2022, I had to stay at home on Wukang Road. It was a hard period for us all. While taking on the volunteer work and handling family cores, I also took the time to re-read Shanghai hospital related historical materials and found that almost a hundred years ago, people in Shanghai were doing the same thing, researching highly contagious viruses, producing vaccines, building quarantine hospitals and popularizing knowledge on how to prevent infectious diseases. It occurred to me that I might do something more to help encouraging the city's morale in fighting the epidemic by restarting my Shanghai hospital book project.

The book idea was initiated after the outbreak of the Covid 19 pandemic in early 2020. At that time, I had planned to write a column on "The Second Facade of the Bund" mainly about historical buildings behind the waterfront bund. Unfortunately, all these buildings closed doors after the epidemic. Meanwhile medical workers' fight against the pandemic turned my attention to Shanghai hospitals and medical institutions.

I had written about the Country Hospital (Huadong Hospital) and Tungchee Hospital (Changzheng Hospital) both designed by famous architect L. E. Hudec. After preliminary research, I discovered many historical buildings concealed in the city's major hospitals. They were built in different eras for hospitals of different backgrounds, showing a variety of architectural styles. These old buildings mirrored the medical history of modern Shanghai and witnessed the hardships and difficulties of medical professionals a century ago.

As of myself, I am always quite interested in the topic of Shanghai hospital architecture. My grandmothes, my mother and several aunts were all doctors. When I was a child, I often followed my mother to the hospital on her duty, and spent many days and nights in the white hospital buildings.

Before writing this book, I happened to read about my grandparents' experience with Shanghai hospitals from grandma Yu Ling's biography. She and my grandpa Qiao Xinming were both veterans of the New Fourth Army.

In October 1942, my grandma, then only 25 years old, took on a boat carrying pickled pork meat to escort my grandpa to seek medical treatment in Shanghai. Grandpa had suffered a serious leg injury after being put in a water prison of Kuomintang government for years. They went all the way to the Red Cross General Hospital (Huashan Hospital), the Third Hospital of the Red Cross and Ste. Marie's Hospital (Ruijin Hospital) to seek medical treatment. After the liberation of Shanghai in 1949, they came to Shanghai again and finally received a successful surgical treatment from famous orthopedist Tu Kaiyuan at Sino-US Hospital (original-ly Tung Chee Hospital, today's Changzheng Hospital). Grandpa was able to walk on crutches and returned to work after that.

Though an interesting topic to me, further research revealed only limited information of Shanghai hospital buildings, which had received little attention in the study of Shanghai architectural history. Hospital buildings are often functional and built with limited budget, so they are not as gorgeous and delicate as banks on the Bund, shops on Nanjing Road and garden villas along Wukang Road. Apart from several exquisite works, there is a lack of systematic research on the historical buildings scattered around Shanghai's major hospitals.

Fortunately, I found many first-hand archival materials in the old Shanghai English newspapers and other documents. With the help of the Shanghai Medical Association, I also met Lu Ming, the former director of the library of Shanghai No. 4 People's Hospital. An expert of Shanghai medical history, he kindly provided me historical materials and helped to contact some hospitals. Professor Gao Xi from the Department of History of Fudan University, Professor Hua Xiahong, Professor Zhang Xiaochun and Dr. Huang Yuting from the College of Architecture and Urban Planning of Tongji University also provided guidance and assistance for the research and writing of this book.

In March 2020, when the pandemic was still serious, I began to interview Shanghai hospital buildings, revisit the hospitals that my grandparents visited in the 1940s. During the exploration, I received support and help from many local hospitals and the experiences were unforgettable.

When I interviewed Shanghai General Hospital, I happened to attend one of its annals compilation meetings and provided a 1914 English newspaper report for their references. While writing about the Woman's Hospital, I discovered that its founder, Dr. Sun Keji delivered an American boy named Peter Raven in 1936. With the help of the Chinese Academy of Sciences, I got in touch with Peter Raven who is now resided in the United States. He is a world-renowned botanist, an academician of the American Academy of Sciences and the first foreign academician of the Chinese Academy of Sciences. Moreover, he's a descendant

of Frank Raven, a legendary financial and real estate tycoon active in old Shanghai. Peter Raven Kept his love for Shanghai, his born city all his life. The Raven family album still preserves the photos of Dr. Sun holding the newborn Peter.

In April 2020, my column "Shanghai Hospitals" started to publish on English newspaper Shanghai Daily.

The column started with the first Western hospital in Shanghai, and then wrote about hospitals founded by the foreigners with different backgrounds: Renji Hospital opened by a British medical missionary, Foo Ming Hospital (Shanghai No. 4 People's Hospital) run by a Japanese doctor, Country Hospital donated by a wealthy British businessman, Tung Chee Hospital established by a German doctor and two hospitals founded by the French Catholic Church, General Hospital and Ste. Marie's Hospital (Ruijin Hospital) etc.

After the 1900s, more hospitals founded by Chinese entered the stage of history: Chinese Red Cross General Hospital (Huashan Hospital), Chung Shan Hospital (Zhongshan Hospital), Shanghai Mercy Hospital (Shanghai

Mental Health Center), Sacred Heart Hospital (First Rehabilitation Hospital), Hongqiao Sanatorium (Xuhui District Hospital) and Woman's Hospital (C. N. Maternity & Infant Health Hospital) etc.

I have written about Shanghai architecture for 18 years, "Shanghai Hospitals" being the most difficult and significant topic.

After anonymously donated to build the Country Hospital in 1926, British merchant Charles Rayer told The China Press that "the comforts of the Country Hospital are extended without distinction of nationalities, race or religion, to all may be afflicted with ill health." He asked for "no greater reward than that this same spirit of cheerful goodwill for all and malice towards none may gradually and firmly unite all those whose lot it is to dwell in this city."

The "cheerful kindness" that transcends nationalities and races is exactly what we need most in a world shadowed by virus and crisis today. China has also called for the building of a community of common health for mankind amid the mounting global public health crises caused by COVID019 pandemic.

The most fascinating part of history is the touching stories. I was enamored of the architectural stories of Shanghai hospitals. The history of medical architecture in Shanghai is a treasure trove with rich content, and there are still many dusty archives at home and abroad waiting for researchers. This book shares the results of the current research, and I look forward to more discoveries in the future.

The day that I finished the last sentence of this book coincided with the new stage of "Great Shanghai Defense " against the epidemic of Omicron in the city since March 2022. Wukang Road, a popular historical street where I live began to revive its vitality. The city is in for a fresh start and it will take some time to heal and to regain its vigor and radiance. Looking back at the medical history of modern Shanghai through these great Shanghai hospital buildings, reading these ingenious and benevolent stories will surely bring some confidence and strength.

Michelle Qiao
June 1, 2022
Moon Atelier on Wukang Road, Shanghai

参考书目

西风东渐与晚清社会　熊月之 著　上海教育出版社 2019

上海卫生——中国保健之注意事项　［英］韩雅各 著　赵婧 译　中华书局 2021

颜福庆传　钱益民、颜志渊 著　复旦大学出版社 2019

近代上海科技先驱之仁济医院与格致书院　王尔敏 著　广西师范大学出版社 2011

仁济医院早期故事　苏精 著　上海交通大学出版社 2019

中外医学文化交流史　马伯英、高晞、洪中立 著　文汇出版社 1993

上海市第一人民医院志　上海市地方志编纂委员会 编　上海科学技术文献出版社 2020

瑞金医院志　上海市地方志编纂委员会 编　上海科学技术文献出版社 2017

上海市肺科医院八十周年院志（1933—2013）

走近上海医院深处的老建筑　陆韵、陶祎珺 编著　同济大学出版社 2017

上海宗教史　阮仁泽、高振农 主编　上海人民出版社 1991

寻访犹太人——犹太文化精英在上海　许步曾 著　上海社会科学院出版社 2007

旧上海的外商与买办 上海文史资料选辑第五十六辑　上海人民出版社 1987

遗产与记忆——雷士德、雷士德工学院和她的学生们　房芸芳 编著　上海古籍出版社 2007

括囊大典 网罗众家——上海市杨浦区图书馆　上海市杨浦区图书馆 编　上海人民美术出版社 2019

董大酉上海建筑作品评析同济大学硕士学位论文　杜超瑜 2018

上海近代基督教堂研究（1843—1949）同济大学硕士论文　周进 2008

异国事物的转译 近代上海的跑马、跑狗和回力球赛　张宁 著　社会科学文献出版社 2020

上海史 The History of Shanghai　［英］兰宁、库寿龄 著　朱华 译　上海书店出版社 2020

上海百年建筑史 1840—1949（第二版）　伍江 著　同济大学出版社，2008

上海近代建筑风格（新版）　郑时龄 著　同济大学出版社，2020

上海建筑指南　罗小未 主编　上海人民美术出版社，1996

上海近代建筑史稿　陈从周、章明 著　上海三联书店，1988

上海邬达克建筑地图　华霞虹、乔争月等 著　同济大学出版社 2013

邬达克　［意］卢卡·彭切里尼、［匈］尤利娅·切伊迪 著　华霞虹、乔争月 译　同济大学出版社 2013

上海邬达克建筑　上海市城市规划管理局、上海市城市建设档案馆 编　上海科学普及出版社 2008

Art Deco 的源与流——中西"摩登建筑"关系研究　许乙弘 著　东南大学出版社 2006

静安历史文化图录　龚德庆、张仁良 主编　同济大学出版社 2011

上海的日本文化地图　陈祖恩 著　上海锦绣文章出版社 2010

上海的德国文化地图　吕澍、王维江 著　上海锦绣文章出版社 2011

上海的俄国文化地图　汪之成 著　上海锦绣文章出版社 2010

上海的英国文化地图　熊月之、高俊 著　上海锦绣文章出版社 2011

我在上海修历史建筑 1997—2017　上海章明建筑设计事务所　上海远东出版社 2017

犹太人在上海　潘光 主编　上海画报出版社 2005 年

同济老照片　陆敏恂 主编　同济大学宣传部 编　同济大学出版社 2007 年

德国对华政策中的同济大学 1907—1941　李乐曾 著　同济大学出版社 2007 年

老上海百业指南，道路机构厂商住宅分布图　吴健熙 选编　上海社会科学院出版社 2008 年

Twentieth Century Impression of Hongkong, Shanghai and other Treaty Ports of China 1908 Lloyd's Greater Britain Publishing Company, Ltd.

A Short History of Shanghai by F. L. Hawks Pott, D.D China Intercontinental Press, 2008

Shanghai's Art Deco Master by Spencer Dodington & Charles Lagrange Earnshaw Books, 2014

Deutsche Architektur in China by Torsten Warner Ernst & Sohn 1994

X-Ray Architecture by Beatriz Colomina Lars Muller Publishers 2019

近现代英文报刊

《字林西报》及其周末版《北华捷报》the North China Daily News & North China Herald

《大陆报》The China Press

《密勒氏评论》Milliard's Review

《社交上海》Social Shanghai

《上海泰晤士报》及其周日版 Shanghai Times & Shanghai Sunday Times

《大美晚报》Shanghai Evening Post

《以色列信使报》Israel's Messengers

《文汇报》《解放日报》《新民晚报》

《中国建筑》

《大众画报》

The China Builder

图书在版编目（CIP）数据

阅读上海医院建筑 /乔争月著. -- 上海:上海三联书店, 2023.7

ISBN 978 - 7 - 5426 - 8095-2

Ⅰ.①阅… Ⅱ.①乔… Ⅲ.①医院－建筑史－上海 Ⅳ.①R199.2

中国国家版本馆CIP数据核字(2023)第069061号

阅读上海医院建筑

著　　者 / 乔争月

责任编辑 / 杜　鹃
封面设计 / 0214_Studio
版式设计 / 一本好书
监　　制 / 姚　军
责任校对 / 王凌霄

出版发行 / 上海三联书店
　　　　　（ 200030 ）中国上海市漕溪北路331号A座6楼
邮　　箱 / sdxsanlian@sina.com
邮购电话 / 021-22895540
印　　刷 / 上海艾登印刷有限公司

版　　次 / 2023年7月第1版
印　　次 / 2023年7月第1次印刷
开　　本 / 787mm X 1092mm　1/32
字　　数 / 340 千字
印　　张 / 14.125
书　　号 / ISBN 978-7-5426-8095-2 / R·132
定　　价 / 79.00 元

敬启读者，如发现本书有印装质量问题，请与印刷厂联系 021-62213990